RL
85
.S56

30449100081143
Skin disorders sou

WEST GEORGIA TECH LIBRARY
FORT DRIVE
LAGRANGE, GA 30240

SKIN DISORDERS SOURCEBOOK

RL
85
.S56

30449100081143
Skin disorders sourceboo

Health Reference Series

Volume Twenty-two

SKIN DISORDERS SOURCEBOOK

LIBRARY
WEST GEORGIA TECHNICAL COLLEGE
303 FORT DRIVE
LAGRANGE, GA 30240

Basic Information about Common Skin and Scalp Conditions Caused by Aging, Allergies, Immune Reactions, Sun Exposure, Infectious Organisms, Parasites, Cosmetics, and Skin Traumas Including Abrasions, Cuts, and Pressure Sores Along With Information on Prevention and Treatment

Edited by
Allan R. Cook

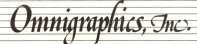

Penobscot Building / Detroit, MI 48226

BIBLIOGRAPHIC NOTE

This volume contains individual publications issued by the National Institutes of Health (NIH), its sister agencies, and sub-agencies. Numbered publications are: NIH 80-8239, 84-663, 92-909K, 92-0048, 92-3193, 93-5012, 93-5013, 93-3442, 94-0178P, 94-5014, 95-0654. Also included are selected articles from the Food and Drug Administration's *FDA Consumer*, CDC's *Morbidity and Mortality Weekly Report*, the *NCRR Reporter*, and *Research Resources Reporter*. In addition, the volume includes copyrighted articles from *American Family Physician*, the American Hair Loss Council, the American Academy for Dermatologic Surgery, the *Baltimore Sun*, Foundation for Ichthyosis and Related Skin Types, the *Journal of the Academy of Dermatology*, the Lupus Foundation of America, the *Mayo Clinic Health Letter*, the *Merck Manual*, the National Jewish Center for Immunology and Respiratory Medicine, the National Psoriasis Foundation, the *New York Times*, *Parents*, *Patient Care*, *Pediatric Clinics of North America*, *Scientific American*, the Skin Cancer Foundation, the United Scleroderma Foundation, and the *Washington Post*. All copyrighted documents are used with the permission of the copyright holder. Document numbers, where applicable, and specific source citations appear on the first page of each chapter.

Edited by
Allan R. Cook

Peter D. Dresser, Managing Editor, Health Reference Series
Karen Bellenir, Series Editor, Health Reference Series

Omnigraphics, Inc.

Matthew P. Barbour, Production Manager
Laurie Lanzen Harris, Vice President, Editorial
Peter E. Ruffner, Vice President, Administration
James A. Sellgren, Vice President, Operations and Finance
Jane J. Steele, Marketing Consultant

Frederick G. Ruffner, Jr., Publisher

Copyright © 1997, Omnigraphics, Inc.

Library of Congress Cataloging-in-Publication Data

Skin disorders sourcebook: basic information about common skin and scalp conditions caused by aging, allergies, immune reactions, sun exposure, infectious organisms, parasites, cosmetics, and skin traumas including abrasions, cuts, and pressure sores along with information on prevention and treatment/edited by Allan R. Cook.
     p.   cm. — (Health reference series; v.22)
Includes bibliographical references and index.
ISBN 0-7808-0080-X (lib.bdg.: alk.paper)
  1. Skin — Diseases — Popular works.   I. Cook, Allan R.   II. Series.
RL85.S56 1997
616.5 — dc21   97-6570
                                                                      CIP

∞

This book is printed on acid-free paper meeting the ANSI Z39.48 Standard. The infinity symbol that appears above indicates that the paper in this book meets that standard.

Printed in the United States of America

Contents

Preface ix
Introduction—Anatomy of the Skin xiii

Part I: Caring for the Skin Through Life's Changes

Chapter 1—Protecting Baby's New Skin 3
Chapter 2—"Strep" Demands Immediate Care 13
Chapter 3—Acne: Taming That Age-Old Adolescent
　　　　　　Affliction 21
Chapter 4—*Candida*: An Itch Like No Other 29
Chapter 5—Treatment Pales Rosacea's Red Face 35
Chapter 6—Pruritus: Persistent Itching 41
Chapter 7—Psychodermatology: Psychological Factors
　　　　　　in Skin Disorders 57
Chapter 8—Wrinkles: Smile Lines and Facial Fissures 71
Chapter 9—Caring for Corns, Bunions, and Other
　　　　　　Agonies of De-Feet 81
Chapter 10—Getting a Leg Up on Varicose Veins 89
Chapter 11—Tips for Treating Aging Skin 99
Chapter 12—Cosmetic Surgery 111

Part II: Psoriasis

Chapter 13—A Guide to Understanding Psoriasis:
        Relieving That Miserable Itch 123
Chapter 14—The Immune Factor: When Friends Become
        Foes 139
Chapter 15—Nail Psoriasis: Questions and Answers............. 143
Chapter 16—Research into Psoriasis 147

Part III: Skin Conditions as Allergic or Immune Responses

Chapter 17—Diagnosis and Management of Atopic
        Dermatitis 157
Chapter 18—Atopic Dermatitis: Is It an Allergic Disease?..... 167
Chapter 19—All About Contact Dermatitis 189
Chapter 20—The Itch of the Great Outdoors 197
Chapter 21—Living with Epidermolysis Bullosa..................... 205
Chapter 22—Ichthyosis: An Overview...................................... 227
Chapter 23—Lichen Planus and Lichen Sclerosus 239
Chapter 24—Skin Diseases in Lupus 243
Chapter 25—McCune-Albright Syndrome 253
Chapter 26—Pityriasis Rosea.. 259
Chapter 27—Scleroderma 261
Chapter 28—Chronic Idiopathic Urticaria 275
Chapter 29—Vitiligo 293

Part IV: The Hazards of Sun Exposure

Chapter 30—Cancerous Skin Mutation from Solar Rays........ 299
Chapter 31—Deaths from Melanoma in the United
        States, 1973-1992 309
Chapter 32—Judging the Risks: Tips for Safer Tanning 315
Chapter 33—Actinic Keratosis: What You Should Know
        About This Common Pre-Cancer 327
Chapter 34—Understanding Xeroderma Pigmentosum 333

Part V: Infectious Organisms, Parasites, and Fungi

Chapter 35—Fever Blisters and Canker Sores 341
Chapter 36—Scabies 351
Chapter 37—Dermatophyte Infections: The Tinea
             Fungus (Ringworm) 359
Chapter 38—Shingles—or Chicken Pox, Part II 363
Chapter 39—New Treatment Helps Ease Pain of Shingles 369
Chapter 40—Group A Streptococcal Infections 375
Chapter 41—Warts 385
Chapter 42—Herpes Simplex Virus and Genital Herpes 389
Chapter 43—Human Papillomavirus and Genital Warts 399

Part VI: Skin Traumas and Treatments

Chapter 44—Anatomy of a Scar 409
Chapter 45—Help for Cuts, Scrapes, and Burns 415
Chapter 46—Keloids and Hypertrophic Scars: When Skin
             Repairs Run Amok 423
Chapter 47—Dog, Cat, and Human Bites 429
Chapter 48—Preventing Pressure Ulcers 447
Chapter 49—Treating Pressure Sores 457
Chapter 50—Dermatologic Surgery 477
Chapter 51—Test-Tube Skin and Other High-Tech
             Treatments for Burns 503

Part VII: Hair, Scalp, and Nail Disorders

Chapter 52—Hair: From Personal Statement to Personal
             Problem 509
Chapter 53—Controlling Dandruff: Over-the-Counter
             Options 515
Chapter 54—Hair Dye Dilemmas 521
Chapter 55—Alopecia Areata and Other Hair-Loss
             Disorders 527
Chapter 56—Hair Loss in Men, Women, and Children 533
Chapter 57—Minoxidil: Hair Apparent? For Some, a New
             Solution to Baldness 543

Chapter 58—Hair Replacement Surgery 549
Chapter 59—Of Lice and Children: Going to the Head of
            the Class 553
Chapter 60—Fingernails: Looking Good While Playing
            Safe 559

Part VIII: Cosmetics and the Skin

Chapter 61—Cosmetic Ingredients: Understanding the
            Puffery 571
Chapter 62—The Collagen Connection 579
Chapter 63—Cosmetic Safety: More Complex Than First
            Blush 585
Chapter 64—Decoding the Cosmetic Label 595
Chapter 65—Tattooing in the '90s 605

Index **615**

Preface

About This Book

One of the body's largest organs, the skin performs important regulatory functions. It allows movement, maintains body moisture and temperature, and provides a physical barrier to foreign materials and organisms. A complex instrument, it contains tiny blood vessels which dilate and contract to control temperature with the help of sweat glands and sebaceous glands. Millions of tiny nerve endings buried within the skin transmit important information about the environment to the brain through the senses of touch, pressure, heat, cold, and pain. But the skin's direct contact with the outside world means the outermost skin cells are constantly worn away and need to be replaced with younger cells from below. Not surprisingly, the skin can suffer from many assaults. Most disorders change the expected appearance of the skin or cause itching, swelling, or pain. A few cause destructive blistering or, in the case of cancer, cell mutation and even death.

This book contains basic information for the layperson on a wide range of common skin complaints, their triggers, and some methods of treating, avoiding, and coping with them. Patients, friends, family members, and the interested general public will find this volume a good place to begin to understand skin reactions.

Some topics, however, are handled in more detail in other volumes of the Omnigraphics' *Health Reference Series*. For more information on cancer, see the *New Cancer Sourcebook* and the *Cancer Sourcebook for Women*. For more information on allergies and the immune system, see the *Allergies Sourcebook* and the *Immune Disorders Sourcebook*. For more information on infectious diseases, see the *Contagious and Non-Contagious Infectious Diseases Sourcebook* and the *Food and Animal Borne Diseases Sourcebook*. Information on reconstructive surgery and burns, will be provided in an upcoming volume.

How To Use This Book

This book is divided into parts and chapters. Parts focus on broad areas of interest and chapters on specific topics within those areas.

Introduction: *Anatomy of the Skin* gives a brief overview of the construction and function of the skin.

Part I: *Caring for the Skin Through Life's Changes* looks at common skin disorders and complaints which tend to occur at specific ages and generally affect most people.

Part II: *Psoriasis* describes the particular chronic skin condition characterized by red, scaly, easily bleeding skin which affects 1 to 3 percent of the population of the United States.

Part III: *Skin Conditions as Allergic or Immune Responses* considers skin complaints that seem to be triggered by the body's response to specific allergens.

Part IV: *The Hazards of Sun Exposure* examines the relationship between sun exposure and cancer. It details the mechanics of mutation and provides helpful hints to assist in avoiding sun damage.

Part V: *Infectious Organisms, Parasites, and Fungi* widens the scope to include biologic triggers for skin disorders.

Part VI: *Skin Traumas and Treatments* discuses the ways in which the skin attempts to repair physical damage and the complications that can arise.

Part VII: *Hair, Scalp, and Nail Disorders* goes beyond the skin itself to include disorders centered on head hair and finger and toe nails.

Part VIII: *Cosmetics and the Skin* asks what happens when we place cosmetic products on the skin and why.

Index: gives page references and cross-references for key words and phrases used in the various articles.

Acknowledgements

The editor gratefully acknowledges the assistance of the many people who helped produce this volume and the private organizations that agreed to grant permission to reprint their articles: *American Family Physician*, the American Hair Loss Council, the American Society for Dermatologic Surgery, *Baltimore Sun*, the Foundation for Ichthyosis and Related Skin Types, the Lupus Foundation of America, the *Mayo Clinic Health Letter*, *Merck Manual*, National Jewish Center for Immunology and Respiratory Medicine, the National Psoriasis Foundation, *New York Times*, *Parents*, *Patient Care*, Pediatric Clinics of North America, *Scientific American*, the Skin Cancer Foundation, the United Scleroderma Foundation, and the *Washington Post*. Special thanks to Margaret Mary Missar for her patient search for the documents that make up this volume, Karen Bellenir for her technical assistance and advice, Bruce the Scanman and special assistant Mike for their optical resurrections and Valerie Cook for her sharp-eyed text verification.

Note from the Editor

This book is part of Omnigraphics' *Health Reference Series*. The series provides basic information about a broad range of medical concerns. It is not intended to serve as a tool for diagnosing illness, in prescribing treatments, or as a substitute for the physician/patient relationship. All persons concerned about medical symptoms or the possibility of disease are encouraged to seek professional care from an appropriate health care provider.

ANATOMY OF THE SKIN

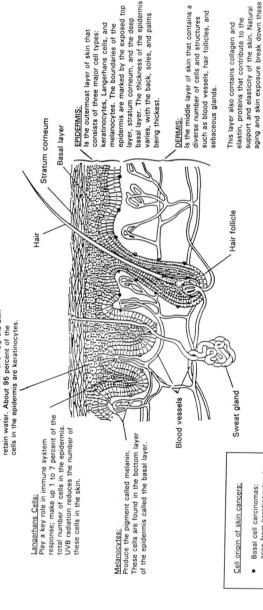

Keratinocytes:
Make the protein keratin and help the skin retain water. About 95 percent of the cells in the epidermis are keratinocytes.

Langerhans Cells:
Play a key role in immune system response; make up 1 to 7 percent of the total number of cells in the epidermis. UVB radiation reduces the number of these cells in the skin.

Melanocytes:
Produce the pigment called melanin. These cells are found in the bottom layer of the epidermis called the basal layer.

Cell origin of skin cancers:
- Basal cell carcinomas: arise from keratinocytes in the basal layer of the epidermis.
- Squamous cell carcinomas: arise from keratinocytes above the basal layer.
- Melanomas: develop from melanocytes.

EPIDERMIS:
Is the outermost layer of skin that consists of three major cell types: keratinocytes, Langerhans cells, and melanocytes. The boundaries of the epidermis are marked by the exposed top layer, stratum corneum, and the deep basal layer. The thickness of the epidermis varies, with the back, soles, and palms being thickest.

DERMIS:
Is the middle layer of skin that contains a diverse number of cells and structures such as blood vessels, hair follicles, and sebaceous glands.

This layer also contains collagen and elastin, proteins that contribute to the support and elasticity of the skin. Natural aging and skin exposure break down these proteins, causing the skin to wrinkle and sag.

HYPODERMIS:
Is the layer of fatty tissue underlying the dermis. It provides nourishment to upper layers and has blood vessels, nerves, sweat glands, and, sometimes, deeper hair follicles. This fatty tissue normally thins with age.

Source: National Institute of Arthritis and Musculoskeletal and Skin Diseases

Introduction

Anatomy of the Skin

Structure and Function of the Skin

Though it's scratched, scrubbed, sat on, and trod on repeatedly, skin wears well.

Skin is flexible and elastic. It stretches smoothly around knobby corners and snuggles comfortably under hairy hollows and along moist passageways.

To properly protect the body, skin is a tattletale. It reveals inner secrets by coloring the face—anemic white or sick-liver yellow, for instance—and alerts its owner when it senses pain, itching, heat and cold.

Normal human skin, not counting the underlying fat, is between about one-fiftieth and one-quarter inch deep, depending on what part of the body it's covering. Yet it's our largest organ: roughly two square yards of it envelop the body to protect against bumps, wounds, chemicals, disease, extremes in temperature, and excessive water loss. Skin also protects against harmful radiation from the sun, while at the same time allowing the body to use the energy in sunlight to make vitamin D.

Skin is actually layers of different types of tissue. The outermost layer, the epidermis, rests upon the dermis, and under that is the hypodermis. (Some experts describe the hypodermis as tissue under the skin, rather than as an actual part of the skin.)

FDA Consumer, June 1987, and the National Institute of Arthritis and Musculoskeletal and Skin Diseases.

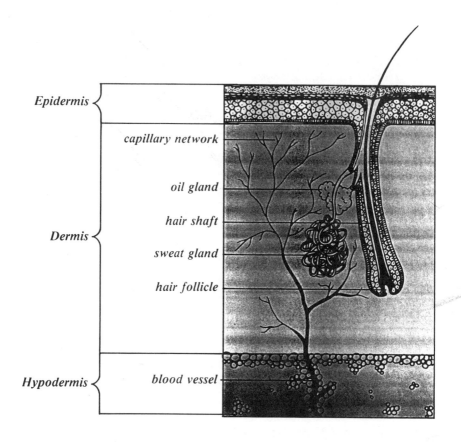

Figure 0.2. Cross Section of Human Skin

The epidermis is the thinnest layer and it, too, favors the layered look—exhibiting, as it does, its own sub-layers of various epithelial cells. Cells residing at the epidermis's inner layers eventually die and, as new cells form, are pushed to the outer layer, or stratum corneum, where they're shed in flakes. Those dead cells are what make the skin waterproof and firm, even hard, as on the feet.

Some cells in the epidermis produce dark-colored granules called melanosomes, which protect against the damaging ultraviolet rays of the sun. The greater the number and the larger the size of a person's melanosomes, the darker the skin is, and the greater the protection.

Introduction: Anatomy of the Skin

How Skin Heals

For repair of minor wounds, skin depends on regeneration by its epithelial cells and on activities by other structures of the body. Suppose, for instance, that a youngster scrapes his knee in a fall. At first, the boy sees blood and other fluid seep from his injury. The area becomes inflamed. Blood vessels there expand, and blood flow increases. The blood vessels become so permeable that plasma (the fluid part of blood) leaks through to swell the spaces outside the vessels with water, proteins, and such cells as white corpuscles, which destroy and dispose of bacteria and dead cells. The area is red, warm and painful. Lymph vessels clot with protein to keep the inflammation from spreading. When the clot subsequently dissolves, resumed lymph flow carries off dead germs and dead cells, and the swelling subsides.

Within 24 hours of the boy's fall, epithelial cells have begun their work. From the normal epidermis around the wound and from hair and other structures embedded in the dermis below, the cells migrate onto the wound surface and start reproducing. The wound's seeping

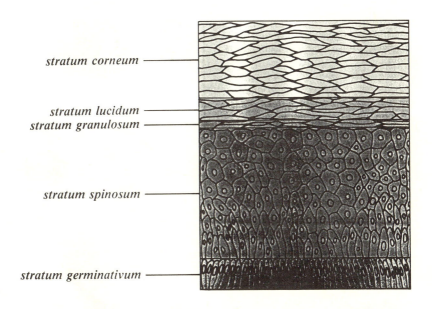

Figure 0.3. Detail of Epidermis

fluids, with all the dead bacteria and skin cells they contain, ultimately clot and dry, forming a scab. After a week or so, a layer of epithelial cells covers the entire wound under the scab as thin new skin. The cells continue reproducing to thicken the new skin, which eventually forces the scab off. The stratum corneum firms up. And finally, the once wounded area becomes nearly perfect skin. On the dense, fibrous tissue known as a scar, though, the skin won't sweat and hair won't grow. If the wound is so severe that a great deal of tissue is lost, proper healing is threatened.

A major protective characteristic of the epidermis is its fairly impenetrable barrier against invasion by organisms. Some germs do make it through, but additional protection is offered by a film known as the basement membrane (a fitting name, in view of its position underneath the epidermis). The basement membrane connects the epidermis to the dermis and allows certain cells and fluids to pass between the two layers. Many an invader is imprisoned there until the body can organize its white blood cells into a defensive attack or until the germ simply starves to death.

Supporting the epidermis is the dermis, which is mainly collagen, elastin proteins and fibroblast cells (which produce connective tissue), all nestled in a thick, gel-like material.

Here in the dermis, blood and lymph perform their infection-fighting, clean-up work and nourish the skin and its appendages—hair follicles, nails, and oil and sweat glands—which are situated in the dermis. There are also tiny muscles that hold the hair erect ("gooseflesh") to reduce heat loss when a person is cold or frightened. And nerve endings tell the brain what the skin feels so that the person can take appropriate actions: add a sweater, move away from the fire, or scratch.

The hypodermis, a mass of loose connective tissue, makes the skin pliable. In most parts of this underlying area, there is also fat, which stores extra food and provides insulation and padding.

Part One

Caring for the Skin Through Life's Changes

Chapter 1

Protecting Baby's New Skin

Skin Problems and Birthmarks

A brief outline of the most common types of skin irritations and marks.

"Her skin is like a baby's" is a compliment we give a woman with a perfect complexion because we think of a baby's skin as smooth and flawless.

But any parent soon learns that babies are prone to rashes, blotches, and blisters that irritate their tender new skin and often cause them acute discomfort. In some cases, rashes are created or made worse by overzealous parental attention. A few need to be checked by your baby's doctor.

We asked Sidney Hurwitz, M.D., about the most common skin problems affecting babies. Dr. Hurwitz is clinical professor of pediatrics and dermatology at Yale University School of Medicine.

Newborn Acne

Newborn acne occurs primarily in male babies, probably because of an increased response to hormones from the mother while the baby was in utero, and shows up as whiteheads, blackheads, and pimples.

Newborn acne can be one of two kinds: neonatal or infantile. Neonatal acne usually disappears in the first six months. Infantile acne may persist for a year or two.

©1985, 1986, and 1990 *Parents*. Reprinted with permission.

Prickly Heat

Prickly heat (miliaria), also known as heat rash, is caused by a temporary blockage of the sweat pores. The sweat can't reach the skin surface to evaporate and breaks through the walls of the pore.

Prickly heat rash usually looks like tiny pink or white pimples with a little redness around them, but it can also resemble fine grains of sand or form pinhead-size water blisters. In more severe cases, the rash can become infected.

Prickly heat usually occurs around the neck, under the arms, and around the diaper area, areas of irritation where skin folds rub together or are constricted by clothing. Sweat and moisture aggravate the condition.

Parents often put baby oil on prickly heat. But that's just the wrong thing to do because the oil keeps the sweat pores blocked and irritated rather than allowing the sweat to evaporate normally. The way to treat prickly heat is to avoid overdressing and overheating the baby. Keep the skin cool by bathing your baby in cool water in hot or humid weather. Pat—don't rub—your baby dry and use lightweight loose-fitting clothing.

Prickly heat can appear suddenly after a hot day, or it can sneak up on you gradually before you realize what is happening. If you are treating it correctly but it seems to be getting worse or if it persists for more than a week without improvement, it is best to have the baby's doctor look at it to be sure it is not infected.

Diaper Rash

Almost all babies develop diaper rash at some time. Most commonly, diaper rash shows up as patches of rough, red, scaly skin and areas of small, red pimples, which may become infected. The rash can also be open and oozing.

Diaper rash is typically caused by prolonged contact with the chemicals and bacteria normally present in urine and in stool. Disposable diapers may aggravate the problem by doing their job too well. The diaper's plastic covering holds moisture in, making the diaper area a tropical mini-environment where the bacteria overgrow and the chemicals become irritating.

In some cases, women who have vaginal yeast infections can transmit the infection to the infant either during birth, as the infant passes through the birth canal, or in handling the baby afterward.

The yeast-like organism is harbored in the baby's lower bowel, where it is harmless. But, some of the yeast fungus is passed out when the baby has a bowel movement. If the diaper area is closed off and the skin is already irritated, the yeast organism proliferates and can cause an infection known as *monilia diaper rash*.

Almost all babies develop a slight diaper rash at some point in infancy. The best way to treat it is to leave the diaper area open to the air as much as possible. Until the rash clears up, switch from plastic-covered disposable diapers to cloth diapers, which should be washed in a mild soap and dried in a dryer. Diaper ointments may help clear up the rash. Avoid talcum powder. It can irritate the skin and cause chafing. Cornstarch is an acceptable and inexpensive alternative, although it has a tendency to cake.

Diaper rash isn't just one condition; it is a set of symptoms that may result from a number of causes. But the same symptoms may be caused by eczema or secondary infections, which must be treated differently. If the diaper rash doesn't respond to treatment after a week or two, have the baby's doctor check it.

Eczema

Eczema (also called atopic dermatitis) is a red, scaly or weeping rash that appears in patches. It is very itchy. The rash usually develops when the baby is about two or three months old. Eczema is more likely to appear in babies whose parents have a history of allergies, such as hay fever, asthma, or eczema. When babies are young, eczema patches typically appear on the face. As they get older and start crawling, the patches extend to the arms and legs, from rubbing and crawling on carpeting. When they get older still, it characteristically appears in the creases at the elbows and knees.

Babies with eczema usually have an inherited tendency toward allergies, although there is still disagreement among specialists as to whether eczema is actually an allergy.

Just how often an allergic reaction to food is responsible for eczema is still not clear, but pediatricians have suspected specific foods were one of the triggering factors of eczema, so they usually recommend that certain foods be removed from the baby's diet or that the formula be changed.

Effective treatment of eczema includes limited baths with gentle soap. After you pat your baby's skin dry, apply a moisturizer often. Use clothing of smooth-textured cotton wherever possible. Babies who have eczema should not be allowed to crawl on wool carpeting. Put a cotton blanket over the carpeting for your baby to crawl on. Do not use a cortisone cream on the rash unless the baby's doctor recommends it.

Babies with eczema often cannot fight off certain skin infections as readily as other babies. These infections—certain streptococcal and staphylococcal infections—seem to aggravate eczema breakouts. Herpes is one such infection, so be careful not to allow anyone with a cold sore to kiss your baby or you may have to cope with a flare up of eczema.

Cradle Cap.

Cradle cap is a patchy, scaly disorder of the scalp. It doesn't itch and is usually easy to manage by using petroleum jelly or mineral oil to soften the scaliness which is then loose enough to be combed out with a fine-toothed comb. If the scalp doesn't respond to treatment, you could first ask your pediatrician for an effective anti-seborrheic shampoo or, if that does not work, a cortisone medication. Most infants will outgrow cradle cap by the time they are a year old.

No one knows whether cradle cap is associated with adult dandruff, but there may be some relationship between cradle cap and eczema.

Contact Dermatitis

Contact dermatitis is an irritant reaction or an allergic reaction of the skin to contact with a variety of substances, such as saliva, bubble bath, strong soaps, and detergents. Babies commonly react to saliva, orange juice, orange rind, tomatoes, and tomato sauce. Woolen clothing, liquid fabric softeners used in the washer, and fabric-softener sheets used in the dryer may also cause irritation. Baby lotions designed to make babies smell better and baby powders designed to make them feel soft are also possible irritants. If your baby has sensitive skin, wash with a gentle soap, pat the skin dry, and use a moisturizer.

Although anything that mars a baby's perfect skin is alarming, most rashes, bumps, and irritations look far worse than they are. With simple and attentive care, most will usually disappear and leave your baby's skin as soft as before.

—*by Nissa Simon*

Nissa Simon is a free-lance writer specializing in medical and related topics.

Protecting Baby's New Skin

Birthmarks

Many babies have, or will have, some type of birthmark. Most marks are nothing to worry about. Some disappear entirely as your infant grows older, and most require no treatment whatsoever.

But because such marks are not usually shown in magazines and books, they can be worrisome to new parents. So we outline here a few of the more common types of birthmarks. Of course, if you are concerned about any marking or discoloration of your infant's skin, the best policy is to consult your doctor.

Dr. Alvin H. Jacobs, professor of dermatology and pediatrics at Stanford University School of Medicine, points out that a true birthmark is the result of an error in early growth. Usually the recipe for combining cells or parts of cells to form the skin was not followed precisely. The result may be a discoloration or a benign tumor-like growth, which is either present at birth or which may not become apparent until some time later.

Red Birthmarks

Dr. Jacobs describes two general kinds of errors. For example, if the error in prenatal development involves tiny blood vessels, the result is a red marking of some sort. Doctors call these vascular nevi: "vascular" meaning blood vessel and "nevi" meaning birthmarks.

The most common birthmark of this kind is the salmon patch, also called a stork bite or an angel's kiss. About four babies in ten are born with these dull-pink markings. They occur most often at the back of the neck, as if the stork bit or nibbled your infant.

They also occur on the face between the eyebrows just above the nose or on the upper eyelids, appearing as if an angel kissed your infant and left a little hickey. Infants often have salmon patches in more than one of these locations.

These marks disappear within the first year of life, especially those on the face. Salmon patches on the neck, however, may take longer to fade away, and about 5 percent are permanent. These are often masked by clothing or hair, and are not noticeable most of the time anyway.

Strawberry marks occur in approximately one in ten infants, but only 1 to 3 percent of babies are born with them. Usually they develop within the first three or four weeks of life.

The most common form does look like a strawberry, because it is solid red and slightly raised. But strawberry marks can take a variety of shapes, and they can occur almost any place on the body.

Usually these marks gradually subside within the first few years of life, thereby requiring no treatment and leaving no permanent trace on the skin. Sometimes, however, strawberry marks may occur on vital organs and interfere with sucking, breathing, or vision, or they may be excessively large. In these rare cases, some treatment may be required and some discoloration or scar may remain.

An unusual birthmark of this type is the port wine stain which occurs in approximately 3 of every 1,000 newborns. In contrast to the strawberry mark, the port wine stain is present at birth, when it is pink and the skin is smooth. Later, it will become more purple and the skin may thicken. It can occur on any area, but it is most common on the face and neck.

Port wine stains are permanent and although research is continuing, there is no, totally satisfactory medical treatment for removing them. Cosmetics with opaque bases are still the best approach.

Brown Birthmarks

Sometimes the error in prenatal development involves the coloring or pigment of the skin rather than the blood vessels, notes Dr. Jacobs. In this case, tan, brown, or black marks may result.

Freckles are the most common type of pigmented marking among whites, especially blond and red-haired persons; who are most likely to have the combination of genes that produce these inherited tan or brownish spots.

Freckles do not usually appear until after five years of age. They become more pronounced following exposure to the sun and may fade away during winter. For the most part, freckles are nothing to worry about, but sunscreens may be used to protect the skin from unusual amounts of ultraviolet light.

Moles are another type of pigmented birthmark. The average person has 20 to 30 of them.

Like freckles, moles are not usually present at birth but develop between the ages of two and six years or at puberty. However, moles that are present at birth should be pointed out to your physician.

Café-au-lait spots take their name from the French words meaning "coffee with milk" because they resemble the light-tan color of creamed coffee. In contrast to freckles and moles, café-au-lait spots are usually present at birth, but they may also appear in early childhood.

They usually have an oval outline, and approximately 10 percent of the population has from one to three such marks. But if your child has more than five or one or more are larger than a half inch, you should consult your physician.

Among darker-skinned individuals, mongolian spots (which have nothing to do with mongolism or Down's syndrome) are the most common mark. More than 90 percent of black and Asian infants have them, while only 10 percent of white babies do.

Mongolian spots are present at birth, tend to be blue-gray, bruise-like, round or oval spots located on the lower back or buttocks. They progressively fade away and are almost always completely gone by adolescence.

The birthmarks described above are among the most common and, except as noted, are nothing to worry about. Almost everyone has one or another of these marks, and usually no treatment is required. Of course, there are other kinds of birthmarks, some of which may need treatment. If you have any doubts about a mark on your infant, discuss it with your pediatrician.

—by Robert B. McCall

Robert B. McCall, Ph.D., is a senior scientist at the Boys Town Center, near Omaha, Nebraska, and author of "Infants: The New Knowledge" (Harvard University Press).

Treating Newborn Infections

Your baby may be prone to some common infections that are not serious if treated promptly.

Newborns not only are susceptible to all the infections to which adults are prey—from ordinary colds to far more serious illnesses—but also are especially prone to particular infections. Fortunately, the most frequent ones aren't likely to be critical, assuming they're treated promptly. The following are among the most common.

Staph. Staphylococci are bacteria that reside on all human skin; any wound or even an irritation provides an opportunity for them to multiply. Staph infections tend to be transmitted in hospital nurseries, and the longer a newborn remains there, the greater the baby's chance of exposure.

Body areas especially subject to staph infection include the healing navel, the circumcision site, as well as the diaper area (which offers the moist, dark, warm conditions ideal for the growth of bacteria). If you notice a rash consisting of multiple "pimples," some containing pus, call your doctor; either vigorous topical treatment or an oral antibiotic will be needed.

Conjunctivitis. An inflammation of the conjunctiva—the mucous membrane around the eye—may be chemical, bacterial, or viral in nature.

The chemical kind appears within the first day of life and is essentially an irritation from the drops—typically silver nitrate—put in the baby's eyes to prevent infection from vaginal bacteria encountered during delivery. The reaction usually subsides by itself within a few days.

Bacterial conjunctivitis. Again staph heads the list of culprits. Bacterial conjunctivitis typically shows up between the second and fifth days, sometimes accompanied by a purulent discharge. Warm compresses and antibiotic treatment prescribed by a physician usually work quickly.

Viral conjunctivitis. The symptoms of viral conjunctivitis are like those of the bacterial infection, except that they tend to appear a few days later. Because taking a culture to find the cause of the infection is time-consuming and expensive, many physicians will instead prescribe an antibiotic as if the infection were bacterial. Antibiotics have no effect on a viral infection.

Candida. The fungus many call yeast is often found in the vagina and may be picked up by a baby during delivery. Common sites are the mouth, where the infection is known as thrush, and the diaper area.

The lesions associated with **thrush** resemble small clumps of cottage cheese on the insides of the cheeks and on the gums. The clumps are hard to wipe away, and the tissue beneath them is reddish. Feeding will be painful for the infant, and a breast-feeding mother may catch the infection from her baby, resulting in cracked and irritated nipples—perhaps even bleeding.

Candida diaper rash, **monilia**, consists of redness around the labia or scrotum, surrounded by a wider red-spotted area. It's not unusual to see this rash and thrush occurring together.

Protecting Baby's New Skin

Again, your physician can prescribe specific antifungal medications for the infected area.

—by Katherine Karlsrud, M.D., with Dodi Schultz.

Katherine Karlsrud, M.D., is clinical instructor in pediatrics at Cornell University Medical College and practices in New York City. Dodi Schultz is co-author of *The First Five Years* (St. Martin's).

Chapter 2

"Strep" Demands Immediate Care

Signs of Group A Streptococcus Infection

- sore throat accompanied by fever
- shortness of breath
- red rash accompanied by fever
- involuntary, jerky movements
- yellow flaky crusts on the skin
- chest pain
- shock
- tender joints
- blood in urine
- puffy face and malaise

Persons developing any of these symptoms should seek immediate medical care.

"Vanishing Disease" Makes a Curtain Call

Few childhoods go by without the tell-tale fever and sore throat of a *Streptococcus,* or "strep," infection. Although these throat infections are common and easily treated, the recent rise of particularly deadly or troublesome strains of Group A *Streptococcus* has pushed the bacterium into the medical limelight—again.

FDA Consumer, October 1991.

In the past, Group A strep has played a starring role in a number of deadly medical epidemics, particularly the scourges of rheumatic fever that swept across the nation in the first half of this century, killing or debilitating thousands of children each year.

After World War II, the number of cases of rheumatic fever dramatically declined until, during the 20 years between 1965 and 1985 alone, the yearly number of cases of rheumatic fever among school-age children dropped by more than 90 percent. The medical community had assumed that less crowded living conditions and the use of antibiotics were keeping the disease at bay. Some physicians even went so far as to call rheumatic fever a "vanishing disease in suburbia."

That complacency was shaken in the mid-1980s when outbreaks of rheumatic fever were reported among children and young adults in various cities scattered throughout the country. Those reports were followed by others of a new and deadly form of strep infection that was afflicting adults. This disease, which is called **toxic streptococcal syndrome**, made the headlines when public television's "Sesame Street" puppeteer Jim Henson was reported to have died of it last year. There's also evidence to suggest that blood infections caused by Group A strep are on the rise.

"Group A *Streptococcus* seems to have taken a little twist again," says Rosemary Roberts, M.D., a medical officer with the Food and Drug Administration's division of anti-infective drug products. "We're seeing manifestations like rheumatic fever that we haven't seen for a while, as well as more invasive strains of Group A strep that are making people sicker much more quickly."

The jury isn't in yet on why Americans are experiencing such a boost in the severity of strep infections. Preliminary findings by researchers at the national Centers for Disease Control in Atlanta suggest that a population increase among previously rare strep types may be behind both the recent rheumatic fever outbreaks and cases of the new toxic streptococcal syndrome. Heightened production of disease-causing toxins by more common strep types may also be responsible for the latest strep casualties.

There are more than 80 known types of Group A *Streptococcus*, which can cause more than a dozen different illnesses. Group A *Streptococcus*, in turn, is part of a broader category of strep organisms that cause an even larger number of diseases.

Some of the more well-known Group A strep afflictions include upper respiratory diseases such as strep throat and scarlet fever, skin disorders such as impetigo, and inflammatory diseases such as rheumatic fever or kidney disease. In addition, blood infections due to Group A strep are a serious and frequent complication of wounds or surgery.

Group A strep infections are treatable with antibiotics, the drug of choice being penicillin. Other antibiotics, such as erythromycin and various cephalosporins, are effective alternatives for patients allergic to penicillin. FDA is responsible for ensuring the safety and effectiveness of these drugs.

Strep Throat

Strep throat (streptococcal pharyngitis) is probably the most well-known Group A strep infection. Although strep throat can occur at any age and at any time of the year, it mainly afflicts school-age children during the winter and spring. The many symptoms of strep throat include an extremely red and painful sore throat, ear pain, fever, enlarged and tender lymph nodes in the neck, white spots on the tonsils, or dark red spots on the soft palette. However, about one out of five people who has strep throat experiences no symptoms.

Because nearly all the symptoms of strep throat can also occur with viral infections, laboratory tests are used to confirm a doctor's suspicion that a patient's sore throat is caused by Group A strep. The traditional laboratory test to identify strep is a throat culture. To isolate and identify Group A strep from a throat swab takes from one to three days using the culture method. In recent years, a number of tests have become available that use antibodies to detect the presence of Group A strep directly on a throat swab, and these devices can provide test results in a matter of minutes. Many physicians feel that the rapid tests do not detect as many positive results as the culture method, so if the rapid test results are negative, a follow-up throat culture is recommended.

Strep throat is highly contagious among children because they are in close contact with one another. In addition, they have not yet developed resistance to any of the strains, as adults have.

The incubation period for strep throat is two to five days. During epidemics, siblings of a strep throat patient have a fifty-fifty chance of also succumbing to the disease, whereas only 20 percent of the parents of such patients will develop strep throat. Children with strep throat should not return to school until their fever returns to normal and they've had at least a day's worth of antibiotics.

Strep throat is easily treated with antibiotics. Treatment is usually not necessary for those individuals who harbor the strep throat microbe but show no signs of an active infection. These people are unlikely to spread infection to others, according to the American Academy of Pediatrics, or experience the complications of a strep infection, which include rheumatic fever and kidney disease.

Scarlet Fever

One of the more colorful variants of a strep infection is scarlet fever. The hallmarks of this disease include a bright red tongue, a brilliant scarlet rash (particularly on the trunk, arms and thighs), a flushed face, sore throat, and fever.

"Scarlet fever is simply strep throat with a rash," says Roberts. The red rash that typifies this disease is prompted by a toxin generated by the *Streptococcus* bacterium. The striking symptoms of scarlet fever make it easy to diagnose, but most physicians confirm their clinical diagnosis with laboratory tests.

Like strep throat, scarlet fever primarily afflicts school-aged children during the winter and spring months. Scarlet fever is easily treated with antibiotics, and, if left untended, the disease can foster the same complications prompted by strep throat.

Rheumatic Fever

Lurking behind several types of strep infections is the possibility of rheumatic fever. Although a relatively uncommon disease, the effects of rheumatic fever are serious enough to warrant concern. Signs of rheumatic fever include a red rash, pea-sized lumps under the skin, tender joints, fever, involuntary jerky movements, heart palpitations, chest pain, and, in severe cases, heart failure. Although most symptoms disappear within weeks to months, about half the time the disease leaves behind deformed heart valves that may limit patients' physical activities and foster premature death from heart failure.

Diagnosis of rheumatic fever is based on its symptoms in conjunction with a history of a recent strep infection, which can be confirmed by tests for strep antibodies in the blood.

Rheumatic fever is thought to be triggered by an overly active immune system, which inadvertently destroys body tissues in its zeal to rid the body of a strep infection. Most symptoms of rheumatic fever crop up one to four weeks after a strep infection, although involuntary jerky movements may not surface for as long as six months after infection. About half of the recent cases of rheumatic fever, however, developed with mild to no previous signs of a strep throat infection, such as a sore throat with fever.

It's these signs of a strep infection that physicians rely on to prevent rheumatic fever. As many as 3 percent of untreated cases of strep throat can develop into rheumatic fever. But antibiotic treatment, even if it's not started until several days after the onset of symptoms, can squelch the possibility of rheumatic fever.

Once rheumatic fever occurs, doctors can do little to prevent its damage in the body. Anti-inflammatory drugs (such as aspirin or steroids) can ease many of the symptoms and possibly prevent some of rheumatic fever's more serious developments. Antibiotics are also used to treat any lingering strep infections. But even with such therapies, the disease often wreaks such damage on heart valves that they have to be surgically repaired or replaced with synthetic or animal implants.

Rheumatic fever usually recurs whenever its victims experience any new strep infections. To prevent such flare-ups, the American Heart Association recommends that anyone who has experienced rheumatic fever take prophylactic (preventive) doses of antibiotics. How long rheumatic fever patients require such a preventive drug regime depends on whether they experienced heart damage and whether they're likely to develop a future strep infection. Children who've had rheumatic fever, for example, generally take antibiotics on a daily basis until they reach adulthood, when the risk of a strep infection greatly diminishes.

Skin Infection

When Group A *Streptococci* literally get under the skin, they can foster a common skin disease known as impetigo. This contagious disease frequently afflicts mainly children during the summer when insect bites, cuts and scrapes are prevalent. These skin infringements serve as portals of entry for the *Streptococci*.

Impetigo starts out as a rash of pinhead-sized blisters or pimples that rapidly run together to form yellow, flaky crusts. The impetigo rash may itch or burn, but rarely causes pain. The disease is diagnosed with the aid of cultures of the fluid lodged beneath the crusts. If large numbers of strep bacteria crop up in these cultures, their guilt in causing the disease is firmly established. Impetigo can also be caused by other bacteria, including *Staphylococcus* or by mixtures of staphylococcal and streptococcal bacteria.

Impetigo is combated with the use of topical or oral antibiotics, depending on its severity and frequency within a given population. Doctors advise impetigo patients to remove the skin crusts and wash their rash with soap on a regular basis. Occasionally, if not treated, streptococcal impetigo develops into a blood infection, and it can also foster kidney disease.

Kidney Disease

All kinds of strep infections can foster an inflammation of the kidneys (acute glomerulonephritis), although the disease most often follows impetigo. Less than 1 percent of all strep infections foster kidney disease, but because certain strains of strep are particularly prone to causing this complication, small epidemics of acute glomerulonephritis can crop up in private homes or in schools.

Symptoms of the disorder include a puffy face due to water retention, blood in the urine, pain in the loins, malaise, nausea, headache, and high blood pressure. These symptoms usually surface one to three weeks following a strep infection and subside within the same amount of time.

Diagnosis of acute post-streptococcal glomerulonephritis is based on symptoms, a history of a recent strep infection, and elevated levels of antibodies to strep in the blood. This form of kidney disease, like rheumatic fever, is thought to stem from an overactive immune response to strep.

Little can be done to prevent this heightened immune response once it's begun, although various drugs (such as diuretics) and dietary measures (such as restricted salt or protein intake) can ease many of its symptoms. Most patients recover without any permanent problems, although occasionally kidney damage inflicted by the disease may require dialysis or a kidney transplant.

Patients rarely experience a recurrence of acute glomerulonephritis following additional strep infections because of the immunity they develop to the specific type of strep bacterium that caused their disorder. (Only a handful of strep types can cause glomerulonephritis, and most cases of the disorder can be traced to a specific Group A streptococcal strain known as Type 12.)

"Strep" Demands Immediate Care

Blood Infection

Although the number of bloodstream infections (septicemia) of Group A strep appears to be on the rise, they are still extremely rare. Only about 4 to 5 people out of 100,000 develop these infections each year, according to the national Centers for Disease Control in Atlanta. But nearly one-third of all patients with *Streptoccocus* blood infections will die of them.

Septicemia usually gets its start when *streptococcal* bacteria on the skin delve into an opening as large as a surgical or battle wound or as small as a minor cut or scrape. Normally, the body's immune system checks these bloodstream invaders before they wreak havoc in the body. In those individuals whose resistance is lowered, however, *Streptoccocus* travels far and wide, causing such symptoms as fever, low blood pressure, chills, confusion, diarrhea, vomiting, or a red skin rash. Septicemia usually afflicts people over 60 who have an underlying disease such as diabetes or renal failure that compromises their immune defenses.

In addition to relying on clinical signs to diagnose septicemia, physicians use laboratory findings, including positive blood cultures, positive antibody tests, and extremely high numbers of white blood cells in the blood.

Toxic Streptococcal Syndrome

The new toxic streptococcal syndrome, first described in 1987 in this country, is similar to septicemia. Patients with this disorder have many of the same symptoms as those of septicemia, but because of the disease's rapid progression, by the time they seek treatment they are often gravely ill. Toxic streptococcal syndrome patients frequently go into shock and experience multi-organ failure, as well as complications such as the pneumonia that reportedly killed Jim Henson.

Only 1 or 2 people out of 100,000 fall prey to toxic streptococcal syndrome each year. Unlike septicemics, most of these patients don't have any underlying diseases hampering their immune defenses. Of 21 cases studied extensively by researchers, most patients were in their 30s and the youngest was 25 years old.

"The individuals who are getting strep septicemia and toxic strep syndrome," points out CDC epidemiologist Walter Straus, "are not the same ones who are getting strep throat."

Patients with toxic streptococcal syndrome are treated with antibiotics as well as with medical measures aimed at curbing the severe complications of the disease. The sooner patients are treated with antibiotics, the more likely they will recover from the syndrome, which kills about one-third of its victims.

Whether Group A *Streptococcus* infects the skin, blood, internal organs, or the throat, it is usually checked by prompt and appropriate antibiotic therapy. This is why, though recent outbreaks of serious strep infections are cause for some concern, they are not likely to prompt the extensive death or debilitation once tied to them.

Streptococci Family

The streptococcal bacteria are extremely versatile and common. Able to invade almost any part of the body, streptococci cause a host of diseases. These microbes are divided into more than a dozen different groups, based on the proteins they harbor in their cell walls and their performance on various laboratory tests. Here's a list of some of the more troublesome categories or species of *Streptococcus* and the diseases for which they are well known:

- **Group A:** strep throat, scarlet fever, rheumatic fever, impetigo, toxic streptococcal syndrome, streptococcal kidney disease, blood infections;

- **Group B:** blood infections in newborns, meningitis, childbed fever;

- **Groups C, D, G, H, K:** urinary tract infections, heart infections, meningitis, upper and lower respiratory tract infections;

- *Streptococcus mutans*: dental caries (cavities);

- *Streptococcus pneumoniae*: pneumonia, ear infections, meningitis, sinus infections.

—by Margie Patlak

Margie Patlak is a free-lance writer in Elkins Park. Pa.

Chapter 3

Acne: Taming That Age-Old Adolescent Affliction

Pimples. Nearly everyone has suffered through them—some more than others. They are an almost universal affliction of adolescence. Even one or two "zits" can cause much posturing and worrying in front of a mirror. A handful may cause panic, and a face full can result in permanent scarring—both of the skin and the psyche.

Describing 17-year-old acne sufferer Pimples Carson in his book *The Wayward Bus*, John Steinbeck wrote that the boy's face was "riveted and rotted and eroded with acne," and medicines sold to treat it "do no good whatsoever."

While acne today looks the same as it did in the 1930s, Steinbeck's assessment of the usefulness of acne medicine no longer holds true.

Although acne can't be cured, it can be treated successfully in the vast majority of people. Some cases, especially the mild types, can be cleared up completely. Vigorous treatment of the more severe types of acne can help prevent facial scarring.

Technically called acne vulgaris; this skin disease affects millions of Americans annually. It can vary from quite mild to extremely severe. About 80 percent of all teenagers develop acne, but the disease may also start as late as age 25 or 30, particularly in women.

What Causes Acne?

No one knows for sure exactly what causes acne, or why it usually begins in adolescence. But a number of factors, most importantly

---

FDA Consumer, October 1990.

heredity, play a role. If one of your parents had acne, there's a good chance you will, too. If both had it, "the gun is pointed directly at you," says FDA dermatologist Carnot Evans, M.D.

Acne develops when the sebaceous glands and the lining of the skin duct begin to work overtime, as they do in adolescence (see accompanying diagram). The glands produce more sebum, making the skin more oily. Normally the lining of the duct sheds cells that are carried to the surface of the skin by the sebum.

When the duct is blocked, cells and sebum accumulate, forming a plug (comedo). If the plug stays below the surface of the skin, it is called a "closed" comedo or whitehead. If the plug enlarges and pops

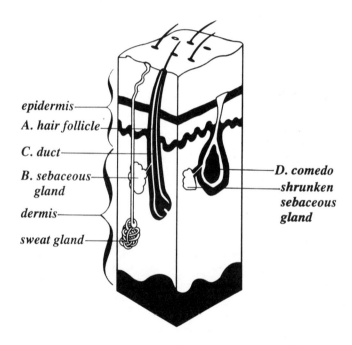

Figure 3.1. *Technically, acne is a disease of the pilosebaceous unit in the skin. This unit is composed of a hair follicle (A) and a sebaceous gland (B), which is connected to the surface of the skin by a duct (C) through which the hair passes. The sebaceous gland produces sebum, a mixture of fats and waxes, which travels through the duct and spreads over the surface of the skin to help keep the skin and hair moist. When acne develops, cells shed from the lining of the duct stick together to form a thick layer that blocks the duct. More cells and sebum pile up behind this layer and form a plug called a comedo (D).*

Acne: Taming That Age-Old Adolescent Affliction

out of the duct, it is called an "open" comedo or blackhead because the tip is dark. This is not dirt and will not wash away. The discoloration is due to a buildup of melanin, the dark pigment in the skin.

Pilosebaceous units are found all over the body, but there are more on the face, upper chest, and back, which explains why acne usually occurs in these places.

There are two main types of acne: non-inflammatory and inflammatory. In non-inflammatory acne, there are usually just a few whiteheads and blackheads on the face. A relatively mild type of acne, it can be treated effectively with nonprescription medicines or, in the case of blackheads, with the prescription drug Retin-A. The majority of people with acne have this type.

With inflammatory acne, the whiteheads become inflamed, and pimples and pustules develop. In its most severe form, inflammatory acne can cause disfiguring cysts and deep, pitting scars of the face, neck, back, chest, and groin. Prescription drugs and sometimes surgery are needed to treat inflammatory acne.

Advent of Adolescence

Acne almost always starts when the body begins to mature—at about age 11 for girls and 13 for boys. Acne tends to be more severe among boys because their bodies begin increased production of male hormones called androgens that, among other things, stimulate the activity of the sebaceous gland. Girls also produce these hormones, but only one-tenth as much. The exact role hormones play in the development of acne is not known. However, studies have found that many teenage girls and women with acne have higher than normal androgen levels. These findings suggest that acne in women may be associated with increased androgen production.

Additional Triggers

In addition to puberty, a number of other factors can cause, trigger or contribute to the development of acne.

- Some drugs (including certain hormones, epilepsy drugs, and anti-tuberculosis medicines) can cause acne.

- Exposure to industrial oils and grease and chemicals, such as PCBs, can cause acne.

- The bacteria corynebacterium acnes can indirectly contribute to the development of acne by causing skin fats to break down into irritating chemicals.

- Stress and strong emotions, such as guilt, anxiety and fear, can trigger acne in people who have a predisposition to the disease.

- The onset of the menstrual period each month can trigger or worsen acne. Some 60 to 70 percent of women notice that acne gets worse the week before menstruation.

- Birth control pills appear to have an effect on acne in some women. Perplexingly, they cause acne in some cases and clear it up in others.

- Some oily cosmetics and shampoos can, on rare occasion, trigger acne in people who have a predisposition to it.

Dispelling the Myths

Contrary to earlier belief, there is no scientific evidence that foods such as chocolate, nuts, cola drinks, potato chips, french fries, and other fatty "junk food" cause acne or make it worse. Nonetheless, some people do notice that certain things they eat or drink or do seem to trigger their acne, says FDA's Evans.

Oily skin and hair do not cause acne either. Although there is an association between the severity of acne and the amount of oil produced by the skin, not all people with oily skin have acne—and some people with dry skin do.

Acne sufferers often report that their acne improves in the summer, leading to the belief that the sun has a modifying effect. A recent Swedish study on the influence of sunlight on skin found that the majority of people with acne experienced improvement after exposure to sun.

However, medical opinion on the value of sunlight varies. "It's hard to say whether it's the sun or psyche that has an effect on acne," says Evans. "The sun may have a modest effect in some people, but the relaxation usually associated with summer is also probably a factor."

One thing is certain, though. The idea that the sun improves acne by drying out greasy skin is incorrect. Sun increases oil production, which is why people tend to have oilier skin in the summer.

Acne: Taming That Age-Old Adolescent Affliction

Clearing up Acne

What can you do to clear up mild acne? Evans advises the following:

- Get a nonprescription acne medicine and apply regularly. Over-the-counter drugs containing sulfur, resorcinol, salicylic acid, and benzoyl peroxide are all effective for treating mild acne.

- Use ordinary hygiene on affected areas, washing your face once or twice daily with your usual soap or cleanser. Deodorant soaps may be used, but they are of no particular value for acne.

- Avoid any food or drink you know is a trigger.

If these measures don't work, Evans advises, see a dermatologist.
While it might be tempting to pick at pimples and squeeze blackheads, this can injure the skin and underlying tissues. Doctors advise patients not to pick pimples. Medical instruments called comedo extractors are used to remove blackheads. Some doctors may suggest that their patients use such an instrument themselves. Other doctors would rather remove the blackheads in their office or clinic because of a risk of scarring.

Treating Serious Acne

One drug dermatologists sometimes prescribe for serious acne is tretinoin, commonly known as Retin-A. A derivative of vitamin A, Retin-A comes in cream, gel and liquid forms and is rubbed onto the skin once nightly. It is highly effective for treating blackhead acne and modestly effective for treating pimples and pustules. Retin-A usually begins to clear up acne in two to three weeks, although in some cases it's more than six weeks before any improvement is noticed.

Scientists do not know exactly how Retin-A works, but research suggests that it both pushes out the comedo plugs beneath the skin and helps prevent their re-formation.

One of the main side effects of Retin-A—one that occurs in all users—is a heightened susceptibility to sunlight. Therefore, those who use Retin-A should stay out of the sun as much as possible, and when in the sun should minimize its effects with sunscreens and protective clothing. Retin-A users should also avoid sun lamps because their ultraviolet rays mimic those of the sun.

Another common side-effect of Retin-A is drying, irritation or peeling of the skin. When this occurs, the doctor may suggest patients cut back use to two or three times a week.

Some antibiotics are effective for treating and preventing pustules and cysts of severe acne. Tetracyclines and erythromycin are the most commonly prescribed.

Treating Severe Cystic Acne

For very severe, disfiguring acne unresponsive to the treatments mentioned, the doctor may prescribe isotretinoin, commonly known as Accutane. Also a vitamin A derivative, Accutane is taken orally in capsule form. It is highly effective for treating severe cystic acne and preventing the deep pits and scars that result.

Scientists do not know exactly how Accutane works, but evidence suggests that it reduces the size of the sebaceous gland and the amount of sebum secreted. In any case, it completely clears up the disease in many people.

Women should use Accutane with extreme caution, however, because it can cause miscarriage and birth defects. If a woman becomes pregnant while taking the drug, there is a great possibility her baby will be born deformed. Therefore, Accutane's use is tightly regulated by FDA. Doctors may only prescribe it for a woman who has had a negative pregnancy test and does not intend to become pregnant while taking it, and who has signed a consent form that she has been fully informed of its side effects. (See "New Warning About Accutane and Birth Defects," in the October 1988 *FDA Consumer*.)

In addition to the danger of fetal malformation and miscarriage, there are a number of minor side effects associated with Accutane. Ninety percent of those who take the drug experience inflammation of the lips (and less frequently of the eyes), and 80 percent experience drying of the skin, nose or mouth.

In severe cases of acne, the dermatologist may surgically drain large pustules or abscesses. In addition, plastic surgery is sometimes used to smooth over deeply pitted and scarred skin. Dermabrasion (a technique to remove scars that is like sandpapering the skin) is being used less frequently. Dermabrasion has become less popular because it can discolor the face and because new acne medicines have made it increasingly less necessary.

However unpleasant and embarrassing acne is, it usually begins, peaks, and runs its course in adolescence, slowly fading away in early

Acne: Taming That Age-Old Adolescent Affliction

adulthood. During those critical teen years, modern medicines and treatment can do much to ease the discomfort and embarrassment of the acne sufferer.

—by Sharon Snider

Sharon Snider is a staff writer for *FDA Consumer*.

Chapter 4

Candida: An Itch like No Other

It's an itchy feeling you might hardly notice at first.

Maybe, you muse, it's just that your jeans are too tight.

Actually, tight jeans may have something to do with it. But if the itch keeps getting itchier, even when your jeans have been off for a while, then there's something else involved.

That something else could very well be a fungus whose technical name is *Candida*, and which causes what is often called a "yeast" infection. Such infections are most common in teenage girls and women aged 16 to 35, although they can occur in girls as young as 10 or 11 and in older women (and less often, in men and boys as well). You do not have to be sexually active to get a yeast infection.

The Food and Drug Administration now allows medicines that used to be prescription-only to be sold without a prescription to treat vaginal yeast infections that keep coming back. But before you run out and buy one, if you've never been treated for a yeast infection you should see a doctor. Your doctor may advise you to use one of the over-the-counter products or may prescribe a drug called Diflucan (fluconazole). FDA recently approved the drug, a tablet taken by mouth, for clearing up yeast infections with just one dose.

Though itchiness is a main symptom of yeast infections, if you've never had one before, it's hard to be sure just what's causing your discomfort. After a doctor makes a diagnosis of vaginal yeast infection, if you should have one again, you can more easily recognize the

---

FDA Consumer, April 1996.

symptoms that make it different from similar problems. If you have any doubts, though, you should contact your doctor.

In addition to intense itching, another symptom of a vaginal yeast infection is a white curdy or thick discharge that is mostly odorless. Although some women have discharges midway between their menstrual periods, these are usually not yeast infections, especially if there's no itching.

Other symptoms of a vaginal yeast infection include:

- soreness
- rash on outer lips of the vagina
- burning, especially during urination.

It's important to remember that not all girls and women experience all these symptoms, and if intense itching is not present it's probably something else.

Candida is a fungus often present in the human body. It only causes problems when there's too much of it. Then infections can occur not only in the vagina but in other parts of the body as well—and in both sexes. Though there are four different types of *Candida* that can cause these infections, nearly 80 percent are caused by a variety called *Candida albicans*.

Many Causes

The biggest cause of *Candida* infections is lowered immunity. This can happen when you get run down from doing too much and not getting enough rest. Or it can happen as a result of illness.

Though not usual, repeated yeast infections, especially if they don't clear up with proper treatment, may sometimes be the first sign that a woman is infected with HIV, the virus that causes AIDS.

FDA requires that over-the-counter (OTC) products to treat yeast infections carry the following warning:

"If you experience vaginal yeast infections frequently (they recur within a two-month period) or if you have vaginal yeast infections that do not clear up easily with proper treatment, you should see your doctor promptly to determine the cause and receive proper medical care."

Candida: An Itch like No Other

Repeated yeast infections can also be caused by other, less serious, illnesses or physical and mental stress. Other causes include:

- use of antibiotics and some other medications, including birth control pills
- significant change in the diet
- poor nutrition
- diabetes
- pregnancy.

Some women get mild yeast infections toward the end of their menstrual periods, possibly in response to the body's hormonal changes. These mild infections sometimes go away without treatment as the menstrual cycle progresses. Pregnant women are also more prone to develop yeast infections.

Sometimes hot, humid weather can make it easier for yeast infections to develop. And wearing layers of clothing in the winter that make you too warm indoors can also increase the likelihood of infection.

"*Candida* infections are not usually thought of as sexually transmitted diseases," says Renata Albrecht, M.D., of FDA's division of anti-infective drug products. But, she adds, they can be transmitted during sex.

The best way not to have to worry about getting yeast infections this way is not to have sex. But if you do have sex, using a condom will help prevent transmission of yeast infections, just as it helps prevent transmission of more commonly sexually transmitted diseases, including HIV infection, and helps prevent pregnancy. Teens should always use a latex condom if they have sex, even if they are also using other forms of birth control. (See "On the Teen Scene: Preventing STDs" in the June 1993 *FDA Consumer*.)

If one partner has a yeast infection, the other partner should also be treated for it. A man is less likely than a woman to be aware of having a yeast infection because he may not have any symptoms. When symptoms do occur, they may include a moist, white, scaling rash on the penis, and itchiness or redness under the foreskin. As with females, lowered immunity, rather than sexual transmission, is the most frequent cause of genital yeast infections in males.

OTC Products

The OTC products for vaginal yeast infections have one of three active ingredients:

- butoconazole nitrate (Femstat 3),
- clotrimazole (Gyne-Lotrimin and others), or
- miconazole (Monistat 7 and others).

These drugs are in the same anti-fungal family and work in similar ways to break down the cell wall of the *Candida* organism until it dissolves. FDA approved the switch of Femstat 3 from prescription to OTC status in December 1995. The others have been available OTC for a few years.

When you visit the doctor the first time you have a yeast infection, you can ask which product may be best for you and discuss the advantages of the different forms the products come in: vaginal suppositories (inserts) and creams with special applicators. Remember to read the warnings on the product's labeling carefully and follow the directions.

Symptoms usually improve within a few days, but it's important to continue using the medication for the number of days directed, even if you no longer have symptoms.

Contact your doctor if you have the following:

- abdominal pain, fever, or a foul-smelling discharge
- no improvement within three days
- symptoms that recur within two months.

OTC products are only for vaginal yeast infections. They should not be used by men or for yeast infections in other areas of the body, such as the mouth or under the fingernails.

Candida infections in the mouth are often called "thrush." Symptoms include creamy white patches that cover painful areas in the mouth, throat, or on the tongue. Because other infections cause similar symptoms, it's important to go to a doctor for an accurate diagnosis.

Wearing artificial fingernails increases the chance of getting yeast infections under the natural fingernails. Fungal infections start in the space between the artificial and natural nails, which become discolored. Treatment for these types of infections—as well as those that occur in other skin folds, such as underarms or between toes—require different products, most of which are available only with a doctor's prescription.

Knowing the causes and symptoms of yeast infections can help you take steps, such as giving those tight jeans a rest, to greatly reduce the chances of getting an infection.

And, if sometimes prevention isn't enough, help is easily at hand from your doctor and pharmacy.

How to Avoid Infection

Here are some steps young women can take to make vaginal yeast infections less likely:

- Wear loose, natural fiber clothing and underwear with a cotton crotch.
- Limit wearing of panty hose, tights, leggings, nylon underwear, and tight jeans.
- Don't use deodorant tampons and feminine deodorant sprays, especially if you feel an infection beginning.
- Dry off quickly and thoroughly after bathing and swimming; don't stay in a wet swimsuit for hours.
- It's better not to have sex in your teens, but if you're sexually active, always use a latex condom.

—by Judith Levine Willis

Judith Levine Willis is editor of *FDA Consumer*.

Chapter 5

Treatment Pales Rosacea's Red Face

When she was a teenager and her friends were bemoaning the whiteheads and blackheads erupting on their faces, Marcia Meyer of Kensington, Md., had a clear, ruddy complexion. She was surprised, then, when her face broke out in pimples for the first time when she was in her twenties. Feeling she was "too old for this," Meyer says, and upset over her appearance, she went to see her dermatologist, who told her she had a skin disorder known as rosacea.

Although few people are familiar with the disease, rosacea is a common skin disorder that afflicts about 1 in 20 people in this country, estimates dermatologist and rosacea expert Jonathan Wilkin, M.D., of Ohio State University in Columbus. Despite its prevalence, many people with the condition go undiagnosed, he says.

Wilkin has seen patients who seek care for other skin disorders and don't realize they have rosacea until he points it out to them. "Most people with rosacea are surprised to hear it's something the medical field can help them with," he says, "because they think it's just a complexion problem that runs in their family."

The disorder can be effectively curbed with various drugs, laser treatments, and surgery, including products regulated by the Food and Drug Administration, as well as by preventive measures. Without proper care, in contrast, rosacea may progress to a more disfiguring condition.

Although it can occur among adults of any age and of any skin color, rosacea is more prevalent among fair-skinned people between the ages

---

FDA Consumer, April 1994.

of 30 and 50. The disease is more common in women, but more severe when it strikes men. People who flush easily are more prone to rosacea, as are people with peaches-and-cream complexions, including many with Irish, English, or Eastern European ancestry, a survey by the National Rosacea Society suggests. The tendency toward rosacea appears to be inherited; often several people in a family have the condition.

Red Mask

Rosacea usually begins with frequent flushing of the face, particularly of the nose and cheeks, although sometimes the redness spreads to the chin and forehead as well. The flushing is caused by swelling of the blood vessels under the skin of the face and can last as little as a few minutes to as long as a few hours. In most cases, however, eventually the blood vessels stay dilated and a sunburn-like redness becomes a permanent feature on the central areas of the face.

This red mask can serve as a red flag for attention. Meyer notes that people tend to tease her about being out in the sun too much. "I'm probably the only person who uses makeup to tone down her face, rather than the reverse," she says.

Once the redness becomes permanent, it often is accompanied by pus-filled or solid red pimples. There are no blackheads or whiteheads with rosacea, and the pimples are usually limited to the central portion of the face. Thin red lines that resemble a road map also tend to surface. These lines are actually small blood vessels in the upper layers of the skin that have become enlarged. If rosacea is not treated, a condition called rhinophyma can develop in some people. Rhinophyma occurs much more frequently in males than in females. The hallmark of rhinophyma is a big bulbous red nose like the one sported by the late comedian W.C. Fields, who had rosacea with rhinophyma. The nose can also become thicker at the base.

This disfiguring condition "has never killed anyone," notes Wilkin, "but it has ruined a lot of lives."

Rosacea can also cause a persistent burning and grittiness of the eyes or inflamed and swollen eyelids. In severe cases, vision may become impaired.

Waxing and Waning

Rosacea is a chronic ailment that waxes and wanes. Between flare-ups, some people have no signs of the disorder. But other people still have facial redness or red lines, accompanied by pimples during flare-ups.

Treatment Pales Rosacea's Red Face

Dermatologists usually diagnose rosacea by its symptoms; no tests are available, but on rare occasions skin biopsies can pinpoint the condition. Few people with rosacea have all the symptoms of the disorder, which can make it tricky to diagnose at times, Wilkin admits. He strongly suspects rosacea in people with just a few symptoms of the disorder if other people in their family have the condition.

There is also a condition known as steroid-induced rosacea, which occurs in some people after applying corticosteroid ointments to their face for a long period to treat eczema or other rashes. The onset of this condition is sudden. The same telltale redness, pimples, and thin, wavy red lines appear on the face as in standard rosacea, but people with steroid-induced rosacea usually have these symptoms wherever the steroid ointment was applied-up to the hairline—and not just centrally located on the face, for example. People with steroid-induced rosacea also often have a distinctive shine to their facial skin.

Steroid-induced rosacea is treated first by stopping the steroid and then by taking the same medications as with standard rosacea. Although it can take several months of treatment before symptoms subside, steroid-induced rosacea is not likely to recur unless corticosteroids are applied again on the face. Less commonly, oral or inhaled corticosteroids can also induce rosacea.

Searching for a Cause

Although dermatologists have been speculating about causes for standard rosacea for more than a century, none have been definitively proven. Most experts think the condition can be provoked by several different factors, some of which may work together to cause rosacea.

One might be an underlying vascular disorder that causes blood vessels in the face to expand and fluid to build up in the skin. This fluid can trigger an inflammatory response that manifests as facial pimples or excess tissue growth on the nose.

Wilkin says several findings support this theory. One is that researchers detected structural abnormalities in the small blood vessels in the facial skin of patients with rosacea. Another is that rosacea worsened when people with the condition take drugs such as theophylline and nitroglycerin, which dilate blood vessels. Also, people with rosacea are more likely to suffer from migraines, which are also thought to be caused by a vascular disorder. A vascular cause for rosacea might also explain why the condition is more common in older women, who are more likely to have swelling of the facial blood vessels as part of the menopausal "hot flashes."

In addition to vascular disorders, another factor that might play a role in fostering rosacea is a microscopic mite by the name of Demodex folliculorum. This mite, a normal resident in human skin, lives in hair follicles, where it dines on cast-off skin cells. They have been retrieved from almost every area of human skin, but they have a taste for the face.

Two recent studies revealed that the mites were significantly more numerous in facial skin samples of people with rosacea than of people without the condition. In addition, the mite population peaked on the skin samples of these patients in the spring, when rosacea tends to flare up. The studies were done by Frank Powell, M.D., and colleagues at the Mater Misericordiae Hospital in Dublin, Ireland, and by F. Forton, M.D., and B. Seys, M.D., of the Saint Pierre University Hospital in Brussels, Belgium.

According to Powell, other studies show that patients with steroid-induced rosacea also had a boosted mite population on their faces. This population dropped when the rosacea subsided after treatment with an ointment that kills mites.

Although these findings do not prove that the skin mite causes rosacea, they do suggest that Demodex might play a role in fostering the disorder. The mites may provoke rosacea by clogging skin follicles, which in turn might trigger an inflammatory response. Rosacea may also be triggered by an allergic-like reaction to these skin mites or to the bacteria the mites harbor. Forton proposes that an underlying vascular disorder of the face that fosters flushing could create an environment particularly hospitable to Demodex mites. These mites could then multiply excessively or penetrate more deeply into the skin, triggering an inflammatory response in the form of pimples.

Other Flare-up Triggers

Several other factors have been found to aggravate (but not necessarily cause) rosacea, mainly by triggering flushing. These factors include drinking hot beverages, smoking, certain emotions (such as worry and anxiety), spicy foods, large meals, exposure to temperature extremes, wind, excessive sunlight, and overindulgence in alcohol. (Although alcohol can worsen rosacea, a nondrinker can develop a case of rosacea just as severe as someone fond of alcohol.) Make-up, moisturizers, sunscreens, or other skin products used on the face that contain alcohol or other irritating ingredients can also foster a rosacea flare-up.

Treatment Pales Rosacea's Red Face

What worsens one person's rosacea may not have any effect on another person's symptoms—it's very individual. "Many patients can actually reduce or eliminate the need for medications to control their rosacea," said Wilkin, "by avoiding the factors that trigger it."

Treatment Effective

If preventive measures aren't effective, however, the pimples can often be effectively treated with certain drugs. FDA has approved Metrogel (metronidazole), a topical antiprotozoal and antibacterial, to treat rosacea. Doctors may also use several other approved drugs to treat rosacea-induced acne. Such drugs include oral and topical antibiotics, particularly those in the tetracycline family, and these are also often used to treat eye manifestations of rosacea. (Pregnant women should not take tetracycline because it can discolor the unborn child's teeth.)

Such therapy for acne is effective in about three-quarters of rosacea patients, usually within a few months, according to dermatologist Seymour Rand, M.D., of FDA.

Removing Unsightly Vessels

Wilkin says that some rosacea patients find antibiotic therapy not only relieves their acne, but also decreases facial redness, which had been hiding the spidery red lines of enlarged blood vessels. Dermatologists can usually rid the face of these enlarged blood vessels by destroying them with an electrical needle or a laser. Patients who have this treatment experience little or no discomfort. Their faces may look somewhat bruised for about a week after the procedure, and may scab, peel or crust.

To treat the more extensive facial redness, dermatologists can use lasers to destroy the expanded blood vessels in the skin that cause it. One recent study by San Diego dermatologist Nicholas Lowe, M.D., and associates found laser therapy effective in more than three-quarters of treated patients. In more than half of those, the therapy not only rid the face of the redness or red lines, but also stemmed the acne. This finding further supports a vascular cause for rosacea, according to Wilkin.

Lasers or electrical devices are also used to remove the excess tissue that accumulates on the nose in patients with rhinophyma. The tissue can also be removed with a scalpel or a rapidly rotating wire brush, which is often used by dermatologists to scrape away tissue in a procedure known as dermabrasion. Local anesthesia numbs patients' noses before treatment. The nose looks red for a year or so following tissue removal and then assumes a normal skin color, according to Wilkin. "I've seen people whose noses were the size of baseballs look great after treatment," he says.

One of the most difficult barriers to countering rosacea is convincing people with the disorder to seek care. Even after Meyer knew she had rosacea, for example, she delayed seeking medical treatment for a flare-up because she thought the emotional stress she was experiencing at the time was behind her "acne."

"Even though my personal problems hadn't gone away," she said, "within a week of treatment, my 'acne' did. My appearance improved so quickly, I wished I hadn't waited so long to see my dermatologist. I hope others won't be so slow to go to the doctor."

Many people don't see a doctor because they don't realize they have a condition that can be treated. But, as Wilkin notes, "People with rosacea can be very hopeful, whatever stage they've got, because there's something that can be done for everyone."

—by Margie Patlak

Margie Patlak is a writer in Elkins Park, Pa.

Chapter 6

Pruritus: Persistent Itching

Overview

Pruritus (or itching) is an unpleasant sensation that elicits the desire to scratch. It is a distressing symptom that can cause alterations in comfort and threaten the effectiveness of the skin as a major protective barrier. Because of the subjective nature of pruritus, the lack of a precise definition, and the lack of suitable animal models, pruritus is a disorder that has not been researched adequately.

The skin comprises 15 percent of the body's total weight, and is the largest organ of the body. The skin has significant psychosocial and physical functions. Its function as a protective mechanism is the skin's most important role. But skin is also essential to self image and one's ability to touch and be touched, thereby providing an important component of communication.

Symptoms of generalized itching, without rash or skin lesions, may be related to anything from dry skin to an occult carcinoma, and the etiology of the symptoms should be explored. Common nonmalignant etiologic factors include drug reactions, xerosis, scabies, or primary skin diseases. Pruritus is one of the most common complaints of the elderly patient, but estimates of the significance of pruritic symptoms in the elderly population vary from 10 to 50 percent. The most common diagnosis related to pruritus in this population is simply dry skin.[1]

1995, National Cancer Institute No. 208/00609.

Generalized pruritus is found in about 13 percent of all individuals with chronic renal disease and about 70 to 90 percent of those undergoing hemodialysis for its treatment.[2] Cholestatic liver disease with intrahepatic or posthepatic obstruction, with or without increased serum levels of bile acids, is often associated with pruritus.[3] Other etiologic factors include (but are not limited to) primary biliary cirrhosis, cholestasis related to phenothiazines or oral contraceptives, intrahepatic cholestasis in pregnancy, and posthepatic obstruction.[3]

References:

1. Duncan, W.C.; Fenske, N.A., "Cutaneous Signs of Internal Disease in the Elderly." *Geriatrics* 45(8): 24-30, 1990.
2. Blachley, J.D.; Blankenship, D.M.; Menter, A.; et al. "Uremic Pruritus: Skin Divalent Ion Content and Response to Ultraviolet Phototherapy." *American Journal of Kidney Diseases* 5(5): 237-241, 1985.
3. Abel, E.A.; Farber, E.M. "Malignant Cutaneous Tumors." In: Rubenstein, E.; Federman, D.D. Eds.: *Scientific American. Medicine.* New York: Scientific American, Inc, Chapter 2: Dermatology, Section XII.

Etiology/pathophysiology

Hematologic disorders that cause pruritus include polycythemia vera. Some conditions that cause iron deficiency, including exfoliative skin disorder, also cause pruritus. Diabetes and thyrotoxicosis are endocrine causes of pruritus.[1]

Pruritus is a frequent clinical manifestation of people with AIDS, AIDS-related Kaposi's sarcoma, and AIDS-related opportunistic infections. Pruritus with or without rash has been reported in approximately 84 percent of people with AIDS and 35.5 percent of those with AIDS-related Kaposi's sarcoma. The incidence of pruritus associated with AIDS-related opportunistic infections approaches 100 percent.[2]

Various malignant diseases are known to produce pruritus. Hodgkin's disease causes pruritus in 10 to 25 percent of patients. In some instances, pruritus precedes diagnosis of the lymphoma,[1] and may be an indicator of a less favorable prognosis when associated with significant fever or weight loss ("B" symptoms).[3] Pruritus associated with Hodgkin's disease is characterized by symptoms of burning and intense itching occurring on a localized skin area, frequently on the lower legs. Other lymphomas and leukemias have been associated with a less intense but more generalized pruritus. Adenocarcinomas and squamous cell carcinomas of various organs (i.e., stomach, pancreas, lung, colon, brain, breast, and prostate) sometimes produce generalized pruritus that is more pronounced on the legs, upper trunk, and extensor surfaces of the upper extremities.[1,3] Pruritus associated with malignant diseases has been observed to diminish or disappear with eradication of the tumor and reappear with recurrence of disease.[3]

Drugs associated with secondary pruritus include opium derivatives (cocaine, morphine, butorphanol), phenothiazines, tolbutamide, erythromycin estolate, anabolic hormones, estrogens, Progestins, testosterone and subsequent cholestasis, aspirin, quinidine and other antimalarials, biologics such as monoclonal antibodies, and vitamin B complex. Subclinical sensitivity to any drug may be related to pruritus.[3]

Hypothesized mechanisms of pruritus have been inferred from studies of pain, since pain and itching share common molecular and neurophysiological mechanisms.[4] Both itch and pain sensations result from the activation of a network of free nerve endings at the dermal-epidermal junction. Activation may be the result of internal or external thermal, mechanical, chemical, or electrical stimulation. The cutaneous nerve stimulation is activated or mediated by several substances including histamine, vasoactive peptides, enkephalins, substance P (a tachykinin that affects smooth muscle), and prostaglandins. It is believed that non-anatomic factors (such as psychological stress, tolerance, presence and intensity of other sensations and/or distractions) determine itch sensitivity in different regions of the body.

The itch impulse is transmitted along the same neural pathway as pain impulses, i.e., traveling from peripheral nerves to the dorsal horn of the spinal cord, across the cord via the anterior commissure, and ascending along the spinothalamic tract to the laminar nuclei of the contralateral thalamus. Thalamocortical tracts of tertiary neurons are believed to relay the impulse through the integrating reticular activating system of the thalamus to several areas of the cerebral cortex. Factors that are believed to enhance the sensation of itch include dryness of the epidermis and dermis, anoxia of tissues, dilation of the capillaries, irritating stimuli, and psychological responses.[1,3-5]

The motor response of scratching follows the perception of itch. Scratching is modulated at the corticothalamic center and is a spinal reflex. After scratching, itching may be relieved for 15 to 25 minutes.

The mechanism through which the itch is relieved by scratching is unknown. It is hypothesized that scratching generates sensory impulses, which break circuits in the relay areas of the spinal cord. Scratching may actually enhance the sensation of itching, creating a characteristic itch-scratch-itch cycle. Other physical stimuli such as vibration, heat, cold, and ultraviolet radiation diminish itching and increase the release of proteolytic enzymes, potentially eliciting the itch-scratch-itch cycle.

A pinprick near or in the same dermatome as an itchy point will abolish the itch sensation.[3] It is known that hard scratching may substitute pain for the itch, and in some instances, the patient might find pain the more tolerable sensation. It is thought that spinal modulation of afferent stimuli (Gate theory) and central mechanisms may play a role in the relief of itch.[3]

Hypothesized pathogenesis of pruritus associated with underlying disease states are varied. Biliary, hepatic, renal, and malignant diseases are thought to produce pruritus through circulating toxic substances. Histamine released from circulating basophils and the release of leukopeptidase from white blood cells may trigger pruritus associated with lymphomas and leukemias. Elevated blood levels of kininogen in Hodgkin's disease, release of histamine or bradykinin precursors from solid tumors, and release of serotonin in carcinoid may all be related to pruritus.[1,6]

People receiving cytotoxic chemotherapy, irradiation, and/or biologic response modifiers for treatment of malignancy are likely to experience pruritus. This same population is quite likely to be exposed to many of the other etiologic factors relating to pruritus ranging from nutritionally related xerosis (dry skin) to radiation desquamation, chemotherapy and biologic agent-induced side effects, antibiotic reactions, and other drug sensitivities.

Cytotoxic Chemotherapy

Each of the major classes of antineoplastic agents (alkylating agents, antimetabolites, antibiotics, plant alkaloids, nitrosoureas, and enzymes) include drugs capable of producing cutaneous reactions including pruritus. Patients receiving antineoplastic drugs frequently report dry skin and scaling, thought to be related to effects on sebaceous and sweat glands.[7,8] Many problems are self-limiting and require no active intervention. Other problems warrant anticipation and implementation of preventive measures.

Hypersensitivity to cytotoxic agents can be manifested by pruritus, edema, urticaria, and erythema. Hypersensitivity reactions vary in symptomatology and depend on the drug, the dosage, and the allergy history of the patient. The agents most associated with hypersensitivities include doxorubicin, daunorubicin, cytarabine, L-asparaginase, paclitaxel, and cisplatin. In most reports, these reactions have been localized to the area of the vascular access and dissipate within 30 to 90 minutes.[9,10] More dramatic and even life-threatening reactions can occur, and the development of pruritus may represent an early stage of serious hypersensitivity reactions.[11]

Radiation Therapy

Radiation therapy-related pruritus is usually associated with dry desquamation of skin within the treatment field. Dryness and pruritus may occur at an accumulated dose of 2000 to 2800 cGy,[12] and is caused by obliteration of sebaceous glands within the field. This is an acute phenomenon that correlates with the depletion of actively proliferating basal cells in the epidermal layer of the skin, a fixed percentage of which die with each dose fraction of irradiation. Remaining basal cells undergo cornification and shed at an increased rate, while non-proliferating basal cells are stimulated and their cell cycle shortened. Subsequent peeling of the skin is defined as dry desquamation. The skin becomes dry and the patient may notice itching and burning sensations.[12] Dry skin is susceptible to further injury through scratching and/or formation of fissures, augmenting the risk of infection and tissue necrosis.

If the desquamation process continues, the dermis will eventually be exposed and moist desquamation results. This side effect increases the risk of infection, discomfort, and pain, possibly necessitating interruption of a treatment plan to allow for healing. This can compromise the final outcome of cancer therapy. For this reason, it is desirable to anticipate and prevent the progression of skin reactions to this stage.[13]

External beam therapy with electrons may elicit sore skin reactions than photon therapy since the depth of penetration and linear energy transfer is closer to the skin surface with electrons. Radiation delivery techniques (bolus doses and tangential fields) also influence the degree of reaction. Fields that include skin folds (i.e., the axilla, breast, perineum, and gluteus) are anticipated to have increased reactions because of friction, higher moisture content, and low aeration.[14,15]

Combination Therapy

Therapy combining radiation and chemotherapy plays a significant role in state-of-the-art cancer therapy. The synergism of these cytotoxic modalities enhances normal tissue reaction and can be expected to precipitate higher complication rates.[7] The total combined effects of the drugs and irradiation exceed the individual effects of either modality. Significant cutaneous reactions are thought to occur more frequently when chemotherapy and irradiation are administered concurrently.[16]

Biologic Response Modifiers

Biologic response modifiers used in the treatment of malignant disease are associated with a wide variety of side effects and toxicities. Pruritus has been a side effect associated with several biologics, but has so far been most reported in patients receiving interferons.[17-20] To date, reports of pruritus as a side effect of biologics are primarily anecdotal and have not been a focus of attention.

Bone Marrow Transplantation

Graft-versus-host disease (GVHD) affects 25 to 50 percent of patients who live longer than 100 days after bone marrow transplantation. The incidence of skin GVHD is reported to be 80 to 90 percent and symptoms vary in severity and type.[21] Reported skin changes include dryness and pruritic, erythematous, maculopapular rashes. Onset can be subtle or sudden; skin GVHD can progress to scleroderma and contracture.[22]

Other Pharmacologic Support During Cancer Treatment

Many pharmacologic agents employed at any point during the cancer course, whether in a primary treatment plan or incorporated into a symptom control or supportive care program, are capable of eliciting a pruritic reaction. These drugs include morphine, other opium derivatives, and aspirin used in pain management; corticosteroids; antibiotics; phenothiazines; and to a lesser degree, hormonal agents (estrogen, progestins, and testosterone).[3] Mechanisms of these reactions range from hypersensitivity to chemical interference with neural pathways.[4]

Infection

Pruritus can be a symptom of infection. Pruritus involving anal or vulvar areas might be caused by infections with trichomonas or fungi, local tumors, hemorrhoids, anal fissures, fistula discharge, wound effluent, or surgical wound drainage.

References:

1. Abel, E.A.; Farber, E.M. "Malignant Cutaneous Tumors." In: Rubenstein, E.; Federman, D.D. Eds.: *Scientific American. Medicine*. New York: Scientific American, Inc, Chapter 2: Dermatology, Section XII.
2. Dangel, R.B. "Pruritus and Cancer." *Oncology Nursing Forum* 13(1): 17-21, 1986.
3. Bernhard, J.D. "Clinical Aspects of Pruritus." In: Fitzpatrick, T.B.; Eisen, A.Z.; Wolff, K.; et al. Eds.: *Dermatology in General Medicine*. New York: McGraw-Hill, 3rd ed., 1987, pp 78-90.
4. Greaves, M.U. "Pathophysiology of Pruritus." In: Fitzpatrick, T.B.; Eisen, A.Z.; Wolff, K.; et al. Eds.: *Dermatology in General Medicine*. New York: McGraw-Hill, 3rd ed., 1987, pp 74-78.
5. Duncan, W.C.; Fenske, N.A.; "Cutaneous Signs of Internal Disease in the Elderly." *Geriatrics* 45(8): 24-30, 1990.
6. Abel, E.A.; Farber, E.M.; "Drug Eruptions and Urticaria." In: Rubenstein, E.; Federman, D.D. Eds.: *Scientific American. Medicine*. New York: Scientific American, Inc, Chapter 2: Dermatology, Section VI.
7. Dunagin, W.G. "Clinical Toxicity of Chemotherapeutic Agents: Dermatologic Toxicity." *Seminars in Oncology* 9(1): 14-22, 1982.
8. Hood, A.F. "Cutaneous Side Effects of Cancer Chemotherapy." *Medical Clinics of North America* 70(1): 187-209, 1986.
9. Gullo, S.M. "Adriamycin Extravasation Versus Flare." *Oncology Nursing Forum* 7(4): 7, 1980.
10. Barlock, A.L.; Howser, D.M.; Hubbard, S.M.; "Nursing Management of Adriamycin Flare." *American Journal of Nursing* 79(1): 94-96, 1979.
11. Weiss, R.B. "Hypersensitivity Reactions to Cancer Chemotherapy." In: Perry, M.C.; Yarbro, J.W. Eds.: *Clinical Oncology Monographs: Toxicity of Chemotherapy*. Orlando, FL: Grune and Stratton Inc., 1984, pp 101-123.
12. Hassey, K.M.; Rose C.M. "Altered Skin Integrity in Patients Receiving Radiation Therapy." *Oncology Nursing Forum* 9(4): 44-50, 1982.
13. Miaskowski, C. "Potential and Actual Impairments in Skin Integrity Related to Cancer and Cancer Treatment." *Topics in Clinical Nursing* 5(2): 64-71, 1983.
14. O'Rourke, M.E. "Enhanced Cutaneous Effects in Combined Modality Therapy." *Oncology Nursing Forum* 14(6):31-35, 1987.
15. Hassey, K.M. "Skin Care for Patients Receiving Radiation Therapy for Rectal Cancer." *Journal of Enterostomal Therapy* 14(5): 197-200, 1987.
16. Phillips, T.L.; Fu, K.K. "Quantification of Combined Radiation Therapy and Chemotherapy Effects on Critical Normal Tissues." *Cancer* 37(2 Suppl): 1186-1200, 1976.

17. Mayer, D.K.; Smalley, R.V. "Interferon: Current Status." *Oncology Nursing Forum* 10(4): 14-19, 1983.
18. Krown, S.E.; "Interferons and Interferon Inducers in Cancer Treatment." *Seminars in Oncology* 13(2): 207-217, 1986.
19. Spiegel, R.J. "Intron A (Interferon Alfa-2b): Clinical Overview and Future Directions." *Seminars in Oncology* 13(3, Suppl 2): 89-101, 1986.
20. Irwin, M.M. "Patients Receiving Biological Response Modifiers: Overview of Nursing Care." *Oncology Nursing Forum* 14(Suppl 6): 32-37, 1987.
21. Sullivan, K.M.; Deeg, H.J.; Sanders, J.E.; et al. "Late Complications after Marrow Transplantation." *Seminars in Hematology* 21(1): 53-63, 1984.
22. Nims, J.W.; Strom, S. "Late Complications of Bone Marrow Transplant Recipients: Nursing Care Issues." *Seminars in Oncology Nursing* 4(1): 47-54, 1988.

Assessment

Pruritus is a symptom, not a diagnosis or disease. Generalized pruritus is a "cardinal symptom of medical significance"[1] and should be taken seriously.

Assessment of pruritus must incorporate an accurate and thorough history and physical examination. The history includes the following data: [2,3]

1. location, onset, duration, and intensity of itching
2. previous history of pruritus
3. previous history of malignant disease
4. current malignant disease and treatment
5. nonmalignant systemic diseases
6. use of analgesics
7. use of antibiotics.
8. use of other prescription and nonprescription drugs
9. presence of infection
10. nutritional and fluid level status
11. current skin care practices
12. existence of other pruritic risk factors
13. review of relevant laboratory values (CBC chemistry)
14. factors that relieve and aggravate itching
15. patient's emotional state

Physical examination will provide data from assessment of:

1. all skin surfaces for signs of infection,
2. all skin surfaces for signs of drug reaction,

3. environmental factors (temperature, humidity),
4. physical factors (tight, constrictive clothing),
5. evidence of scratching (erythema, dryness, excoriation),
6. skin turgor, texture, color, temperature, and lesions.

References:

1. Bernhard, J.D. "Clinical Aspects of Pruritus." In: Fitzpatrick, T.B.; Eisen, A.Z.; Wolff, K.; et al., Eds.: *Dermatology in General Medicine*. New York: McGraw-Hill, 3rd ed., 1987, pp 78-90.
2. Lydon, J.; Purl, S.; Goodman, M. "Integumentary and Mucous Membrane Alterations." In: Groenwald, S.L.; Frogge, M.H.; Goodman, M.; et al. Eds.: *Cancer Nursing: Principles and Practice*. Boston: Jones and Bartlett, 2nd ed., 1990, pp 594-635.
3. Pace, K.B.; Bord, M.A.; McCray, N.; et al. "Pruritus." In: McNally, J.C.; Stair, J.C.; Somerville, E.T. Eds.: *Guidelines for Cancer Nursing Practice*. Orlando, FL: Grune and Stratton. Inc., 1985, pp 85-88.

Interventions

Management of pruritus associated with neoplastic disease is directed toward effective management of the underlying malignancy, elimination of actual or potential alterations in skin integrity, and promotion of comfort. Given the subjective nature of itching, the extent to which any therapy is effective may be modified by psychological factors. Multiple approaches and combined efforts may be needed to promote comfort and prevent alterations in the integrity of the skin.

Treatment

Treatment of pruritus can be grouped into four categories: [1,2]

1. patient education and minimizing or eliminating provocative factors;
2. application of topical preparations;
3. systemic therapy; and
4. physical treatment modalities.

Patient Education and Elimination of Provocative Factors

Patients and care-givers must be included in planning care and providing care to the extent possible. Education is an important aspect of symptom control. Skin care regimens incorporate various aspects of the same principles protection from the environment, good cleansing practices, and internal and external hydration.[3] The intensity of the regimen and the techniques employed will vary according to etiologic factors and the degree of distress associated with the pruritus.

Affected individuals (either patients or care-givers) should have a good understanding of factors that promote or aggravate itching. Knowledge of factors that alleviate symptoms provides rationale for the development and implementation of effective and reasonable self-care interventions.

Adequate nutrition is essential to the maintenance of healthy skin. An optimal diet should include a balance of proteins, carbohydrates, fats, vitamins, minerals, and fluids. Daily fluid intake of at least 3,000 cc per day is suggested as a guideline, but may not be possible for some individuals.[4,5]

Aggravating factors should be avoided, including the following:

- Fluid loss secondary to fever, diarrhea, nausea and vomiting, or decreased fluid intake
- Use of ointments (e.g., petroleum mineral oil)
- Bathing with hot water
- Use of soaps that contain detergents
- Frequent bathing or bathing for longer than 1/2 hour
- Adding oil early to a bath
- Genital deodorants or bubble baths
- Dry environment
- Sheets and clothing laundered with detergent
- Tight restrictive clothing or clothing made of wool, synthetics, or other harsh fabric
- Emotional stress
- Use of opium alkaloids, morphine, and antibiotics
- Underarm deodorants or antiperspirants

Alleviating factors should be promoted, as follows:

- Basic skin care
- Application of emollient creams or lotions
- Use of mild soaps or soaps made for sensitive skin
- Limiting bathing to 1/2 hour daily or every other day
- Adding oil at the end of a bath or adding a colloidal oatmeal treatment early to the bath

- Use of cornstarch to areas of irradiated skin following bathing
- Maintenance of a humid environment (e.g., humidifier)
- Use of cotton flannel blankets if needed
- Washing of sheets, clothing, undergarments in mild soaps for infant clothing (e.g., Dreft [TM])
- Wearing of loose-fitting clothing and clothing made of cotton or other soft fabrics
- Use of distraction, relaxation, positive imagery, or cutaneous stimulation
- Use of antibiotics if pruritus is secondary to infection
- Use of oral antihistamines, with increased doses at bedtime
- Use of topical mild corticosteroids (except for pruritus secondary to radiation therapy)

Topical Skin Care

If pruritus is thought to be primarily related to dry skin, interventions to improve skin hydration can be employed. The main source of hydration for skin is moisture from the vasculature of underlying tissues. Water, not lipid, regulates the pliability of the epidermis, providing the rationale for use of emollients.[6] Emollients reduce evaporation by forming occlusive and semi-occlusive films over the skin surface, encouraging the production of moisture in the layer of epidermis beneath the film (hence, the term moisturizer).[3]

Knowledge of the ingredients of skin care products is essential, since many ingredients may enhance skin reactions. Three main ingredients of emollients are petrolatum, lanolin, and mineral oil. Both petrolatum and lanolin may cause allergic sensitization in some individuals.[3]

Petrolatum is poorly absorbed by irradiated skin and is not easily removed. A thick layer could produce an undesired bolus effect when applied within a radiation treatment field.[7] Mineral oil is used in combination with petrolatum and lanolin to create creams and lotions and may be an active ingredient in bath oils. Other ingredients added to these products, such as thickeners, opacifiers, preservatives, fragrances, and colorings, may cause allergic skin reactions.

Product selection and recommendations must be made in consideration of each patient's unique needs and should incorporate such variables as the individual's skin, the desired effect, the consistency and texture of the preparation, its cost, and acceptability to the patient.[3] Emollient creams or lotions should be applied at least two or three times daily and after bathing. Recommended emollient creams include Eucerin (TM) or Nivea (TM) or lotions such as Lubriderm (TM), Alpha Keri (TM), or Nivea (TM).[4] Gels with local anesthetic (0.5 to 2 percent lidocaine) can be used on some areas, as often as every 2 hours if necessary.[8]

Some topical agents including talcum powders, perfumed powders, bubble baths, and cornstarch can irritate the skin and cause pruritus. Cornstarch has been an acceptable intervention for pruritus associated with dry desquamation related to radiation therapy, but should not be applied to moist skin surfaces, areas with hair, sebaceous glands, skin folds or areas close to mucosal surfaces, such as the vagina and rectum.[9,10] Glucose is formed when cornstarch is moistened, providing an excellent medium for fungal growth.[10] Agents with metal ions (i.e., talcum and aluminum used in antiperspirants) enhance skin reactions during external beam radiation therapy and should be avoided throughout the course of radiation therapy. Other common ingredients in over-the-counter lotions and creams that may enhance skin reactions include alcohol or menthol. Topical steroids can reduce itching, but reduce blood flow to the skin, resulting in thinning of the skin and increased susceptibility to injury.[11]

Skin Cleansing

The goal of skin cleansing is to remove dirt and prevent odor, but actual hygienic practices are influenced by skin type, lifestyle, and culture. Extensive bathing aggravates dry skin and hot baths cause vasodilation, which further promotes itching. Many soaps are salts of fatty acids with an alkali base. Soap is a degreaser and can also irritate skin. Older adults or individuals with dry skin should limit use of soaps to those areas with apocrine glands. Plain water should suffice for other skin surfaces. Mild soaps have less soap or detergent content. Super-fatted soaps deposit a film of oil on the skin surface, but there is no proof that they are less drying than other soaps and they may be more expensive.

Tepid baths have an antipruritic effect, possibly resulting from capillary vasoconstriction. The bath should be limited to a half hour every day or every two days. Examples of mild soaps that can be recommended include Dove (TM), Neutrogena (TM), and Basis (TM). Oil can be added to the water at the end of the bath or applied to the skin before towel drying.

Pruritus: Persistent Itching

Environment

Heat increases cutaneous blood flow and may enhance itching. Heat also lowers humidity, and skin loses moisture when the relative humidity is less than 40 percent. A cool, humid environment may reverse these processes.

Residue left by detergents used in laundering clothes and linens, fabric softeners, and anti-static products may aggravate pruritus. Detergent residue can be neutralized by the addition of vinegar (one teaspoon per quart of water) to rinse water. Mild laundry soaps marketed for infant items may offer a solution as well.

Loose fitting, lightweight cotton clothes and cotton bed sheets are suggested. The elimination of heavy bed-covers may alleviate itching by decreasing body heat. Wool and some synthetic fabrics may be irritating. Distraction, music therapy, relaxation, and imagery may be useful to relieve symptoms.[12]

Pharmacologic Therapy

If treatment of the underlying disease and/or control of other aggravating factors provides inadequate relief of pruritus, topical and oral medications may be useful. Topical steroids may provide relief when symptoms are related to a steroid-responsive dermatosis, but anticipated benefits must be weighed against the vasoconstrictive side effects. Topical steroids have no role in the management of pruritus of unknown origin. Topical steroids should not be applied to skin surfaces inside a radiation treatment field.

Systemic medications useful in the management of pruritus include those directed toward the underlying disease or control of symptoms. Antibiotics can reduce symptoms associated with infection. Oral antihistamines may provide symptomatic relief in histamine-related itching. A higher dose of antihistamines at bedtime may produce antipruritic and sedative effects. Diphenhydramine hydrochloride, 25 to 50 mg every 6 hours, has demonstrated effectiveness.[13] Hydroxyzine hydrochloride, 25 to 50 mg every 6 to 8 hours, or cyproheptadine hydrochloride, 4 mg every 6 to 8 hours, may provide symptomatic relief.[14] Oral Chlorpheniramine (4 mg) or hydroxyzine (10 or 25 mg) orally every 4 to 6 hours has been used with good results.[15] If one antihistamine is ineffective, one of another class may provide relief.

Sedative or tranquilizing agents may be indicated, especially if relief is not provided by other agents. Antidepressants can have strong antihistamine and antipruritic effects.[15] Diazepam may be useful in some situations to alleviate anxiety and promote rest.[16]

Sequestrant agents may be effective in relieving pruritus associated with renal or hepatic disease through binding and removing pruritogenic substances in the gut and reducing bile salt concentration. Cholestyramine is not always effective and does produce gastric side effects.[17]

Aspirin seems to have reduced pruritus in some individuals while increasing pruritus in others. Thrombocytopenic cancer patients should be cautioned against using aspirin. Cimetidine alone or in combination with aspirin has been used with some effectiveness for pruritus associated with Hodgkin's disease and polycythemia vera.[18]

Physical Modalities

Alternatives to scratching for the relief of pruritus can help the patient interrupt the itch-scratch-itch cycle. Application of a cool washcloth or ice over the site may be useful. Firm pressure at the site of itching, at a site contralateral to the site of itching, and at accupressure points may break the neural pathway. Rubbing, pressure, and vibration can be used to relieve itching.[2,12]

There are anecdotal reports of the use of Transcutaneous Electronic Nerve Stimulators (TENS) and acupuncture in the management of pruritus.[1] Ultraviolet phototherapy has been used with limited success for pruritus related to uremia.[1]

References

1. Bernhard, J.D. "Clinical Aspects of Pruritus." In: Fitzpatrick T.B.; Eisen A.Z.; Wolff K., et al., Eds. *Dermatology in General Medicine*. New York: McGraw-Hill. 3rd ed., 1987, pp 78-90.
2. Dangel, R.B. "Pruritus and Cancer." *Oncology Nursing Forum* 13(1): 17-21, 1986.
3. Klein, L. "Maintenance of Healthy Skin." *Journal of Enterostomal Therapy* 15(6): 227-231, 1988.
4. Lydon, J.; Purl, S.; Goodman, M. "Integumentary and Mucous Membrane Alterations." In: Groenwald, S.L.; Frogge, M.H.; Goodman, M. et al, Eds. *Cancer Nursing: Principles and Practice*. Boston: Jones and Bartlett, 2nd ed. 1990, pp 594-635.
5. Pace, K.B.; Bord, M.A.; McCray, N., et al. "Pruritus." In: McNally, J.C.; Stair, J.C.; Somerville, E.T., Eds. *Guidelines for Cancer Nursing Practice*. Orlando, FL: Grune and Stratton, Inc., pp 85-88.

6. Blank, L. "Factors Which Influence the Water Content of the Stratum Corneum." *Journal of Investigative Dermatology* 18(2): 133-139, 1952.

7. Hilderley, L. "Skin Care in Radiation Therapy: a Review of the Literature." *Oncology Nursing Forum.* 10(1): 51-56, 1983.

8. De Conno, F; Ventafridda, V.; Saita, L. "Skin Problems in Advanced and Terminal Cancer Patients." *Journal of Pain and Symptom Management* 6(4): 247-256, 1991.

9. Hassey, K.M. "Skin Care for Patients Receiving Radiation Therapy for Rectal Cancer." *Journal of Enterostomal Therapy* 14(5): 197-200, 1987.

10. Maienza, J. "Alternatives to Cornstarch for Itchiness." *Oncology Nursing Forum* 15(2): 199-200, 1988.

11. Hassy, K.M.; Ross, C.M. "Altered Skin Integrity in Patients Receiving Radiation Therapy." *Oncology Nursing Forum* 9(4): 44-50, 1982.

12. Yasko, J.M.; Hogan, C.M. "Pruritus." In: Yasko J., Ed.: Guidelines for Cancer Care: Symptom Management. Reston, VA: Reston Publishing Company, Inc., 1983, pp 125-129.

13. Geltman, R.L.; Paige, R.L. "Symptom Management in Hospice Care." *American Journal of Nursing* 83(1):78-85, 1983.

14. Levy, M. "Symptom Control Manual." In: Cassileth, B.R.; Cassileth, P.A. Eds. *Clinical Care of the Terminal Cancer Patient.* Philadelphia: Lea and Febiger, 1982, pp 214-262.

15. Winkelman, R.D. "Pharmacologic Control of Pruritus." *Medical Clinics of North America* 66(5): 1119-1129, 1982.

16. "Supportive Care." In Casciato, D.A.; Lowitz, B.B. *Manual of Bedside Oncology*, Boston: Little & Brown, 1st ed., 1983, pp 59-95.

17. Abel, E.A.; Farber, E.M. "Malignant Cutaneous Tumors." In Rubenstein E.; Federman D.D., Eds.: *Scientific American.* Medicine. New York: Scientific American, Inc, Chapter 2: Dermatology, Section XII.

18. Daly, B.M.; Shuster, S. "Effect of Aspirin of Pruritus." *British Medical Journal* 293(6552): 907-908, 1986.

Chapter 7

Psychodermatology: Psychological Factors in Skin Disorders

The mind-body connection runs both ways: Psychiatric disorders may have dermatologic symptoms, and cutaneous disease may have devastating emotional consequences. A biopsychosocial approach works best.

At least one third of patients seen in dermatology clinics have a skin problem with an important psychological component.[1] These underlying psychological factors give rise to a wide spectrum of disorders, ranging from patients with bona fide skin disease aggravated by emotional stress to those who have no cutaneous illness but are convinced they do. Psychodermatologic conditions require a multidisciplinary approach that may include psychotherapy, cognitive-behavioral therapy, and psychopharmacotherapy—in addition to dermatologic care and other medical treatment as needed.[2]

Many patients resist referral to a mental health professional, however, and continue to seek treatment from a dermatologist or primary care physician for cutaneous symptoms that are psychologically based.[3] Thus, the clinical management of patients who have mixed psychiatric and dermatologic disorders poses a special challenge to the primary physician. Here are some principles of management.

What Is Psychodermatology?

Psychodermatology integrates psychiatric and neurologic knowledge and therapeutics into the diagnosis and treatment of skin disorders. The goals of this approach are to:

©*Patient Care*, July 1995. Reprinted with permission.

- Elucidate the role of neurotransmitters in the pathophysiology of cutaneous disorders,

- enhance therapeutic efficacy by introducing a biopsychosocial approach to patient management, and to

- expand the therapeutic armamentarium by investigating the use of psychotropic medications in the treatment of selected dermatologic conditions.

Establishing a therapeutic alliance with the patient is the most critical step in successfully managing psychodermatologic disease. Empathy and rapport are especially needed because patients with more serious types of psychopathology, such as delusions of parasitosis, may be defensive and often deny the psychiatric component of their illness. A thorough skin examination is often an effective way to establish a good relationship and gain the patient's trust. It demonstrates that you take the complaint seriously and may also reveal underlying disorders or mistaken diagnoses.

Inevitably, you will need to explain that the dermatologic symptoms may be psychogenic or at least have a strong psychiatric component. Since the patient's main objective is symptomatic relief, emphasize that treating the psychological component is a way of alleviating symptoms. A therapeutic response to an appropriate psychopharmaceutical may enable the patient to deal better with the psychological factors contributing to the dermatologic manifestations. Throughout the encounter, be aware that you may experience negative feelings toward a patient whose condition is primarily psychogenic. Nonetheless, try not to let your feelings adversely affect the therapeutic relationship.

Because of the wide range of skin disorders that may be considered psychodermatologic, a classification scheme is needed (see Table 7.1). Four broad categories form the conceptual framework: psychophysiologic disorders, primary psychiatric disorders, secondary psychiatric disorders, and nonpsychiatric conditions for which psychopharmacology may be effective. The underlying psychopathology—depression, psychosis, obsessive-compulsive disorder, or anxiety—determines the course of therapy.

Psychodermatology: Psychological Factors in Skin Disorders

Drugs Mentioned in this Article

- **Alprazolam** (Xanax)
- **Amitriptyline HCl** (Elavil, Endep)
- **Buspirone HCl** (BuSpar)
- **Clomipramine HCl** (Anafranil)
- **Desipramine HCl** (Norpramin, Pertofrane)
- **Doxepin HCl** (Sinequan)
- **Doxepin HCl Cream 5 percent (topical)** (Zonalon Cream)
- **Fluoxetine HCl** (Prozac)
- **Fluvoxamine maleate** (Luvox)
- **Pimozide** (Orap)

Psychophysiologic Disorders

Psychophysiologic disorders are cutaneous disorders usually precipitated or exacerbated by emotional stress. Familiar examples include chronic, recurrent inflammatory skin conditions such as atopic dermatitis, psoriasis, eczema, and acne (see Table 7.1). Stress is also thought to play a role in chronic urticaria, alopecia areata, rosacea, herpes simplex virus infection, and telogen effluvium (the temporary loss of hair from normal resting follicles). These disorders are not caused by stress but are triggered or worsened by stressful life events. The neuroimmunologic mechanisms by which psychological factors trigger dermatologic flare-ups are not well-understood.[4]

A psychophysiologic disorder may be further classified as psychosomatic or somatopsychic. Skin conditions aggravated by stress from external factors (job difficulties, marital problems, personal loss) are considered to be psychosomatic. Somatopsychic conditions, on the other hand, involve skin disorders that produce psychological symptoms, such as the emotional stress a patient may experience when a skin condition does not seem to improve with treatment.

If the condition is predominantly psychosomatic, psychotherapy or stress-management strategies are usually recommended. Somatopsychic problems may require more dermatologic treatment, such as using stronger topical agents or initiating systemic therapy. In some cases, both psychosomatic and somatopsychic factors may contribute to symptoms, emphasizing the need to attend to the whole patient in the context of life events.

Whether the condition is predominantly psychosomatic or somatopsychic, psychopharmacotherapy can help alleviate the patient's emotional distress. Although stress can manifest itself in a variety of subjective experiences, the underlying diagnosis in this group of patients is most often anxiety and emotional tension caused by situational stress.[5] When both the psychological manifestations of anxiety (excessive worry, tension, agitation) and the physiologic signs of anxiety (hyperventilation, palpitations, sweating) become so severe as to compromise the patient's routine functioning, the use of an antianxiety medication, such as a benzodiazepine or Buspirone HCl, is appropriate.

Unlike other benzodiazepines that have a depressant effect, alprazolam has an antidepressant effect—comparable to that of desipramine HC1 but with an earlier onset of action.[6,7] Although alprazolam may be the best choice for patients with symptoms of both anxiety and depression, the risks of sedation and dependence, particularly when this drug or other benzodiazepines are taken for prolonged periods, must be considered. Alprazolam is most appropriate for short-term treatment of acute situational stress.

Buspirone—a nonbenzodiazepine, nonbarbiturate anxiolytic—has a slow onset of action and minimal side effects during long-term use, which make it a good choice for patients with chronic anxiety. It has minimal sedative effects, and it does not produce withdrawal symptoms or interact with alcohol or benzodiazepines.[8,9] Buspirone cannot be administered as needed: It must be given regularly for at least two weeks before a therapeutic benefit occurs.

Primary Psychiatric Disorders

Essentially normal skin may become the focus of a patient with a primary psychiatric disorder. Either no authentic dermatologic disorder exists, or the condition is a minor one that the patient grossly exaggerates. Once again, it is essential to identify the presence of underlying psychopathology.

Besides anxiety, the most common psychiatric conditions underlying dermatologic symptoms are depression, psychosis, and obsessive-compulsive disorders. Common examples of skin involvement in primary psychiatric disorders are neurotic excoriations, delusions of parasitosis, and trichotillomania (compulsive hair-pulling).

Psychodermatology: Psychological Factors in Skin Disorders

Depression and Skin Disease

Since the skin is easily accessible, it may become a target when self-destructive tendencies are expressed as a manifestation of depression. For instance, excoriation is often encountered in a particular group of depressed patients who exhibit psychomotor agitation or irritability, such as hand-wringing and pacing.[3] While many antidepressants are effective, doxepin HCl, desipramine, and fluoxetine HCl appear to be particularly helpful in specific subgroups of depressed patients with psychodermatologic disorders.

Doxepin, a tricyclic antidepressant, is a good choice for depressed and agitated patients with chronic excoriations. Its potent antihistaminic and anxiolytic effects offer relief from the intense pruritus and anxiety that these patients commonly experience. The drug has a long half-life, permitting administration of the entire dosage at bedtime (up to 160 mg) and enhancing patient compliance. A starting dosage of 10-25 mg/d is suggested; the dosage may be increased by 25 mg every 5-7 days until an optimal dosage of about 100-300 mg/d is achieved. For patients who show no therapeutic response, serum doxepin and nordoxepin levels should be obtained.

As with other tricyclic antidepressants, doxepin's principal side effects are sedation and anticholinergic symptoms, such as dry mouth, blurred vision, chronic constipation, and urinary retention. The drug is usually well tolerated in young patients but should be used with extreme caution in patients with a history of arrhythmias, seizures, or mania.

If a patient becomes too sedated with doxepin, consider desipramine. A therapeutic effect is usually seen at a dosage of 100-150 mg/d. Desipramine has fewer anticholinergic and sedative side effects than doxepin, but it lacks antihistaminic and antipruritic properties.

The antidepressant fluoxetine, at 20 mg/d, is useful in treating both depressive and compulsive symptoms and is further discussed under obsessive-compulsive disorders.

Psychosis Involving Dermatologic Symptoms

The most frequent cutaneous manifestation of a psychotic disorder is delusion of parasitosis, in which patients firmly believe that their skin is infested with ectoparasites. Delusion of parasitosis falls under the psychiatric diagnosis of monosymptomatic hypochondriacal psychosis.[10] This condition differs from schizophrenia by the encapsulated or confined nature of the delusion. Patients may function relatively well in society and seldom suffer general deterioration in personality.[11]

The clinical management of delusional conditions poses significant obstacles, such as gaining the patient's agreement to initiate drug therapy and overcoming resistance to obtaining psychiatric care. Pimozide, a dopamine antagonist, is especially effective in treating delusion of parasitosis and other forms of encapsulated delusional disorder involving the skin, possibly because it is also a powerful opioid antagonist. (This is an unlabeled use of the drug.) The ability to block opiate-mediated neurologic pathways may diminish the formication—crawling and biting sensations—experienced by many patients with delusions of parasitosis.

The starting dosage of pimozide should be low—1 mg/d (a half tablet). The dosage can be increased by 1 mg every 5-7 days until improvement is seen, generally at 4-6 mg/d or lower. When symptoms have abated for 2-3 months, the dosage can be gradually decreased. The short-term use of relatively low dosages helps minimize the risk of pseudo-parkinsonism, dystonia, and tardive dyskinesia. Baseline and midtreatment ECGs are recommended because pimozide has been associated with a prolonged QT interval, T-wave changes, and the presence of U waves.

Obsessive-compulsive Disorders

An obsession is an intrusive, irrational idea or thought that is beyond the patient's conscious control. Compulsion refers to a repetitive, irresistible behavior such as picking acne sores or pulling out one's hair (see "Help for trichotillomania"). In contrast to delusional patients, those with an obsessive-compulsive disorder are aware of their actions and recognize the senseless damage they are inflicting on their skin. Despite this insight, they are unable to control their compulsion.

Several medications have been found effective in diminishing obsessive-compulsive urges. Clomipramine HC1 is a tricyclic antidepressant that selectively blocks the synaptic re-uptake of serotonin, the neurotransmitter thought to be associated with obsessive-compulsive behavior.[12] The initial dosage of clomipramine, 26 mg/d, is increased gradually to a maximum adult dosage of up to 260 mg/d, but most patients respond at lower dosages. The efficacy of clomipramine in children and adolescents 10 years or older has been widely reported;

a titrated dosage not exceeding 3 mg/kg/d has been recommended for pediatric populations. In addition to the side effects of other tricyclics, clomipramine is associated with nausea, seizures, and sexual dysfunction.

The selective serotonin re-uptake inhibitor (SSRI) fluoxetine also has been used for compulsive disorders at dosages of 20 mg/d or higher. Its side effects are minimal and dose-related; the most common are diarrhea, agitation, anxiety, and rash. There have been a few reports of increased anxiety or agitation in depressed patients, so be alert for these adverse effects.

Fluvoxamine maleate, recently approved by the FDA for obsessive-compulsive disorder, is an SSRI that apparently has no active metabolites. The most frequent side effect is nausea, reported in up to 40 percent of subjects in clinical trials. Because of this, the starting dosage is usually low—60 mg/d—and is then slowly titrated upward by 60-mg increments to an average therapeutic dosage of 200-300 mg/d given in two divided doses. Besides nausea, other possible side effects include somnolence, insomnia, nervousness, sexual dysfunction, and asthenia. Anticholinergic side effects such as constipation or dry mouth are less common than with a tricyclic such as clomipramine.

Secondary Psychiatric Disorders

Patients with disfiguring skin diseases may suffer significant secondary psychological symptoms including depression, social phobia, paranoia, panic attacks, and agoraphobia. Much of the emotional response to cutaneous disfigurement involves not only a negative effect on self-image but the stigmatization imposed by society. Historically, people suffering from psoriasis were mistaken for lepers and treated as social outcasts. Even today, some people with psoriasis report being avoided as if they had a contagious disease.

The psychological implications of psoriasis may extend to all domains of a patient's life. When psoriasis occurs on the hands or face, the negative impact can extend to the workplace, particularly for patients with jobs involving public contact or group presentations. In some cases, the embarrassment and stigma of the skin disorder can limit professional achievement (see "The psychological impact of psoriasis").

When cosmetic disfigurement is the key cause of psychological problems, patients often experience low self-esteem, extreme self-consciousness, and mild to moderate symptoms of anxiety and depression.

A small but significant group develops more serious psychiatric disturbances such as social phobia, major depressive episodes, or severe anxiety that interferes with normal life.

The patient's age at the time of disfigurement seems to be a critical factor in determining the intensity and gravity of the emotional response to the cosmetic deformity. Younger patients experience greater psychological trauma, particularly if they are not yet married or are still developing their adult identity. These patients often benefit from psychiatric evaluation and treatment. In general, the underlying pathology in secondary psychiatric disorders is associated with loss of self-esteem, withdrawal, and feelings of inferiority. Often these negative feelings can be just as debilitating as a physical handicap or cosmetic impairment.

Psychotherapy, group therapy, and behavior modification may be appropriate for treating secondary psychiatric disorders. Psychopharmacologic therapy is frequently a useful adjunct, especially for managing anxiety and depression.

Psychopharmacology for Nonpsychiatric Conditions

A growing body of evidence suggests that psychopharmacologic therapy is beneficial in a variety of dermatologic and other medical conditions that do not entail a psychiatric component. For instance, tricyclic antidepressants can play a beneficial role in controlling chronic back pain.

In dermatology, doxepin has been used effectively to treat cholinergic urticaria and certain cases of chronic idiopathic pruritus, and a topical form of doxepin recently received FDA approval for treatment of itching. (Unlabeled use for oral administration.) Amitriptyline HC1 is the therapy of choice for postherpetic neuralgia (unlabeled use). In most nonpsychiatric conditions, the therapeutic dosage of a tricyclic antidepressant is significantly lower than that used for depression.

Monitoring and Follow-up

Frequent follow-up of psychodermatologic patients is important for several reasons. First, the dosage of a psychopharmaceutical may require titration weekly, or even more often, until the optimal dosage is established. When the dosage of a tricyclic antidepressant is increased, side effects may not become obvious until 5-7 days later. Some patients, such as those with delusions, may be highly ambivalent about

Psychodermatology: Psychological Factors in Skin Disorders

Table 7.1. Classification of psychodermatologic disorders

Disorder	Types	Examples	Typical features
Psychophysiologic	Psychosomatic	Atopic dermatitis, psoriasis, eczema	Emotional symptoms contributing to flare-up of skin condition
	Somatopsychic	Anxiety about persistent skin condition	Skin condition giving rise to emotional stress
Primary psychiatric	Depressive	Neurotic excoriation	Self-inflicted skin abrasions; psychomotor agitation
	Psychotic	Delusion of parasitosis	Fixed false belief that skin is infected by parasites; formication (crawling and biting sensation)
	Obsessive-compulsive	Trichotillomania	Compulsive pulling out of one's hair
Secondary psychiatric	Depression, social phobia, anxiety, paranoia	Psoriasis, vitiligo, alopecia areata	Disfigurement accompanied by severe emotional symptoms
Nonpsychiatric (dermatologic) conditions for which psychopharmacologic therapy may be effective	—	Postherpetic neuralgia, cholinergic urticaria, idiopathic pruritus	Painful or itchy skin

drug therapy and need more positive reinforcement than the average patient with acne or psoriasis. Finally, frequently scheduled visits allow the physician to prescribe small amounts of medication each time, thereby minimizing the potential for serious overdose in severely depressed or psychotic patients.

Although psychodermatologic problems pose many challenges, they also offer the physician considerable satisfaction, whether successful treatment results in complete remission, marked improvement, or reduction in symptom severity. Treatment of psychodermatologic disorders should generally not be restricted to drug therapy. Optimal management requires a multidisciplinary approach using an array of adjunctive therapeutic options, including psychotherapy, behavioral modification, and judicious use of psychopharmacologic agents. Referral to a mental health professional, as well as consultation with a dermatologist or psychiatrist, is almost always helpful.

The most essential factors in achieving a successful outcome in psychodermatologic disorders are keeping an open mind, establishing rapport, showing empathy, identifying underlying psychopathology, making a correct diagnosis, and choosing an appropriate psychopharmacologic agent, if indicated. Maintaining a biopsychosocial approach to management of these patients should significantly improve their quality of life.

Case Studies

Depression and Neurotic Excoriation

A 32-year-old white female with a two-year history of excoriations was seen in the dermatology clinic. Examination revealed excoriations on her face, back, extensor aspects of the arms, and anterior thighs. There was a noticeable sparing of the upper lateral back, which she could not reach. Relative sparing was also evident on the medial aspects of the arms and the posterior legs.

This classic distribution, in which the excoriations are seen mainly in easily reachable areas, suggested a diagnosis of neurotic excoriations. Psychological evaluation revealed symptoms of depressed mood, crying spells, insomnia, and feelings of hopelessness, helplessness, and worthlessness.

The patient was referred for psychotherapy. At the same time, she was started on doxepin HCl; the dosage was gradually increased to 100 mg/d. At this dosage, the patient noticed a significant decrease of insomnia, pruritus, and agitation. Eventually, she experienced an antidepressant effect and, once she was no longer depressed, her excoriating behavior stopped. She was maintained on doxepin for two months and then tapered off the drug. She continued with psychotherapy to explore possible psychological issues that may have contributed to her episode of major depression.

Help for Trichotillomania

A 25-year-old white female presented with a three-year history of compulsive hair-pulling. When the behavior started, the patient was experiencing much situational stress. Although the stress had long been resolved, she continued to pull her hair.

The patient had large areas of incomplete alopecia, mainly in the frontal scalp. She said she had tried to stop the hair-pulling by keeping her hands busy or sitting on them. These efforts failed, either because her hair-pulling was so automatic that she was unaware of it; or because conscious efforts at preventing the behavior only increased the intensity of her compulsive urge. This was experienced by the patient as feeling restless and increasingly ill at ease, which could be relieved only by hair-pulling behavior.

First, to increase her awareness of her behavior and to interrupt it, the patient was asked to keep a little notebook with her at all times and to consciously keep vigilant about what her hands were doing. If she noticed that she was pulling out her hair, she was instructed to stop immediately and write down the exact time, date, and any possible environmental or intrapsychic factors that may have precipitated the behavior. Even though the patient could not think of a precipitating factor on all occasions, the mere fact that she had to record a certain amount of information interrupted her hair-pulling behavior and gradually reduced its frequency.

To reduce the compulsive urge, the patient was started on fluoxetine HCl, 20 mg/d. After several weeks, the daily dosage was increased to 40 mg. When the medication was started, she was asked to maintain her motivation and vigilance and to try not to think of the medication as a "magic bullet." Over several months, the compulsive urge gradually diminished, and she was able to stop her destructive hair-pulling. Fluoxetine was discontinued about two months after the hair-pulling ceased, and the patient has not relapsed.

The Psychological Impact of Psoriasis

A 36-year-old white female was admitted to the Psoriasis Treatment Center of the University of California, San Francisco, Medical Center, with severe generalized plaque-type psoriasis covering more than 70 percent of her total body surface. She was unresponsive to various topical corticosteroids and tar preparations, as well as to outpatient therapy with ultraviolet light type B (UVB).

At the time of admission to the Day Treatment Program, the patient described intense feelings of embarrassment, depression, and social phobia, manifested by her reluctance to come into contact with strangers for fear that they might mistake her psoriasis for something else, such as AIDS. She described situations in which people had reacted to her condition as if it were contagious-for example, she was once asked to leave a swimming pool by hotel management. She reported that people either stay away from her or bombard her with questions like "What do you have on your skin?"

She was tired of explaining her condition to strangers, sometimes on a daily basis. She had low self-esteem and also felt "dirty," even though she knew that psoriasis was not a contagious disease. She also felt isolated since she did not know anyone else who had generalized psoriasis.

At the Psoriasis Treatment Center, she was treated with daily applications of black tar all over her body, along with much more intense exposure to UVB. During treatment, which lasted one month, the patient participated in group therapy, where she met other patients with generalized psoriasis and was much encouraged to learn that she was not alone. She was greatly relieved to discover that it is possible to live an enjoyable and productive life, despite occasional flare-ups of psoriasis.

Most important, her psoriasis cleared for the first time in many years. When she left the program, she was overjoyed to find that she had normal-looking skin and that she was able to wear skirts and short sleeves. Although she understood that her psoriasis might return, this did not dampen her enthusiasm, and she was committed to continuing outpatient phototherapy to keep her condition under control.

Psychodermatology: Psychological Factors in Skin Disorders

Article Consultant

John Y.M. Koo, MD, is Director of the Psoriasis Treatment Center and Vice Chairman of the Department of Dermatology at the University of California, San Francisco, Medical Center. Board-certified of psychiatry and dermatology, Dr. Koo is Associate Professor of Dermatology at the University of California, San Francisco, School of Medicine.

Edited by Peter D'Epiro
Special projects editor

References

1. Rook, A; Wilkinson, D.S.; Ebling, F.J.G.; et al. *Textbook of Dermatology*, ed 4. Oxford. Blackwell Scientific Publications, 1986, p 2257.
2. Tsushima, W.T. "Current psychological treatments for stress-related skin disorders." *Cutis* 1988:42, pp 402-404.
3. Koblenzer, C.S. "Psychiatric Syndromes of Interest to Dermatologists." *Int J Dermatol*. 1993:32, pp 82-88.
4. Farber, E.M.; Rein, G; Lanigan, S.W. "Stress and Psoriasis: Psychoneuroimmunologic Mechanisms." *Int J Dermatol*. 1991;30, pp 8-12.
5. Koo, J.Y.M.; Pham, C.T. Psychodermatology: Practical Guidelines on Pharmacotherapy." *Arch Dermatol*. 1992:128, pp 381-388.
6. Fawcett, J; Edwards, J.H.; Kravitz, H.M.; et al. "Alprazolam: An Antidepressant? Alprazolam, Desipramine, and an Alprazolam-desipramine Combination in the Treatment of Adult Depressed Patients." *J Clin Psychopharmacol*. 1987:7, pp 295-310.
7. Remick, R.A.; Keller, F.D.; Buchanan, R.A.; et al. "A Comparison of the Efficacy and Safety of Alprazolam and Desipmamine in Depressed Outpatients." *Can J Psychiatry*. 1988:33, pp 590-594.
8. "Buspirone: A Non-benzodiazepine for Anxiety." *Med Lett Drugs Ther.* 1986:28, pp 117-122.
9. Cohn, J.B.; Wilcox, C.S. "Low-sedation Potential of Buspirone Compared with Alprazolam and Lorazepam in the Treatment of Anxious Patients: A Double-blind Study." *J Clin Psychiatry*. 1986:47, pp 409-412.
10. Munro, A. "Monosymptomatic Hypochondriacal Psychosis." *Br J Psychiatry*. 1988:153(suppl 2), pp 37-40.
11. Baker, P.B.; Cook, B.L.; Wnokur, G. "Delusional Infestation: The Interface of Delusions and Hallucinations." *Psychiatr. Clin North Am*. 1995;18(2), pp 345-361.
12. Rapoport, J.L. "The Neurobiology of Obsessive-Compulsive Disorder." *JAMA*. 1988:260, pp 2888-2890.

Chapter 8

Wrinkles: Smile Lines and Facial Fissures

"When your friends begin to flatter you on how young you look, it's a sure sign you're getting old."

—Mark Twain

Few events are more dreaded—and less serious—than the appearance of that first wrinkle. But, unlike that other infamous sign of aging, the first gray hair, which can be quickly and surreptitiously plucked out, that wrinkle is here to stay.

Or is it? A creamy flood of new cosmetic products seems to promise not only to prevent new wrinkles, but also to erase the old ones. The price tags for these modern fountains of youth are usually high, but many think no price is too dear for an unlined face.

But the truth is, it's never been scientifically proven that any of these cosmetics actually gets rid of wrinkles. So what about all those advertising claims that promise to send those wrinkles packing?

If a company claims that its product can affect the skin below the surface—for example, can repair cells or make the skin "function as if it were young again"—FDA may consider the product a drug for regulatory purposes. If FDA considers it to be a new drug, the manufacturer must prove that it is safe and effective before it can be legally marketed. None of the currently marketed wrinkle-fixers has a new drug approval.

FDA has already determined that several companies are making drug claims on some of their skin treatment products. In *Regulatory*

FDA Consumer, July/August 1987.

Letters sent beginning April 17, the agency told those companies that the claims "represent and suggest that the articles are intended to affect the structure and function of the human body, and that the products are adequate and effective.... Because of such claims the products are regarded as drugs."

"Also, we are unaware of any substantial scientific evidence that demonstrates the safety and effectiveness of these articles for their intended uses, nor are we aware that these drugs are generally recognized as safe and effective for their intended uses. Therefore, the products are new drugs...."

In order to keep making claims that these products alter the skin's functions, the companies must file applications for new drug approval that include data from clinical studies that prove safety and effectiveness. If they don't file applications for new drug approval or stop making the drug claims, FDA is prepared to "take appropriate regulatory sanctions such as seizure or injunction," according to the letters.

As long as the effectiveness of these products is in question, the answer for those who want an unlined face is to not get wrinkles in the first place. Unfortunately, that's impossible. While some wrinkles can be prevented by staying out of the sun, aging skin won't stay unlined forever.

What happens to adult skin to make those wrinkles appear?

In young, undamaged skin, the dermis—the dense layer of tissue beneath the thin, outer epidermis—contains flexible, soft, resilient connective tissue called elastic fibers. But as the skin ages, or is damaged by the sun's ultraviolet rays, the structure of these fibers deteriorates.

The deterioration begins with excessive production of abnormal fibers. This is an inevitable part of aging even without sun exposure. "To get a wrinkle you have to have too much skin," says Dr. Albert Kligman of the University of Pennsylvania's Department of Dermatology. "It's got to sag. That's mainly the result of an excessive amount of tissue."

The elastic fibers eventually break down into a fiberless mass. Once that happens, mechanical stress will cause wrinkles to appear. "You have to use your facial muscles very energetically to work those lines into that sagging tissue," Kligman explains. Unlike young, normal fibers, sagging tissue, when stretched, can't snap back. The tissue remains stretched—and wrinkled. Kligman compares wrinkles of the skin to grooves in an old well-used glove.

Wrinkles: Smile Lines and Facial Fissures

The facial muscles used to inhale a cigarette may cause some wrinkles, according to a study published in the December 1985 *British Medical Journal*. The study said "smoker's face" is characterized by wrinkles that spread out at right angles from the upper or lower lips or corners of the eyes.

Even in skin that has been kept in the dark, the elastic fibers will eventually deteriorate. However, the majority of this deterioration isn't visible until after the age of 70. On the other hand, wrinkles from sun damage can start to appear as early as 30.

The only way to prevent this premature damage is to stay out of the sun or use a strong sunscreen. In fact, a cosmetic's claim that it "prevents new wrinkles" usually means it contains a sunscreen.

In addition to sunscreens, many products contain moisturizers for dry skin. Dry skin doesn't cause wrinkles. But moist, soft skin—even if it is wrinkled—certainly looks better than rough, scaly, dry skin.

Moisturizers form a seal that keeps water from evaporating from the skin's surface cells. More water in the cells means greater flexibility, softness and smoothness. This effect can come with equal success from a $65 bottle of exotically named cream or a plain jar of petroleum jelly.

The important point here is that any moisturizer's results are only temporary. But how temporary differs from product to product.

A 10-year dermatological study led by University of Pennsylvania researchers tested different moisturizers on young women (mainly college students) who had very dry skin on their legs. The study found that using petrolatum (petroleum jelly) for 14 days almost eliminated the roughness, cracks and scales typical signs of common dry skin. The beneficial effects could be seen for about two weeks after the last application. On the other hand, the moderate dry-skin relief from cold cream only lasted three to four days after use was stopped.

The runner-up to petroleum jelly was lanolin. Mineral oil, vegetable oils and lard are at the bottom of the list in terms of major, lasting relief from dry skin. Mineral oil's relief lasted only one day.

The study, presented at the Safety and Efficacy of Topical Drugs and Cosmetics Symposium in 1982 in Philadelphia, was not able to substantiate claims that humectants (moistening agents) attract moisture or improve a moisturizer's effectiveness. Some commonly used humectants include urea, glycerin, pyrollidone, carboxylic acid, lactic acid, and propylene glycol. Vitamins, minerals and organic substances such as elastin, deoxyribonucleic acid, and ribonucleic acid didn't improve effectiveness either.

Despite many claims, collagen-based cosmetics offer no benefits beyond softening and moisturizing the skin. (Collagen, a protein, is the chief constituent of skin, connective tissue and bone. Most of the collagen used in cosmetics comes from cows.) Collagen's molecules are too large to get past the skin's outermost layer. However, collagen injections, done by a physician, can smooth out wrinkles (see "The Collagen Connection" in the June 1985 *FDA Consumer* and reprinted in this volume).

Lotions and creams made with more oil than water always moisturize better than ones made with more water than oil. Of course, the ones with less oil are less messy and feel better, especially ones that promise "no greasy feeling" or that they are "absorbed quickly." The University of Pennsylvania study concluded that "a boon to all sufferers from dry skin would be a product with the efficacy of petrolatum and the hedonic-aesthetic properties of a light oil-in-water cream."

Studies on alleviating dry skin are rare. According to the University of Pennsylvania study, "the ordinary forms of dry skin, sometimes disdainfully called 'cosmetic dry-skin,' do not enjoy high status in the medical establishment."

While some moisturizers can alleviate the symptoms of dry skin, there aren't any products for sale anywhere, from the pharmacy to the fanciest department store, that will actually get rid of wrinkles.

So why would anyone pay the high prices some companies charge for products that do nothing more than a jar of petroleum jelly can do, and sometimes less?

"Cosmetics are fashion products," explains Heinz Eiermann, director of FDA's division of colors and cosmetics. For some people, how the product feels and how it is absorbed is just as important as how well it works, he says. Even the packaging and the availability of salespeople may be an influencing factor, he believes. But he adds that, "There is absolutely no correlation between price and the quality of the product."

And, at least for now, there's no way to get rid of that wrinkle.

Wash and Wear

How often should people wash their faces?

"As little as they can," says University of Pennsylvania dermatologist Albert Kligman.

There aren't any definite rules on how often to wash, says FDA dermatologist John Sanders. He explained that, first, each person's

Wrinkles: Smile Lines and Facial Fissures

needs are different. For example, he said, an office worker doesn't get as dirty as a car mechanic. And second, an individual's washing schedule can be affected by what he or she did on a certain day or the time of year.

But he agrees with Kligman that less is better. "The public has been brainwashed into thinking that they have to be cleaner than clean," he said. "Although the majority of the public can get away with too much washing because their skin is pretty tolerant, people should realize that soaps are irritants."

In addition to irritation, almost all soaps dry the skin because they remove skin lipids (fats) and the skin's own moisturizing substances. "Moist skin contains 10 to 30 percent moisture," says FDA's Heinz Eiermann, director of the division of colors and cosmetics. "Near or below 10 percent, the stratum corneum (the outermost layer of skin) becomes dry and brittle. If repeated use of soap and water leach out too much of the moisturizing material, the skin cannot retain sufficient moisture and becomes dry, particularly in an environment with low relative humidity.

"However, the dry skin syndrome is not permanent because of the normal 20- to 25-day cell turnover. New stratum corneum cells are constantly being formed and the moisturizing material replenished."

When it is time to wash, both Kligman and Sanders recommend a mild soap followed by a moisturizer if needed. While many dermatologists tell patients that applying the moisturizer to damp skin will improve the moisturizer's effectiveness, Kligman says there is no evidence to support this. However, he said it doesn't seem to cause any harm, either.

The advice against washing too much applies to people with oily skin and acne as well as those with dry skin. "There is no evidence whatever that lack of washing worsens acne nor that frequent cleaning is helpful," Kligman said in his book *Acne, Morphogenesis and Treatment*. (See "Stubborn and Vexing, That's Acne" in the May 1980 *FDA Consumer*.)

"We no longer wash to get clean," said Kligman. "We wash to be refreshed. You won't damage the skin by never washing."

Other steps for good skin care include:

- **Use a sunscreen.** The strength of the sunscreen and how often it should be used depend on many factors, including skin color—fair skin requires a stronger sunscreen applied more often than darker skin—and geographical location—the sun's rays are strongest near the equator.

- **Water your environment.** To relieve dry skin, increase the humidity in the air if you live in a dry climate or if you spend the winter months in dry, overheated homes and offices. While humidifiers are the best way to increase humidity, house plants (which should be sprayed with water from time to time) and a pot of water on the radiator can help, too.

—*by Dori Stehlin*

Dori Stehlin is a member of FDA's public affairs staff.

Wrinkles: Cosmetic Treatments Can Rejuvenate Your Face

©1995 *Mayo Clinic Health Letter*.
Reprinted from July 1995 *Mayo Clinic Health Letter* with permission of Mayo Foundation for Medical Education and Research, Rochester, MN 55905. For subscription information, call 1-800-333-9037.

They first appear around your eyes and mouth. Then they spread to your forehead and cheekbones.

Wrinkles. You can't escape them. But cosmetic treatments can help eliminate fine lines or make deep wrinkles less noticeable.

What Causes Wrinkles?

As you age, your skin makes less oil. Its outer layer (epidermis) becomes rough and dry. In the underlying dermis, two fibrous proteins that keep your skin taut (collagen and elastin) gradually diminish. Your skin first starts to wrinkle, then sag.

Secretion of skin pigment (melanin) also becomes irregular, resulting in blotchy skin.

Sun exposure and smoking speed up the aging process.

Ways to Reduce Wrinkles

These medical treatments can noticeably improve the appearance of your skin:

Wrinkles: Smile Lines and Facial Fissures

- **Retin-A:** Daily use of a prescription cream containing retinoic acid (a synthetic derivative of vitamin A) reduces fine wrinkles. Retin-A sloughs off outer layers and exposes smoother skin underneath.

    Retin-A also causes collagen to re-accumulate, thickening the skin fibers that preserve moisture.

    The use of Retin-A causes irritation and redness for about two weeks.

- **Alpha hydroxy acids:** Prescription creams containing acids found in fruits, milk and sugar cane also promote shedding of your skin's outer layer.

    Alpha hydroxy acids are less irritating than Retin-A. However, because they don't penetrate as deeply, anti-aging effects are less noticeable. Alpha hydroxy acids also aren't proven to help rebuild collagen.

- **Chemical peels:** These procedures use stronger acids than prescription creams and are applied by your doctor. One application causes temporary inflammation and noticeable peeling of your skin's outer layer.

    Chemical peels are more effective than prescription creams for deeper wrinkles, but can cause scarring or infection.

    Your skin takes about two weeks to heal and about three months to assume a natural color and texture.

- **Combination programs:** To remove deeper wrinkles, some doctors combine a prescription cream with a chemical peel. Sometimes a bleaching cream is added to help fade age spots and promote even skin color.

- **Injections:** Collagen from the skin of cows or fat from your thigh or abdomen is injected under facial wrinkles. Injections smooth the surfaces of wrinkles to make them less noticeable.

    However, collagen and fat gradually degrade. Depending on the depth of your wrinkles, you may need touch-up injections.

- **Abrasion:** Your doctor uses a machine with a small rotating wheel to gently "sand" the surfaces of fine wrinkles or scars.

    Scabbing and swelling typically last one to two weeks.

- **Surgery:** In a traditional facelift, wrinkles on your face and neck are removed by tightening and removing excess skin. Use of large incisions can cause scarring and temporary numbness from nerve disturbance. It can also take months for the swelling to disappear.

  A new procedure uses minimally invasive surgery to remove wrinkles with little or no scarring or numbness (see Figure 8.1). But it's uncertain whether the results last as long as traditional procedures.

  Because endoscopic surgery doesn't remove excess skin, it works best for people in their forties to mid-fifties without deep wrinkles.

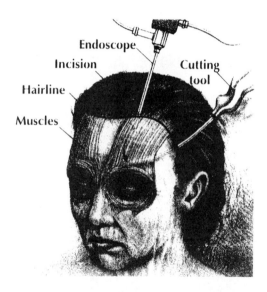

Figure 8.1. In an endoscopic forehead lift, your surgeon makes small incisions behind your hairline. He or she threads an endoscope containing a camera and lighting system through one of the incisions, then inserts small cutting tools into the others.

After loosening facial muscles on your forehead, your surgeon pulls back your tissue and repositions it. Permanent stitches underneath your repositioned tissue keep it in place until the muscles reattach themselves to underlying bony tissues.

Wrinkles: Smile Lines and Facial Fissures

Simple Ways to Save Your Skin

Over-the-counter moisturizers can cover up fine lines. But unlike their prescription counterparts, over-the-counter anti-aging ingredients aren't concentrated enough to reach deeper skin layers where wrinkling begins.

So what is the best way to reduce the signs of aging?

- **Wear a sunscreen:** Products with a sun protection factor (SPF) of 15 or greater can prevent new wrinkles and keep existing ones from getting deeper. Don't rely on cosmetics for sun protection unless they contain sunscreens with an SPF of 15.

- **Moisturize daily:** All moisturizers are combinations of oil and water and work basically the same. They help your skin retain water, smoothing its surface and "plumping up" fine wrinkles.

    For maximum moisturizing qualities, apply a moisturizer after washing your face while it's still damp.

No Fountain of Youth

If you want to rejuvenate your appearance, cosmetic treatments can make a noticeable difference. But they don't eliminate all wrinkles and results may not be permanent. Costs also aren't covered by insurance and can be expensive.

Chapter 9

Caring for Corns, Bunions and Other Agonies of De-feet

How often have you been offered a chair and invited, colloquially speaking, to "take the weight off your feet?" However inelegantly put, the invitation is usually welcome, for the feet bear a tremendous burden in the course of day-to-day living. Considering that an average day of walking subjects the feet to a force equal to several hundred tons, it is little wonder that they ache by nightfall.

Like other parts of the body, the feet are highly specialized structures. Each is made up of 26 bones, laced with ligaments, muscles, nerves and blood vessels. The principal functions of the feet are weight-bearing and locomotion. Their range of motion allows them to move with ease over practically any surface, whether it is rough, uneven or slippery. Their flexibility enables the ballet dancer to stand on one toe, the climber to gain a foothold on a rock face, the circus performer to walk the tight wire, or the small child to gain a few inches to reach the forbidden cookie jar.

But as versatile as they are, our feet are also prey to countless problems. Because of their location and the fact that they must support all our weight, the feet are subject to more pressure and injury than any other part of the body. They can also be affected by congenital or hereditary malformations, such as clubfoot. (Such problems can usually be corrected in infancy with special casts or braces.)

Other foot problems may be an indication of some other underlying health disorder. Circulatory problems, diabetes, anemia and even

FDA Consumer, June 1985.

kidney disorders are often first detected in the feet. Foot joints are frequently the first to be involved when arthritis strikes.

Still other foot problems are brought on by personal habits, sometimes the result of following fashion rather than common sense in choosing shoes. Among the more common foot ailments are corns and calluses, warts, athlete's foot, ingrown nails, and bunions.

Corns and calluses are very much alike. Both have a marked thickening of the top layer of the skin, caused by long periods of pressure or friction against the skin. Calluses can develop anywhere on the weight-bearing areas, such as the sides and soles of the feet. They are usually raised, off-white in color, and have a normal pattern of skin ridges on the surface.

Corns come in two major varieties: hard and soft. Hard corns are the more common, usually occurring on the surfaces of the toes. They appear shiny and polished. Soft corns are whitish in color and are most often found on the web between the fourth and the little toe. Unlike calluses, corns have a central core, which consists of a base on the surface of the skin and an apex pointing inward. Pressure of the core on nerve endings in the skin causes the pain of corns.

Calluses and corns usually develop from wearing ill-fitting shoes, socks or stockings. They may also occur as a result of an underlying foot problem such as a bony growth on the toe.

Calluses and hard corns can be self-treated with over-the-counter (OTC) drug products, according to a panel of experts that assisted FDA in its review of ingredients in these products.

Salicylic acid is the only ingredient the panel found safe and effective for treating calluses and hard corns. The experts recommended it be used in concentrations of 12 to 40 percent in pads, plasters and disks and at concentrations of 12 to 17.6 percent in collodion (a solution of nitrocellulose), which leaves a transparent film when applied to the skin. The panel said there was insufficient data on which to recommend a concentration of salicylic acid that would be safe and effective for treating soft corns. They called for studies on soft corn treatment. (FDA's proposed rules on OTC drug ingredients for callus and corn treatment have not yet been published.)

Other types of treatment include removing some of the thickened skin—something that should be done only by a doctor—and using pads to relieve pressure over bony growths. Occasionally these growths are removed surgically.

Warts on the bottom of the feet, called plantar warts, are often mistaken for calluses, but they have nothing in common. Although

Caring for Corns, Bunions and Other Agonies of De-feet

the pressure of walking on plantar warts can cause pain, pressure does not cause them. Plantar warts, like warts on other parts of the body, are caused by a virus. (See "On Treating Warts With Spunk Water And Other Things" in the October 1983 *FDA Consumer*.)

A plantar wart can grow only on the bottom of the foot and occurs in children as well as adults. It may appear singly or in clusters. The wart is flat and may be either hard or soft. Because they are caused by a virus, warts can be spread from one person to another either directly or indirectly in public areas such as swimming pools or showers. For this reason, many medical experts feel warts should be removed even though most of them will go away by themselves in time.

Salicylic acid is the only safe and effective OTC ingredient the panel found for removal of warts. This ingredient acts as a skin peeler, destroying the wart tissue. Because the drug can harm healthy skin, the panel recommended keeping the product away from surrounding skin, preferably by encircling the wart with a ring of petrolatum.

If there is any doubt about a wart, a doctor should be consulted. Wart treatments that doctors use include freezing the wart with liquid nitrogen, removing it surgically, or using prescription drugs. Single-dose X-ray treatment is another option but is less common today than it once was.

Athlete's foot is a fungal infection that, despite its name, is not exclusive to the locker room. It usually occurs in men between the ages of 14 and 40, but women also may fall prey to the fungus.

Itching, burning and redness are the common symptoms of athlete's foot (known medically as tinea pedis). White scale (flaking skin) develops in the toe web, especially between the fourth and little toe. Blisters may also occur. On the sole of the foot, athlete's foot may appear as irregularly grouped blisters and superficial scale.

The fungi that most commonly cause athlete's foot—*Trichophyton mentagrophytes*, *T. rubrum* and *Epidermophyton floccosum*—are prevalent in homes, offices and athletic facilities, but that doesn't mean everyone passing through will get the affliction. However, the chance of infection increases if there is broken skin or increased moisture from tight shoes, excessive sweating, humid summer weather, or a tropical climate.

To treat athlete's foot, FDA's expert advisory panel on OTC antimicrobial drugs recommended using OTC drugs that contain iodochlorhydroxyquin, tolnaftate, or undecylenic acid and its calcium, copper and zinc salts. Tolnaftate can also be used to prevent, as well as treat, this condition, the panel said.

The panel also recommended that haloprogin and miconazole nitrate be switched from prescription to OTC status for the treatment of athlete's foot. Nystatin, another prescription drug recommended for OTC use, should be used only in combination with other safe and effective OTC ingredients, the panel said. (Proposed rules covering these ingredients have not yet been published by FDA.)

An ingrown toenail almost always afflicts the big toe and occurs when a section of the nail curves into the flesh of the toe corners and becomes imbedded in the soft tissues, causing pain, swelling, inflammation and ulceration.

Incorrect trimming of the nails is usually the cause of ingrown toenails, although pointed-toe shoes and tight shoes and hosiery may also be to blame. People with nails that curl naturally are more likely to develop this condition.

To avoid ingrown toenails, the nails should be cut straight across without tapering the corners.

Unfortunately, FDA's expert advisory panel did not recommend any OTC ingredients as being safe and effective for self-treatment of the discomfort of ingrown nails. Medical treatment is aimed at relieving external pressure and includes prescription medications that will harden the nail groove or help shrink the soft tissue. Hot packs may be applied, as well as topical antiseptics and medications to control infection. In stubborn cases, surgery may be needed to remove part of the nail.

Few foot afflictions are more disfiguring and painful than bunions. Many experts blame ill-fitting shoes for this condition, while others consider this an oversimplification. Bunions have been known to occur in people who don't wear shoes and, conversely, don't always develop in people whose footwear is poorly fitted. Heredity, flat feet, and structural defects resulting from poliomyelitis or cerebral palsy also make some people more prone to bunions.

Bunions are actually misaligned big toe joints that become swollen and tender. The technical name is *hallux valgus* — *hallux* being the Latin name for the great toe and valgus another Latin word meaning bent outward. Normally the bones of the big toe lie more or less in a straight line with the large metatarsal bone of the foot. When a bunion develops, the large metatarsal bone angles outward, away from the other metatarsals, and the big toe bones are forced in the opposite direction (see illustration). Pressure over this joint causes inflammatory swelling of the bursa, a fluid-filled sac that prevents friction between two bones of a joint.

Caring for Corns, Bunions and Other Agonies of De-feet

Bunions may not produce symptoms, but usually they become quite painful, swollen and tender. The skin over the bunion may become thick and rough. There are no topical medications that will make a bunion go away. Use of protective pads and shoes that do not constrict the front part of the foot may help in relieving symptoms. Often the only answer to this deformity is surgery, which ranges from removal of bony outgrowths on the toe to joint resection (cutting away parts of the bone itself), fusion, and toe realignment.

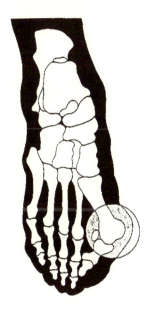

Figure 9.1. Misalignment of the large metatarsal and the bones of the big toe (circled area) is the underlying cause of bunions.

Corns, calluses, warts, athlete's foot, ingrown toenails and sometimes even bunions can, to a large extent, be prevented by proper foot care. This includes selecting shoes that fit correctly, keeping the feet clean and dry, and trimming nails properly.

Good foot care is particularly important in helping the elderly to live useful, satisfying lives. Foot ailments make it difficult for many older people to work or participate in social activities.

To keep older people mobile, the American Podiatric Medical Association (the professional organization of foot doctors) recommends walking as the best exercise for the feet. Shoes with a firm sole and soft upper are best for daily activities, the association says. Socks or stockings should be of the correct size and preferably seamless. Elderly people should not wear constricting garters. Feet should be bathed and inspected daily.

For diabetics of any age, these foot-care recommendations are not only important—they are essential. Any injury to the lower extremities can have serious consequences. Because diabetics tend to have poor circulation, they must avoid anything that will decrease blood flow to the feet, such as wearing tight shoes, constricting socks or garters, or even sitting cross-legged.

Diabetics are more prone to infection; thus any break in the skin is a danger sign. Because they often lose sensation in their feet, diabetics may cut themselves or develop an infection without knowing it. For this reason, it is important that the feet be bathed daily and inspected for cuts, swelling or sores. Bath water should be warm, never hot. And diabetics should never use hot water bottles or electric blankets on their feet.

Commercial corn, callus and wart removers, which are caustic, are not for the diabetic, either. They can destroy tissue and pave the way for infections. Labels on such preparations usually warn against use by diabetics. Finally, diabetics should have a podiatrist remove corns, calluses and warts and trim toenails, rather than doing this themselves. This not only provides an opportunity for a careful foot examination by a doctor but avoids the chance of infection from accidental cuts.

Barefootin'

It's a sure sign that summer's really here when you see children and teenagers walking down the street barefoot, with shoes in hand. Walking barefoot on soft grassy areas is safe enough, but the "concrete jungle of modern cities poses potential hazards to unprotected feet, says the American Podiatric Medical Association.

Concrete breaks down the fat padding on shoeless feet, making them more susceptible to injury from glass, wood and metal fragments. Virus infections, such as plantar warts, and parasitic infections are easily picked up by bare feet, especially since the feet are usually dirty.

Beaches are natural places for barefoot walkers because the surface "gives," putting equal pressure on all parts of the foot. However, caution should be exercised even there, the association warns. Many beaches are veritable "mine fields" of broken glass and other debris.

Caring for Corns, Bunions and Other Agonies of De-feet

On Choosing Shoes

Poorly fitted shoes are a major cause of foot problems. This does not mean that everyone has to wear something akin to an orthopedic shoe. Stylish shoes are not necessarily bad for the feet, according to the American Podiatric Medical Association. The key is fit and variety. A shoe that fits properly, no matter the style, can be worn with no ill effects as long as the feet are in good shape to begin with. By the same token, wearing the same shoes exclusively and for long periods can lead to foot discomfort, the association says.

Wear a shoe that fits the occasion and change heel heights at least once a day. If high heels are worn constantly, the muscles in the back of the legs tend to shorten. Switching to flat heels can then put a strain on these muscles. Wearing flat shoes all the time isn't good either, for this can make the same muscles go slack and the feet will slide forward when high heels are worn.

Unfortunately, many consumers accept poorly fitted shoes in the belief that everything will be fine after a "break-in" period, according to Houston podiatrist David I. Arlen. Writing in the May 1984 *Journal of the American Podiatry Association*, Arlen says there is no such thing as a break-in period and consumers should not accept this condition as a normal part of wearing new shoes.

The feet should be measured each time a new pair of shoes is purchased, Arlen says. Foot size may change because of age, season, physical activity, and time of day. Both feet should be measured and the shoes selected to fit the larger foot. There should be a half-inch of space between the end of the longest toe and the inside end of the shoe's toe box. And don't count on all shoes of a given size being exactly the same. Sizes may vary, depending on where the shoes were made.

Wearing properly fitting shoes is a habit that should begin with baby's first pair. It is especially important to change the size of socks and shoes to keep pace with the growing child. Parents may not realize that a child's foot is flexible and can be crammed into a shoe that is too small without discomfort, though not without harm to the foot.

As children grow older, their shoe preference turns to sneakers or running shoes. There is nothing wrong with this choice provided the fit is good, the podiatry association notes. However, excessive foot perspiration is a common problem for those who wear tennis shoes for prolonged periods. This can set the stage for fungal infections such as athlete's foot. Trench foot, a condition similar to frostbite, can develop when children keep wet sneakers on their feet all day.

These problems can be prevented by common-sense measures such as keeping the feet clean and dry, airing the shoes for 24 hours between wearings, and replacing sneakers often.

—by Annabel Hecht

Annabel Hecht is a member of FDA's communications staff

Chapter 10

Getting a Leg Up on Varicose Veins

During his years in Africa, the renowned British physician Denis Burkitt wondered why he encountered so few cases of varicose veins among his native patients. Being a curious fellow, he sent questionnaires to colleagues in other parts of tropical Africa asking if their experience was similar. It was. In fact, one doctor in Kenya reported that he had seen only three cases of varicose veins in 22 years of practice. That certainly wasn't true for the people back home in England.

It isn't true for Americans, either. It is estimated that 25 percent of adult women and 10 percent of adult men in this country have varicose veins.

For some, varicose veins are merely a cosmetic annoyance that may make them reluctant to wear clothes or participate in sports that show too much leg. Others find them painful, occasionally disabling. At their worst, varicose veins may lead to chronically swollen legs and skin ulcers that never heal. They may become inflamed, a condition known as phlebitis. When a blood clot forms in the inflamed vein, a more serious disease called thrombophlebitis is the result. And though it doesn't happen very often, varicose veins can hemorrhage.

The word varicose means abnormally dilated and twisted. Varicose veins may occur anywhere in the body—hemorrhoids are one example. One of the contributing factors to the development of hemorrhoids is straining during bowel movements, in which increased abdominal pressure is transmitted to veins in the anal area and, according to Dr. Burkitt, to leg veins. Thus, Burkitt theorizes that constipation

---

FDA Consumer, February 1990.

might be the primary reason that varicose veins are more prevalent in urbanized Western countries than in more traditionally living Third World agricultural communities.

However, when people speak of varicose veins, they are usually referring to the surface or superficial veins in the leg. Their appearance varies from person to person, but varicosities are commonly bluish and distended. They may be barely visible in people who have a great deal of subcutaneous (under the skin) fat in their legs. In others, they can swell out to resemble bulging, knotty ropes or even a bunch of grapes. Small groups of tiny blue or red veins under the skin called spiderbursts accompany varicose veins. While spiderbursts are not varicose veins, about 80 percent of those with varicosities will also have some spiderbursts.

Vein Construction

Why veins become varicosed has to do with the way veins are constructed and how they function. Veins are thin-walled, hollow tubes with only a small amount of elastic and muscle tissue. They are different from arteries, the workhorses of the vascular system. The thick, muscular walls of arteries throb with every heartbeat, conveying oxygenated blood under pressure to every cell in the body. The more fragile veins operate at a more leisurely pace, carrying blood containing carbon dioxide back to the heart, where it will be pumped to the lungs for reoxygenation.

Blood pressure, though lower in the veins than the arteries, is still the main driving force in circulation. But in the areas farthest from the heart—the feet and legs—venous blood needs assistance in returning uphill against the force of gravity. The body has a few mechanisms to help out.

Veins have tiny folds of tissue called valves in their inner walls. These cup-like structures open when blood flowing upward pushes through, but close tightly if blood from above falls back, thus insuring a one-way flow. Valves are spaced at irregular intervals along the veins' inside walls. The number of vein valves varies from person to person. Up to 20 may be found in the long saphenous vein, the main surface vein that runs along the whole length of the leg; and there are from 9 to 12 in the short saphenous vein, which runs from the foot up to the back of the knee. The veins that branch off from the saphenous veins, called tributaries, are the ones that most frequently become varicosed.

Getting a Leg Up on Varicose Veins

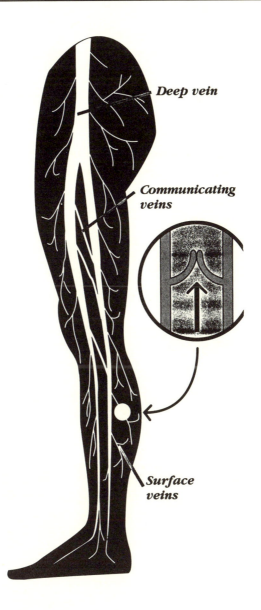

Figure 10.1. A cross-section of a vein showing the cup-like structure called a valve. Valves open to let blood flow upward toward the heart and close to keep blood from dropping backwards toward the feet. The arrow indicates the direction of the flow.

Blood also gets a boost upward by the actions of leg muscles, which squeeze the deep veins in the leg during exercise, pumping blood toward the heart. These groups of muscles in the foot, calf, thigh and abdomen are so effective that they have been called a peripheral heart. Their strength also helps support the heavy column of blood from ankle to the heart.

Another factor that assists in returning blood to the heart is the act of inhaling, which creates a negative pressure in the chest that draws the blood upward.

The surface veins are linked with the deep veins in the leg through a set of connecting veins called perforators. Thus, venous blood normally flows from the surface veins through the connectors to the deep veins, where it is pumped upward by the action of the leg muscles.

Disorderly Conduct

Sometimes, however, things happen that disrupt this orderly sequence. It is thought that a defective valve may start the process. Experts don't know where the first valve fails, though some believe this occurs in one or more of the connecting veins in the lower leg. Others think valve failure begins higher up in the groin, where the large saphenous vein meets the femoral vein. Still others theorize that weak vein walls cause valves to fail.

A weakened valve that doesn't close properly permits blood to flow the wrong way—from the deep veins to the surface veins instead of the other way around. This extra weight of blood presses on the surface vein walls, stretching them. Valves in this stretched area may be pulled apart one by one by pressure from above, causing blood to fall backward and pool in the veins. More pressure is put on the remaining healthy valves and the vein wall, which must now support a longer column of blood. This pressure eventually causes some of the surface vein walls to balloon out into varicose veins.

The severity of varicose veins often has no relationship to the symptoms. People with unsightly veins may have no discomfort, while others with minor varicosities suffer torments. Many experience aching, tired legs, especially after being on their feet a long time. Other common symptoms are a feeling of fullness or a burning sensation. Others may have swollen or itchy ankles, leg cramps at night, stabbing pains that become worse at the end of the day, or tenderness along the veins. Women may feel more discomfort during their menstrual periods.

Getting a Leg Up on Varicose Veins

When legs ache or are painful, a visit to the doctor is in order to rule out other possible problems. A condition called intermittent claudication, due to obstructions of the leg arteries, may cause pain during exertion and relief with rest. An irritated nerve in the back may cause an aching sensation in the calf. But it's probably varicose veins if pain is relieved when legs are elevated.

Treatment

The most conservative treatment is no treatment. If varicose veins cause no problems, and a physician determines that the deep vein system is healthy, nothing needs to be done. When legs ache slightly, elevating them to drain pooled venous blood may give all the relief that is needed.

Sometimes the doctor will prescribe the use of graduated compression stockings. This type of elastic stocking exerts the greatest pressure at the ankle, with gradually lessening pressure as it goes up the leg, and can be knee-high, thigh-high, even waist-high. Elastic stockings put pressure on vein walls, forcing blood from the superficial veins back into the deep veins and squeezing valves closer together. When combined with regular leg elevation and exercise such as walking or swimming, elastic stockings may be a good choice for people who must be on their feet all day long and for those with mild varicosities. Sometimes they are the only treatment advisable for those too ill or too old to tolerate other forms of therapy. They can be uncomfortable, though, in warm weather.

Another type of nonsurgical treatment is sclerotherapy, or injection therapy, which can be done in the doctor's office. In this procedure, a mild solution of a sclerosing (sclero = hard) agent, such as sodium tetradecyl sulfate, is injected into the vein. The solution irritates the inner vein walls so that scar tissue forms and closes it off. Pressure bandages applied on the leg after injection keep the vein walls together and prevent blood flow. The shrunken vein remains in the leg, and blood flow is routed to other veins.

Injection therapy works best on smaller veins, spiderbursts, and on people with relatively few varicosities, but it can be used on almost all varicose veins. However, sclerotherapy is never used on people who have many incompetent valves or deep vein disease, which can usually be determined by simple tests performed in the doctor's office.

After a year's follow-up, about 90 percent of patients report good to excellent results, providing that appropriate selection for sclerotherapy has been made, according to Andrew M. Gage, M.D., and Andrew A. Gage, M.D., in the September 1987 issue of *Hospital Medicine*. One disadvantage is that the procedure sometimes causes a brown discoloration of the skin that may or may not fade. Another drawback is that in some cases the closed-off veins reopen in a few years. If this happens, injection therapy can be safely repeated.

Surgery

Sometimes varicose veins need more aggressive treatment. Valves in the long saphenous vein may fail, causing its tributaries and smaller veins to varicose. Or the long saphenous vein itself may become varicosed. Such cases may call for a surgical procedure called "stripping." The saphenous vein is removed with a device called a vein stripper that actually pulls the vein out of the body. With the diseased vein gone, the blood is forced to find new channels to the deep vein system and circulation is improved.

"Varicose vein surgery is quite safe," says David Calcagno, M.D., assistant professor of surgery at Georgetown University School of Medicine, Washington, D.C., and co-director of Georgetown's Center for Vascular Disease. "We use epidural anesthesia, so the patient isn't put to sleep. We make two incisions, one at the level of the groin and one at the ankle level, separate out the saphenous vein, and then take it out. But then we usually have to make multiple other incisions in the leg to take out the remaining varicose veins."

The incisions are tiny and heal rapidly, usually with little or no scarring. The main tributaries of the saphenous vein, which are cut and tied off during surgery, eventually dry up and disappear. Many of the smaller tributaries tear and bleed when the vein is pulled out, though they quickly seal themselves off. The leg is then wrapped with Ace bandages and elevated.

Many people have a choice of treatment. "We do both injection therapy and surgery," says Calcagno. "It depends on the anatomic situation and the patient's preference. Surgery is better if there's a lot of underlying valvular incompetence or just a very large number of varicose veins. In the last instance, surgery may be more expeditious in that it takes care of the problem in one sitting rather than in multiple visits for vein injection."

After surgery, most doctors recommend walking to help the circulation and wearing elastic stockings or bandages for a short time. Injection therapy can be used on the remaining small varicosities.

When deep veins are blocked or have been damaged by accidents or diseases, such as phlebitis or thrombophlebitis, they cannot pump blood to the heart efficiently enough to compensate for the removal of superficial veins. In these cases, varicose veins should not be removed.

"If we are at all suspicious that the trouble lies in the deep veins, we perform non-invasive vascular testing in the vascular lab. We use both the Doppler probe and IPG (impedance plethysmography)." These techniques are used to determine if the deep leg veins are obstructed and to evaluate the extent of the obstruction.

Easing the Pain

People predisposed to varicose veins may not be able to prevent them, but they can do a number of things to prevent symptoms or complications:

- Elevate the feet whenever possible, such as when watching television or reading.

- Try to avoid prolonged periods of sitting or standing, which cause blood to accumulate in the lower legs, and cause ankles and veins to swell.

- On long trips, walk up and down the aisles of the plane or train every hour or so or stop the car occasionally to stretch the legs. If elastic stockings have been prescribed, be sure to wear them while traveling.

- Walk, run or swim regularly to get the leg muscles pumping and blood moving up the veins.

- Avoid constricting clothing. Tight garters, girdles, pantyhose, and high boots can impede the circulation in the legs.

- Lose weight, if necessary.

The "Haves" and "Have Nots"

Experts find it hard to say exactly what predisposes some people to varicose veins, though heredity is probably the most important factor. Some people are born with veins or valves that have a tendency to weaken. Others have too few valves, so that the individual valve must support more than its share of stress. Many families have more than one member with varicose veins.

Is aging a factor?

Definitely. Just as skin becomes less elastic with age, veins also lose elasticity and muscles weaken. Varicose veins are not common in people under 25, except for women who have had multiple pregnancies. According to the results of the Framingham Study, which keeps track of the development of cardiovascular disease among residents of Framingham, Mass., varicose veins most often develop in women between 40 and 49 years and in men between 70 and 79.

Is inactivity an accelerator?

Leg veins need the pumping action of the muscles to return blood efficiently to the heart. Varicose veins are rare in developing countries where people work hard physically. The Framingham Study confirmed that varicose veins were more common in men and women who were not physically active.

Is pregnancy a precipitator?

One woman interviewed for this article told of her experience. "Varicose veins run in my family so I wasn't too surprised when veins started to pop out early in my pregnancy, but only in one leg," she said. "When I was pregnant with my second child, they popped out in the other leg."

Pregnant women have about 20 percent more blood in their bodies than nonpregnant women. This extra volume of blood, combined with the weight of the unborn baby pressing down on the pelvic veins can stress vein walls and impede circulation. Hormone levels, which rise during pregnancy, may relax the muscles in vein walls, causing veins to dilate and valves to separate. Varicose veins often improve after delivery.

Does flab figure in?

Overweight people have a higher proportion of fat to muscle, which means less muscular support for the veins and less muscle to do the pumping. As in pregnancy, extra poundage in the abdominal area puts pressure on vein walls and may aggravate existing cases of varicose veins. A number of population studies have reported that both women and men with varicose veins are more often obese.

Is it a dietary deficiency?

Dr. Burkitt thought so. Low dietary fiber may cause constipation, which in turn leads to abdominal straining that may damage vein valves in the leg, or so Burkitt theorized. He postulated that one reason varicose veins were rare in Africa is that diets in developing countries are generally high in fiber, as opposed to Western diets. However, this doesn't explain why the African Masai, who subsist on a diet of milk and blood (which contains plenty of fiber in the form of fibrin, an insoluble material that is the basic component of a blood clot), have few leg varicosities though as many as 45 percent of the Masai complain of constipation.

Is the chair the culprit?

People who squat or sit on the ground, as in some African and Asian agricultural communities, have stronger leg vein walls than people in more industrialized communities. It will be interesting to see how Westernization and affluence affect the leg veins of the Japanese, who had few varicose veins in the past when they were accustomed to sitting on the floor.

— by Evelyn Zamula

Evelyn Zamula is a free-lance writer in Potomac, Md.

Chapter 11

Tips for Treating Aging Skin

How the Skin Ages

As the skin loses its regenerative capabilities, cumulative damage from ultraviolet radiation mounts up. Intrinsic aging may be unavoidable, but lifelong care can limit the harm.

Intrinsic Aging

Numerous structural and functional changes combine to age the skin, resulting in thinning, fragility, and loss of elasticity. Circulation and innervation decrease, and the structural attachment between the dermis and epidermis deteriorates. A variety of neoplasia appears on the skin as part of the aging process. Benign growths include seborrheic keratoses, cherry angiomas, and skin tags. A common premalignant lesion is the actinic keratosis, which appears on areas of chronic sun exposure.

Aging of the skin is a process involving intrinsic structural and functional changes in combination with extrinsic factors such as exposure to ultraviolet (UV) light, wind, or thermal extremes (see Figure 11.1). As it ages, the skin becomes thinner—at times almost like parchment—and inelastic. Because the structural attachments between epidermis and dermis break down, the epidermis can actually tear away with slight trauma, as when a person is pulled across a bed

---

©1992 *Medical Economics*. Reprinted with permission of Patient Care.

or adhesive tape is removed abruptly. With age, dermal circulation becomes less efficient and vascular walls become thinner. As a result, elderly people tend to bruise easily.

Cutaneous innervation also diminishes, increasing the likelihood of mechanical injury, and thinning of subcutaneous tissue lessens the skin's insulating capacity and increases the risk of hypothermia. Malnutrition, to which older persons are prone because of poor eating habits (especially after the death of a spouse) and untreated dental problems, can further exacerbate skin deterioration.

Problems in Aging Skin

Among the most common benign lesions of aging skin are acrochordons, also known as skin tags. These are found in areas of skin laxity and friction such as the armpits and groin, and beneath the breasts in women. In a tendency that runs in families, women may also develop crops of skin tags on the neck. Skin tags generally develop before age 40 in women, but after age 50 in men. Seborrheic keratoses are wart-like growths that first appear as flat, brown lesions, but may become large, verrucous, and cosmetically compromising. They are harmless, however, and can simply be scraped off with a curette or removed with liquid nitrogen.

Cherry angiomas (De Morgan's spots) are benign proliferations of the capillaries, usually seen on the trunk. Areas of mottled pigmentation most often found on the lateral aspects of the neck, known as poikiloderma of Civatte, typically result from a combination of excessive sun exposure and the use of fragrances. This discoloration is most common among women who play golf or other outdoor games.

A common premalignant skin lesion is actinic keratosis, which develops on areas of the body that have been chronically sun-exposed. Solar lentigines, though usually considered benign, may occasionally develop into malignant melanoma. Some patients today are concerned by the small red papules of senile ectasia, mistaking these harmless lesions for Kaposi's sarcoma. Senile ectasia is not premalignant.

Skin Cancer

The aging process predisposes the skin to development of carcinoma. Melanocytes decrease at a rate of 20 percent per decade after age 30, decreasing the skin's ability to protect itself from ultraviolet (UV) light. T-cell function is diminished, Langerhans' cells are lost,

Tips for Treating Aging Skin

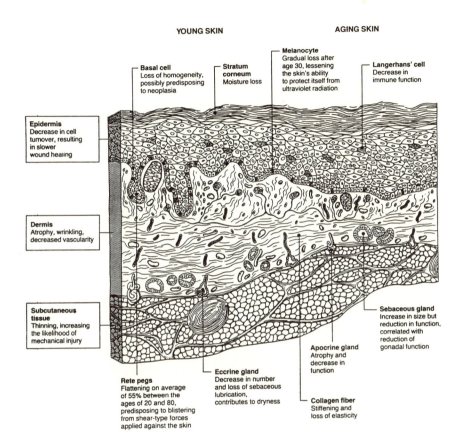

Figure 11.1. How the Skin Ages: Human skin normally acts as a barrier between the exterior environment and the homeostatic environment of the body, providing mechanical and sensory protection. By the time people are in their 80s, however, there has been a 15 to 20 percent reduction in over all skin function. Thinning of the skin, structural breakdown, and loss of vascularity contribute to this functional deterioration.

and the overall inflammatory response is muffled. Sun exposure is responsible for 90 percent of all skin cancer, but risk also depends on skin color, sex, and geographic location. Basal cell carcinoma usually remains localized, but squamous cell carcinoma may metastasize.

The development of skin cancer is a dose-related phenomenon that relies on this intrinsic predisposition in combination with the extrinsic effects of photoaging. A lifetime of actinic assault places a person at considerable risk, particularly if he is fair-skinned or lives in an area of great sun intensity. Photoaging is responsible for many of the ordinary wrinkles and brown spots common in older people, but it is also responsible for 90 percent of skin cancers.

After age 30, people lose approximately 20 percent of their epidermal melanocytes per decade. These cells produce pigment—leading to a suntan—in response to UV light to protect the skin from further assault. The inevitable concomitant of decreased melanocyte population is increased susceptibility to UV-induced damage. Moreover, older people are often unable to acquire an even suntan because the remaining melanocytes tend to form irregular aggregates (clumps which are visible in some persons as solar lentigines).

As we age, T-cell function decreases and Langerhans' cells die off. Loss of these immunocompetent cells increases a person's risk of systemic and dermatologic infection and cancer. Even without sun exposure, older skin apparently is simply more likely to become cancerous than younger skin. Contact with a known carcinogen such as 3,4-benzpyrene results in cancer more often in older than in younger skin, apparently because of an intrinsic cellular heterogeneity inherent in aging.

This muffled inflammatory response of the skin allows an older person to sit out in the sun without becoming sunburned for a longer period of time than when he or she was younger, but not without incurring significant UV-induced damage. Because a person may think he or she does not burn as easily as before, he is likely to assume mistakenly that he can tolerate the sun better. The cellular insult is as bad or worse, the defense capability is less, and the body's warning signs are less effective.

Specific factors that contribute to a person's likelihood of developing skin cancer include ethnic origin, sex, and geographic location. Fair-skinned persons of Celtic or Scandinavian origin are at the greatest risk, particularly those with red or blond hair and blue eyes. Similarly, whites in general develop skin cancer 27 times more frequently than blacks. Males are more commonly affected, probably because

Tips for Treating Aging Skin

they more commonly work outdoors. Makeup and lipstick may provide some protection for women, who are less prone to develop malignancies involving the lips and other parts of the face.

The most common cancer of aging skin is basal cell carcinoma, which accounts for 80 percent of all skin cancers. Basal cell carcinoma only rarely spreads, and the lesion is usually removed before it can destroy any surrounding tissue. These are the warning signs of basal cell carcinoma:

- An open sore that persists for three weeks or more
- An irritated red area that may be painful or itchy
- A smooth growth with an elevated border
- A pearly or translucent nodule that resembles a mole (red, pink, white, black, or brown)
- A white or yellow lesion that is similar to scar tissue.

Squamous cell carcinoma is more dangerous, since it can metastasize. The lesion itself may be irregular, scaly, or bleeding. Although squamous cell carcinoma often develops from a preexisting actinic keratosis, it can also arise in an area of chronic trauma or irritation. The lower lip is a common site, especially in cigarette smokers. The nose may protect the upper lip from UV exposure, and hence from malignancy. Melanoma, which is the most lethal of the common skin cancers, can also occur in younger people.

The incidence of skin cancer doubles with every four degrees of proximity to the equator and is thus 5.7 times more common in Texas than in Minnesota. A given patient would be expected to develop skin cancer about 10 years earlier and would be prone to multiple lesions if he lived in an area of high, rather than low, UV intensity. High altitude also can increase the hazard of intense UV exposure.

Dermatologists recommend a thorough skin examination once a year for all older people. This examination should include both exposed and non-exposed areas of the body. A person with a history of skin cancer should be examined every six months. People of all ages need to watch their skin for development of any new spots and especially for any change in an old lesion. Also, if one small area of skin cancer is found, a careful examination for other lesions is in order.

Elderly patients should understand that a change in a skin lesion or mole need not be dramatic or quick. Most cancerous lesions on the skin of older people tend to develop slowly, in contrast to cancerous lesions in younger people, which tend to develop and spread more quickly.

Preventing Photoaging

Avoiding sun exposure is the single most significant measure a person can take to protect skin. Long-sleeved clothing, sunglasses, and hats should be worn, and sunscreen with a sun protection factor of at least 15 should be used routinely. Conventional sunscreens containing para-aminobenzoic acid are useful for UV-B radiation. It now appears that UV-A may be harmful as well; newer sunscreens block both. Protection should begin early in life, and sunscreens must be used generously and consistently to be effective.

Avoidance of sun exposure can greatly reduce the effects of photoaging. Dermatologists recommend that individuals of all ages, particularly those who are fair-skinned and live in areas of intense sun, restrict outdoor activities as much as possible to times of least intense sun, before 10 a.m. or after 4 p.m. Clothing should be loose, light-colored, and made of tightly woven fabric. A man's long-sleeved shirt can filter out approximately 50 percent of the UV rays, and an undershirt can increase this to 70 percent for the body and shoulders. A hat with a large brim or flap covering the neck is also important.

These measures will not eliminate exposure to UV radiation, or the risk of skin cancer. Even with proper clothing, and even in the shade or on an overcast day, a person who spends significant time outdoors needs to use a sunscreen with a sun protection factor of at least 15.

It was previously thought that only UV-B radiation was significant in causing sun damage, but now it appears that UV-A may also play a part, and possibly infrared radiation as well. UV-A is present in sunlight year round, and is more penetrating and abundant than UV-B. Newer sunscreens have been developed that contain oxybenzone and Parsol 1789, which block both UV-A and UV-B. Some authorities believe that these formulations will be much more effective in preventing photoaging and skin cancer, and should now be used routinely. Others, however, feel that sunscreens containing para-aminobenzoic acid, which filter only UV-B, still can be helpful if used consistently.

To be effective, any sunscreen must be used correctly. A sunscreen that has a sun protection factor of 15 when tested in the laboratory will provide a factor of 7 if only half the required amount is used. And in fact, studies show that the average person uses only about half the proper amount of sunscreen.

In some patients, tretinoin (Retin-A) appears to alleviate the effects of photoaging (unlabeled use). It is worth reminding some patients that the photoaging that takes place during the summer can be repaired, to some extent, by a winter of little sun exposure. Continuing the UV exposure at a tanning parlor during the winter is a foolhardy practice that can contribute to hastening of photo-damage and aging of the skin.

What to Expect from Tretinoin

Long-term use of tretinoin (Retin-A) in some patients appears to improve the texture of the skin and smooth the fine wrinkles characteristic of photoaging(unlabelled use). Skin color also improves and some small premalignant lesions disappear. Deep wrinkles and expression lines are usually not affected by tretinoin.

A double-blind study evaluating the response of 30 patients to tretinoin therapy found that after 12 weeks of treatment 93 percent of patients showed at least some cosmetic improvement particularly in fine wrinkling and facial color. The main adverse consequence was a dermatitis characterized by erythema swelling and scaling which generally improved with emollients. The investigators acknowledge that their study participants were relatively young (mean age 50, age range 35 to 70) and that further studies are needed to determine the long-term success of the treatment for reversal of photoaging.

Not all clinicians are finding equivalent success with tretinoin however and they furthermore caution that patients must be very careful to avoid sun exposure during treatment. Patients must also avoid sun-sensitizing substances such as products containing sulfur resorcinol salicylic acid and benzoyl peroxide. More recent evidence suggests that abrasive preparations may be somewhat more effective than tretinoin on photoaging.

Dry Skin

The majority of older people are afflicted by some degree of xerosis and itching, particularly during the winter. Hydrocortisone cream and a thick emollient may be applied if inflammation is severe; the emollient alone may be used when inflammation is absent. Therapeutic moisturizers are usually more effective for the severe dryness of aged skin than are cosmetic moisturizers. Super-fatted soaps can also be beneficial. Moisturizing products need not be exotic to be effective, plain petrolatum is very useful if applied to damp skin.

Xerosis is the most common problem that develops as skin ages. The exact cause of skin dryness or roughness with aging is unknown, but the decrease in the moisture content of the stratum corneum and altered function of the eccrine and sebaceous glands probably contribute. The problem is generally worse in winter, with dry air and heat helping to deplete what little moisture the skin may have. In some circumstances, however, there may be an underlying cause such as thyroid dysfunction. Itching may result if the dryness is severe, and if the person scratches inflammation may ensue. The itching can be worsened by ingestion of coffee, alcohol, or spicy foods, and by some medications often used by older people, such as diuretics.

Although some dermatologists suggest that elderly people bathe less to avoid drying out the skin, others feel that many patients find this practice unacceptable. With minimal use of soap and sufficient use of emollients, the elderly can bathe every day if they wish. After the bath or shower, the person should blot the skin nonabrasively with a towel, not wipe it completely dry. If the dryness is so severe as to have caused cracking and inflammation, a hydrocortisone cream can be applied to the damp skin, followed by an emollient that will seal in moisture. If there is no inflammation, an emollient such as mineral oil, lanolin, or jojoba oil can be used alone over the damp skin to seal in moisture.

Moisturizers and emollients do not need exotic ingredients or an impressive price tag to be effective. One of the best emollients to use on damp skin after bathing (though many patients find it cosmetically unacceptable) is plain white petrolatum (Vaseline). In general, unscented products are preferable because the added fragrances can have an irritant effect. Some dermatologists recommend the substitution of cleansing cream for soap, but others prefer super-fatted, non-sudsing soaps, which clean the skin without removing the natural oils.

Therapeutic moisturizers with lactic acid or urea are more effective for the severe dryness of aged skin than are cosmetic moisturizers. These products are intended to alleviate the causes of dryness, rather than simply make the skin temporarily feel lubricated. Some authorities believe that ordinary cosmetic moisturizers actually worsen the dryness, although they may provide a temporary moisturizing sensation. Caution patients not to overuse therapeutic moisturizers, however, because they can cause perioral or rosacea-like dermatitis on the face.

Increasing the humidity of the house during the winter may be beneficial. Some authorities also recommend bath oils for dry skin, but others consider this too hazardous for the elderly person, because of the danger of falling in the slippery tub.

Tips for Treating Aging Skin

Keeping Your Skin Healthy

You probably know that a healthy-looking tan isn't healthy at all. Too much sun over too long a period of time will make your skin leathery and wrinkled and greatly increase your chances of skin cancer. These guidelines will help you keep your skin healthy and younger-looking.

Sun Exposure

- Stay out of the sun as much as possible during the midday hours of 10 a.m. to 4 p.m., especially if you are fair-skinned and blond or redheaded. Avoid tanning parlors and other artificial tanning methods.

- Wear protective clothing when you are exposed to sunlight. Long sleeves, long pants, and a hat will shield your skin from much of the dangerous ultraviolet (UV) radiation. Sunglasses that filter UV-A and UV-B rays are important for preventing damage to your eyes.

- Always use sunscreen with a sun protection factor (SPF) of 15 or more when you are in the sun. Apply it generously, and replace it after swimming. If you use a waterproof sunscreen, let it dry for 30 minutes before you go in the water. You need sunscreen even on overcast days or when sitting in the shade. Winter outdoor activities such as skiing also can expose you to high-intensity UV radiation.

- If you are taking any medication, check with your physician before you go out into the sun. Many drugs can cause the skin to be overly sensitive to sunlight.

Skin Cancer

In most instances, skin cancer is curable, if it is caught early enough. Examine your skin thoroughly on a regular basis, and have a complete yearly skin examination. If you have ever had skin cancer before, have a checkup every six months. Watch for these warning signs in particular:

- An open sore that lasts for three weeks or more
- An irritated red area that is painful or itchy
- A smooth growth with an elevated border
- A pearly or translucent spot that resembles a mole; this can be red, pink, white, black, or brown
- A white or yellow area that resembles scar tissue.

The most common types of skin cancer, basal cell carcinoma and squamous cell carcinoma, don't usually spread throughout the body. But a third type, melanoma, can spread rapidly and kill. The most common early warning sign of melanoma is a change in the shape, size, or surface texture of a mole.

All three of these skin cancers have been increasing in recent years, possibly because of depletion of the ozone layer of the atmosphere. The increase may also reflect the fact that many people today have more leisure time than in the past-time which is often spent in the sun in scanty clothing. Sixty years ago, only 1 person in 1,500 developed melanoma. In another decade, however, 1 person in 90 is expected to be affected.

Dry Skin

Natural changes of aging tend to result in drying of the skin. To keep your skin from drying out excessively, avoid harsh soaps and use a good moisturizer after bathing.

Moisturizers don't have to be expensive to be effective. A petrolatum jelly such as Vaseline, for example, helps seal in the skin's natural moisture. Apply the moisturizer when your skin is slightly damp. If your skin is so dry that it itches, avoid spicy foods, caffeine, and alcohol. Keep in mind, however, that itching can be a sign of a serious underlying condition such as diabetes or kidney disease.

References

1. Bickers DR: Sun-induced disorders. Emerge Med Cain North Am 1985; 3: 659-676.
2. Elias PM: Epidermal effects of retinoids: Supramolecular observations and clinical implications J Am Acad Dermatol 1986;15(4 pt 2): 797-809.
3. Fenske NA, Lober CW: Structural and functional changes of normal aging skin J Am Acad Dermatol 1986; 15(4 pt 1): 571-585.
4. Katz SI: The skin as an immunologic organ J Am Acad Dermatol 1985; 13: 530-536.

5. Kligman AM, Grove GL, Hirose R, et al: Topical tretinoin for photoaged skin J Am Acad Dermatol 1986; 15(4 pt 2) 836-859.
6. Kligman LH: Photoaging: Manifestations, prevention and treatment Dermatol Ct/n 1986; 4: 517-528.
7. Kripke ML: Immunology and photocarcinogenesis New light on an old problem. J Am Acad Dermatol 1986; 14: 149-155.
8. Marks R, Hill S, Barton SP: The effects of an abrasive agent on normal skin and on photoaged skin in comparison with topical tretinoin. Br J Dermatol 1990; 123: 457-466.
9. Potts RO, Buras EM Jr, Chrisman DA Jr: Changes with age in the moisture content of human skin. J Invest Dermatol 1984; 82: 97-100.
10. Richey HK, Fenske NA: Nonmelanomatous skin cancer: New concepts in pathogenesis South Med J 1987; 80: 362-365.
11. Staberg B, Wulf HC, Klemp P, et al: The carcinogenic effect of UVA irradiation J Invest Dermatol 1983; 81: 517-519.
12. Stern RS, Weinstein MC, Baker SG: Risk reduction for nonmelanoma skin cancer with childhood sunscreen use. Arch Dermatol 1986; 122: 537-545.
13. Weiss JS, Ellis CN, Headington JT, et al: Topical tretinoin improves photoaged skin: A double-blind vehicle-controlled study. JAMA 1988; 259: 527-532.

—by Neil A. Fenske, MD;
Leonard D. Grayson, MD;
and Victor D. Newcomer, MD

Neil A. Fenske, MD is a professor of internal medicine and pathology and director, division of dermatology, University of South Florida College of Medicine, Tampa, and chief of dermatology, H. Lee Moffitt Cancer Center and Research Institute and James A. Haley Veterans Hospital, Tampa, Fla.

Leonard D. Grayson, MD is a clinical assistant, department of medicine, Southern Illinois University School of Medicine; and chief, department of allergy, QP&S Clinic, Quincy, Ill.

Victor D. Newcomer, MD is a professor of dermatology, University of California, Los Angeles, UCLA School of Medicine, Los Angelos.

Chapter 12

Cosmetic Surgery

Fast Facts

- As with all surgical procedures, cosmetic surgery carries with it certain risks.
- Select a doctor who is well trained and experienced in performing the specific procedure you want. (For help, use the questions listed below.)
- Find out beforehand any possible side effects, risks, and complications of the surgery you want.
- Early on, discuss with your doctor what goals you hope to accomplish with cosmetic surgery and whether these goals are realistic.
- Remember that insurance usually does not cover costs for elective cosmetic surgery.

In the quest to look better, millions of Americans are turning to cosmetic surgery. Each year, more consumers elect to have their faces lifted, their stomachs "tucked," or their thighs slimmed.

In response to this growing demand, many doctors now widely advertise their ability to surgically correct the less-than-perfect parts of one's anatomy. The majority of surgeons performing cosmetic surgery are qualified and perform successful operations. However, doctors

---

Bureau of Consumer Protection. Office of Consumer & Business Education (202) 326-3650. *Facts for Consumers*. Federal Trade Commission, September 1992.

with insufficient training or experience or questionable credentials also are attracted to this field because of the millions of consumer dollars spent annually on cosmetic surgery.

As with all surgical procedures, cosmetic surgery carries with it certain risks. If performed poorly, it can be disfiguring or even life-threatening. It is essential, therefore, to select a doctor who is well trained and experienced in performing the specific procedure you want. The following information may help you if you are considering cosmetic surgery.

How Do You Choose the Right Doctor?

Before beginning your search, you may want to learn more about surgical options by reviewing books on cosmetic surgery that can be found in your local library and discussing your plans with your family physician. If you decide to pursue cosmetic surgery, ask your physician for the names of qualified surgeons. You also can obtain names of appropriate physicians by calling your local hospital or consulting the *ABMS Compendium of Certified Medical Specialists* or the *Directory of Medical Specialists* available in most libraries.

Plan to consult with several surgeons who specialize in the type of cosmetic surgery procedure you want. While this may seem a considerable investment of time and money (most physicians will charge a consultation fee), remember that if the operation is not performed properly, you could carry the scars for life.

Be wary of physicians who suggest that you have features "fixed" that do not bother you, use a hard sell to obtain your business, or brush aside your concerns about safety. In addition, no responsible doctor should mind your asking the following questions.

What is your area of specialty and what training do you have in the specific cosmetic surgery procedure I want?

Make sure the doctor you choose is well trained to perform the type of surgery you want. Ask where the doctor earned a medical degree and in what specialty the doctor completed an accredited residency program. Ask for information on how this training relates to the specific procedure you want, as well as what fellowships, workshops, and other education programs pertinent to your operation the physician has completed.

Finally, find out if the doctor is certified by an appropriate medical board. A board tests the level of physicians' knowledge in specific specialties. Normally, before qualifying to take the exams in a particular specialty, physicians must first complete a formal residency training program in that field. Those who pass the voluntary exams are considered "certified" in that area of expertise. Confirm the physician's credentials and board affiliation with your county medical society or state medical board.

Do you have hospital privileges?

Even if the surgery you want will be performed in the doctor's office or clinic, ask if the doctor is on staff at a local hospital and has privileges there to perform that procedure. Hospital privileges generally assure that the physician you select has been reviewed by his or her peers.

How many operations like mine have you performed in the past year? During your career?

No matter how good the doctor's credentials, a doctor skilled in facial surgery may not be the best one to perform breast surgery or hair transplants. Find a doctor who has experience specifically in the procedure you want.

How many of your patients have needed additional surgery?

Additional surgery is sometimes needed to correct problems arising from the original operation. An ethical surgeon will answer this question. He or she also will answer questions about the probability of problems and tell you whether there will be an additional charge in the event more surgery is required.

How safe is this operation?

Nobody can guarantee an absolutely successful outcome to any surgical procedure—and you should be suspicious of anyone who does. All surgery involves some risk and unpredictability. Although rare, people have been known to die or suffer from life-limiting disabilities after cosmetic surgery. The physician should explain all the possible risks and complications associated with the procedure, as well as their degree of probability.

What are the potential side effects of my surgical procedure? How long will these last?

Many doctors agree that patients are often unprepared for the side effects that may occur after cosmetic surgery. These include pain, scarring, swelling, bruising, bleeding, infection or worse. Some patients may not be able to resume their normal activities for weeks after their operation. Be certain to have the physician you choose explain the potential side effects of your procedure.

What should I expect before, during, and after my operation?

Have your doctor and nursing staff explain in detail what to expect at every stage of the procedure. If they are not willing to spend the time needed to address all of your questions and concerns, then you should probably look elsewhere.

Information materials such as brochures and videotapes should be available for you to read or view. If your physician uses "computer imaging" to show what changes you can expect from surgery, note that drawing on a "TV screen" can be very different from working with real flesh and bone. The computerized image you see may not be exactly what you get.

The same is true of pre- and post-operative photographs of other patients. Before-and-after photos may give you some feel for the surgeon's skill, but every patient's physical characteristics and experience are different.

Will you perform the operation yourself ? Who will administer the anesthesia? Where will my operation take place?

Make sure that you talk to the doctor who will perform your surgery and ask who will take care of you after the operation. Find out what type of anesthesia will be used and who will administer it. Be certain the individual is qualified to administer the anesthesia.

Where will your surgery take place?

If your physician suggests his or her office or clinic, ask about the facility's equipment for life-support and other emergencies. If you are having major surgery, you may want to seek extra protection by making sure the facility is approved by one of the three accrediting organizations listed under "For More Information."

Cosmetic Surgery

What are your fees?

Find out in advance what the procedure and follow-up care will cost. If your surgery will be performed in a hospital or ambulatory surgical center, remember that in addition to your doctor's fee, there will be a charge for use of the facility and the services of the anesthesiologist.

Insurance usually does not cover costs for elective cosmetic surgery, and many doctors require payment in advance. Therefore, you may want to compare fees. But just because a surgeon charges higher prices does not mean he or she is better than other physicians.

How realistic are my own expectations for this operation?

Most doctors consider the best candidates for elective cosmetic surgery to be those who are well adjusted and emotionally secure. Ideal patients desire the operation to enhance their own self-esteem—not to influence the opinions of others. Although greater self-confidence may lead to other enhancements in life, consumers who hope cosmetic surgery will help add excitement to their social lives, win back a spouse, or obtain a promotion at work are often disappointed. Discuss with your doctor what you hope to accomplish with surgery and whether your goals are realistic.

Can I contact former patients who have had the same surgical procedure I want?

Talking to former patients who have had the same procedure you desire is one way to learn more about the operation and your doctor. But keep in mind that each patient has different physical characteristics and expectations. Although a physician may have good results with one person, that does not guarantee your surgery will turn out the same.

What Are Some Common Cosmetic Surgery Procedures and Their Potential Risks?

Before having any operation, it is important to have realistic expectations about the benefits that can be achieved and understand the possible risks and side effects. Those issues should be discussed thoroughly with your surgeon. Below is a brief, simplified overview of some of the potential complications and side effects of common cosmetic surgery procedures. It cannot substitute for a consultation with a properly-trained physician.

Any of these operations can result in infection or blood collecting beneath the skin, conditions requiring additional treatment and, in a few cases, further hospitalization. In rare instances, permanent and conspicuous scarring can result. Further, although many of these operations are not done under general anesthesia, those that are carry additional risks.

Face lift (rhytidectomy): Although a face lift can improve some signs of aging, surgery will not stop the aging process. Following the operation, there may be significant puffiness and bruising for several weeks, and some individuals may feel a temporary numbness or tightness in the face or neck. Nerve damage that causes permanent loss of sensation or movement in the facial muscles can occur in rare instances.

The scars resulting from a face lift are normally in the hairline and folds of the ear, and usually lighten with time until they are barely visible. The kind of scars cannot be predicted with total accuracy, because everyone heals differently.

Nose surgery (rhinoplasty): Changing the shape of the nose is one of the most complex procedures, even for a skilled surgeon. If too much cartilage or bone is removed, the nose can look misshapen. Additionally, if care is not taken with the internal structure of the nose, you can end up with a nose that does not function correctly. Before the operation, make sure you and your doctor thoroughly discuss what kinds of changes you would like and how the changes will "fit in" with your other facial features.

It can take several weeks for bruising around the eyes to go away and several months for any swelling that occurs to completely disappear. You may experience some difficulty breathing for some weeks following the procedure.

Eyelid surgery (blepharoplasty): Performed to remove excess skin and fat above and below the eyes, this procedure usually causes bruising that fades within a week to ten days. However, discoloration can last for several weeks. The physician must be very careful not to remove too much skin, which could cause too much "white of the eye" to show. In addition, though rare, risks include dry eye syndrome (the eyes stop making tears) and drooping of the lower lid.

Hair transplants: The most common of these procedures, called punch grafting, is performed by transplanting small pieces of skin with healthy hair follicles to bald spots. This process may be repeated several times over a period of 8 to 18 months. Common temporary aftereffects include pain, swelling, bruising, and the formation of crusts on the scalp. In another technique, called scalp reduction, part of the bald scalp's skin is removed, and the skin with hair is stretched and sutured together over this area. Some discomfort, including headaches and scalp tightening, may follow for a short time. Less frequently, flap surgery is performed by rotating wide strips of skin with hair to cover areas where bald skin has been removed. In another procedure, the hair-bearing scalp tissue may be expanded so that the enlarged tissue can replace the bald area. The latter two procedures require general anesthesia, and more serious complications, such as damage to tissue, can result.

Breast augmentation (enlargement): In this procedure, silicone envelopes filled with salt water (saline solution), silicone gel, or a combination of both can be implanted to enlarge the breasts. In April 1992, the FDA announced that because it continues to be concerned about the safety of silicone gel-filled breast implants, all patients to receive these implants must be enrolled in clinical studies. Silicone implants for the purpose of breast augmentation will be available only to a very limited number of women. (Women who need the implants for breast reconstruction will be assured access to the studies.) The FDA made this decision because it determined that manufacturers of silicone implants have not proven that these devices are safe.

As of May 1992, saline-filled implants continue to be freely available. In the future, manufacturers of saline-implants will be required to submit data to the FDA to prove that these devices are safe and effective in order to continue marketing these devices. Known risks of saline-filled implants include the possibility of infection, hardening of the scar tissue surrounding the implant, formation of calcium deposits in the surrounding tissues, implant rupture, and interference with the detection of early breast cancer. Evaluating the risks and benefits of breast implants can be a difficult issue. Discuss this issue thoroughly with your doctor. You also may want to contact the FDA at the address or telephone number listed under "For More Information."

Breast reduction: With breast reduction or lift surgery (mastopexy), there will be some degree of scarring, and there may be unevenness in breast size. You will want to ask your physician about this and other possible effects, such as a temporary or permanent change in nipple sensation or a decreased ability to breast-feed.

"Tummy tuck" (abdominoplasty): The common nickname for this procedure—which removes excess, sagging skin and underlying fat from the abdomen—belies the fact that it is major surgery normally done under general anesthesia. An incision is made from hip bone to hip bone and, although it is located low along the "bikini line," a significant scar results. Full recovery, as with other major surgery, may take a couple of months or longer.

Injections: Facial wrinkles may be treated by injecting them with collagen or fat. Neither substance produces permanent results, and the longevity of the results depends on the patient's skin and reaction to the substance. People may be allergic to collagen and not know it. Also, the FDA is investigating whether there is a cause-and-effect relationship between having collagen treatments and later developing "PM/DM" (chronic, progressive, sometimes fatal inflammatory disorders) or similar diseases. The injection of liquid silicone has not been approved by the FDA for any purpose, and the FDA prohibits manufacturers and doctors from marketing or promoting this product.

Chemical Peels and Dermabrasion: These two techniques may be used to treat scarring (such as those from acne or skin injury), skin wrinkles, or splotchy pigmentation. To perform chemical peels, an acid or other agent is applied to destroy the top layers of skin. Temporary pain, swelling, and redness may result. Dermabrasion is performed by using machines that remove the top layers of skin. This helps smooth skin irregularities. Treated skin may be sensitive to sunlight. Risks include scarring and uneven pigmentation which, in rare cases, may be long-term or permanent.

Liposuction (suction-assisted lipectomy): To perform this very popular procedure, a doctor inserts a thin tube into a fatty part of the body and, using a special vacuum pump, suctions out unwanted fat, leaving a flattened area with little scarring. The growing popularity of the procedure has attracted many physicians with widely varying

Cosmetic Surgery

training and experience. There have been reports of blood clots, fluid loss, infection, and even death following liposuction. Make certain the doctor you choose is well trained and experienced in performing this procedure.

Contrary to popular belief, liposuction is:

- Not a substitute for good routines of diet and exercise. Ideal candidates are close to their ideal weight, but have pockets of resistant fat on their hips, thighs, abdomens, or chin.

- Not a cure for "cellulite," the popular term for the dimpled skin often found on the thighs.

- Not a solution for people with stretched-out, inelastic skin that cannot redrape around body contours.

If you are a good candidate and proceed with the surgery, you will need to wear a girdle or other compression garment until any bruising and swelling disappear.

For More Information

The FDA can provide further detailed information about breast implants, collagen injections, and liquid silicone injections. To obtain this information, send a postcard to: "Breast Implants" or "Collagen and Liquid Silicone Injections," FDA, HFE-88, 5600 Fishers Lane, Rockville, MD 20857. The FDA also has a toll-free hotline on breast implants: 1-800-532-1110. For the hearing impaired, the number is 1-800-688-6167.

If the physician you choose suggests that your operation be performed in his or her office, check with one of the following organizations to see if the facility has passed an inspection:

- the Accreditation Association for Ambulatory Health Care, Inc. (708-676-9610);
- the American Association for Accreditation of Ambulatory Plastic Surgery Facilities (708-949-6058); or
- the Joint Commission for the Accreditation of Healthcare Organizations (312-642-6061).

After surgery, if you have a problem that cannot be resolved with the physician, contact your county medical society, state medical board, or your local consumer protection agency.

You may also report any problems to the Federal Trade Commission. Write:

Service Industry Practices, FTC,
6th and Pennsylvania Avenue, NW,
Washington, DC 20580.

Although the FTC does not generally intervene in individual disputes, the information you provide may indicate a pattern of possible law violations requiring action by the Commission or referral to state authorities.

Part Two

Psoriasis

Chapter 13

A Guide to Understanding Psoriasis: Relieving That Miserable Itch

Introduction

The National Psoriasis Foundation (NPF) of the United States is dedicated to educating people about psoriasis. The NPF published "A Guide to Understanding Psoriasis" to give you a basic awareness of psoriasis and its treatments. That booklet is reproduced here as this chapter. But each person's psoriasis is unique, and it is difficult to address every issue in this chapter. Most likely, you will discover topics that you wish to explore further and new questions will arise. That's why the NPF offers numerous educational booklets to answer your questions. Most of these booklets are highlighted throughout the "Guide" so that you are aware of this supplemental information. The NPF welcomes your inquiries and stands ready to assist you.

What is psoriasis?

The word psoriasis comes from a Greek word meaning to itch. It is a disease that rarely kills but can cause untold misery. The writer John Updike, who suffered from it, called it a curse.

©1995 National Psoriasis Foundation. Reprinted with permission of National Psoriasis Foundation/USA booklet, *Guide to Understanding Psoriasis*, 6600 SW 92nd Avenue, Suite 300, Portland, Oregon 97223. For subscription information, call 1-800-723-9166. Also extracted from *FDA Consumer*, April 1995. "Psoriasis Treatments: Relieving That Miserable Itch."

Thick, reddened, itchy patches of skin covered with flaky, silver scales. A chronic skin condition that tends to improve in warm summer weather and worsen in cold winter weather. Skin cell reproduction gone crazy. These are all descriptions of psoriasis.

The Food and Drug Administration regulates products used to treat psoriasis, which affects between 4 million and 6 million Americans.

About 150,000 new cases of psoriasis are diagnosed every year, 10,000 of them in children and most in people under 40. Men and women are equally affected. The disease is not contagious— you cannot catch psoriasis from anyone.

Most people with psoriasis have a mild to moderate form of the disease. But because of its disfiguring nature, even mild psoriasis can cause severe psychological and emotional distress.

Psoriasis is a chronic skin disorder and no one knows what causes it. We do know, however, that you cannot "catch" psoriasis; psoriasis is not contagious. There are many treatments for psoriasis but, to date, there isn't a cure. Psoriasis affects 1 to 2 percent of the population in the United States.

The most common form of psoriasis is called plaque psoriasis. It is characterized by raised, inflamed (red) lesions covered with a silvery white buildup of dead skin cells, called scale. The technical name for plaque psoriasis is psoriasis vulgaris (vulgaris means common). Though this chapter's focus is on plaque psoriasis, there are other forms of psoriasis. They are pustular, guttate, inverse, and erythrodermic psoriasis. The NPF publishes a booklet "Specific Forms of Psoriasis" that describes these forms of psoriasis.

What does psoriasis look like?

The initial lesions of plaque psoriasis might appear as red, dot-like spots and may be very small. These initial eruptions gradually enlarge and produce a silvery white surface scale. Surface scales come off easily and are shed constantly, but those below the surface of the skin are quite adherent. When forcibly removed, they may leave tiny bleeding points known as the Auspitz's sign. The plaques may cover large areas of skin and merge into each other. Often, the lesions appear in the same place on the right and left sides of the body. Lesions vary in size and in shape from individual to individual.

A Guide to Understanding Psoriasis

How is psoriasis diagnosed?

Typically, psoriasis is diagnosed simply through observation—the inflamed lesion topped with silvery white scale. There are no blood tests for psoriasis; the diagnosis is made by a physician's examination of the skin lesions and occasionally by looking at a skin biopsy under a microscope. Sometimes, small pits in the fingernails can aid in diagnosing psoriasis.

African-Americans may not have the typical red, scaly patches. Their psoriasis may be the same color as the rest of their skin. The treatment is the same, however, for all races.

Who gets psoriasis?

Anyone can develop psoriasis, though heredity seems to play a role. There is a family association in one out of three cases.

Psoriasis appears in men and women in equal number. It can appear at any age, but appears most often between the ages of 15 and 35. In approximately 10-15 percent of individuals with psoriasis, the disease first appears before the age of ten. The disease is also reported in infants.

There are no personality types that have been identified as being more likely to develop psoriasis.

What causes psoriasis?

The cause of psoriasis is unknown. It is thought that some type of biochemical stimulus triggers the abnormal cell growth that characterizes psoriasis.

A normal skin cell matures in 28-30 days. In psoriasis, cells move to the top of the skin in three or four days. The excessive skin cells that are produced "heap up" and form the elevated, red, scaly lesions that characterize psoriasis. The white scale that covers the red lesion is composed of dead cells that are continually being cast off. The redness of the plaques is caused by the increased blood supply necessary to feed this area of dividing skin cells.

Skin injury, emotional stress, and some forms of infection are thought to help trigger its development. For example, psoriasis will sometimes appear at the site of a surgical incision, or may follow a drug reaction, or streptococcal throat infection. When injury to the skin leads to the appearance of psoriasis, it is known as the Koebner phenomenon.

The NPF's booklet "Psoriasis Research" provides detailed information on what is known about the biochemical nature of psoriasis and environmental factors that affect its course.

How serious is psoriasis?

The severity of psoriasis is measured in terms of its physical and its emotional impact. In physical terms, psoriasis is evaluated by the extent of body surface affected and its location on the body. If 10 percent of the body surface is involved, the case is usually considered mild. Ten to 30 percent is considered moderate; and more than 30 percent, severe. The palm of the hand equals 1 percent.

However, psoriasis can involve a small area of the body and have a serious impact on the person's ability to function. Psoriasis confined to the palms of the hands and soles of the feet, for example, can be severe enough to be physically disabling.

For most people, psoriasis remains limited to one or a few patches on the skin. The most common areas for psoriasis to appear are the scalp, elbow, knees, and trunk, though it can appear anywhere on the body.

When the disease affects major body surfaces, various physical problems can occur such as intense itching, skin pain, dry and cracking skin, and swelling. Body movement and flexibility can be affected.

In a few cases, severe types of psoriasis, such as pustular or erythrodermic psoriasis, can elevate body temperature to the point of placing strain on internal organs such as the heart and kidneys. In these instances, hospitalization is required to avoid complications which may threaten the person's life.

The emotional impact of psoriasis is as important to understand as the physical impact. Psoriasis can be unsightly and cause, or contribute to, low self-confidence and self-esteem. It may induce feelings of embarrassment, anger, depression, and guilt. Learning about psoriasis is the first step in coping effectively with this skin disorder. The NPF booklet that thoroughly discusses the emotional impact of psoriasis is "Psoriasis: How It Makes You Feel."

What is the normal course of psoriasis?

Normally, psoriasis goes through cycles of improvement and flares. Psoriasis can go into spontaneous remissions for reasons that are not

A Guide to Understanding Psoriasis

understood. One study showed that two out of five patients indicated they had experienced remissions from the disease, lasting from 1 to 64 years.

One other consideration is psoriatic arthritis. About 10 percent of people with psoriasis develop this form of arthritis, which is similar to rheumatoid arthritis but generally milder. It causes inflammation and stiffness and frequently involves the fingers and toes. Psoriatic arthritis is treated by a dermatologist, but sometimes the patient will be referred to a physician who specializes in treating arthritic disorders.

The NPF's booklet "Psoriatic Arthritis" specifically describes the symptoms and treatment for this condition.

Treatments for Psoriasis

also will cause the skin to itch.

There is not a cure for psoriasis at this time, but there are treatments that can, in most cases, temporarily clear the plaques or significantly improve the skin's appearance. The goal of psoriasis treatment is to clear psoriasis lesions from the skin. Once the treatment works, it is generally discontinued and resumed if the psoriasis returns.

The treatment used will depend upon several things: the type of psoriasis, location on the body, severity, the patient's age, and medical history.

Topical medications are used for mild to moderate psoriasis. These include emollients (moisturizers), steroids (cortisone-type medications), anthralin, various coal tar preparations, and vitamin D_3. These may be used alone, in combination, or with ultraviolet light (UVB). Regular sunbathing can clear psoriasis for some people because of the exposure to natural ultraviolet light.

Treatments for moderate to severe psoriasis include the topical medications already mentioned for mild to moderate psoriasis, ultraviolet light type B (UVB); PUVA (an oral or topical medication [psoralen] plus ultraviolet light type A); an oral or injected medication called methotrexate (MTX); and oral retinoid medications (Tegison and Accutane). These treatments may be used alone or in combination with each other. Systemic treatments for severe psoriasis are more toxic than topical treatments and their benefits must be weighed against their risks.

A rule of thumb in psoriasis therapy is to use the most effective therapy for an individual that poses the least amount of side effects.

Generally, physicians will start with the least potent therapy and work up until one is found that will clear the psoriasis for the patient.

There is no single treatment that works for everyone who has psoriasis. Reactions to psoriasis treatments will vary from individual to individual. Often experimentation is required before an effective approach is discovered for the patient.

A treatment regimen may need periodic adjustment. A once-effective treatment can cease working which will necessitate switching to another therapy.

It is important to remember not to give up on treatment because of slow results. A commitment to lengthy treatment may be necessary to achieve clearance.

Emollients

The use of a lubricant on a regular schedule will help to restore moisture and flexibility to psoriatic skin. It can also help to reduce scaling, itching, and inflammation. There are a wide variety of emollients on the market. Generally, people select those that do not contain heavy perfumes, but are very mild.

Topical Steroids

Topical steroids are the most commonly prescribed therapy for treating localized areas of psoriasis. They come in various strengths, from very mild to very potent. The higher the strength the more effective the medication may be, but the possibility of side effects increases as well.

Steroids used to treat psoriasis are prescription medications. There are very low-strength hydrocortisone preparations that can be purchased over-the-counter (OTC) but they are not generally helpful in treating psoriasis.

Steroids are not usually effective in producing remission of severe psoriasis and can result in a "rebound" (the psoriasis comes back as bad or worse than before the treatment) of the disorder if used in large amounts.

Systemic (Internal) Steroids

Systemically administered steroids (internal administration of steroid medication by pill or muscular injection) are generally avoided in the treatment of psoriasis because of potentially serious side effects. Systemic steroids can also cause psoriasis to worsen, and, at times, precipitate life-threatening pustular forms of psoriasis.

Injected Intralesional Steroids

Injections of steroid medication directly into an isolated lesion (plaque) of psoriasis (called Intralesional steroid injections) can be effective in clearing psoriasis lesions and seldom produce side effects. Also, a physician may give small doses of an oral steroid (such as prednisone) for a brief time to control a sudden flare.

Steroid medications are thoroughly discussed in the NPF's booklet of the same name.

Occlusion

Covering psoriasis lesions with a tape dressing, plastic wrap, or a special suit is called occlusion. Occlusion is sometimes used in conjunction with topical steroid medications. Sometimes lesions are covered with just a special tape dressing. Occasionally, if there is extensive psoriasis on the body and limbs, a special suit may be worn to enhance the effects of psoriasis medications or moisturizers.

Coal Tar

Crude coal tar or coal tar solutions are commonly used in the treatment of psoriasis. They may be prescription or over-the-counter medications.

Tar for the body can be applied directly to the affected area or it may be added to bath water to soak the whole body. It can also be used in combination with a topical steroid medication.

The tar preparation may be used in combination with ultraviolet light, type B (UVB). When coal tar is used in conjunction with UVB, the tar is left on the involved skin for a period of time, ranging from a couple of hours to overnight, prior to exposing the skin to the UVB light. The tar is removed from the skin prior to exposing the skin to the UVB light.

The NPF's booklet "Tar" details the use of coal tar for treating psoriasis on the body and scalp. Its use is also discussed in the booklet "Scalp Psoriasis."

Anthralin

Anthralin is a topical prescription compound that can be effective in clearing psoriasis. It is used in different concentrations. The higher strength compounds cause staining of the skin and irritation, effects which make it difficult to use in the home. But lower-strength anthralin compounds have been developed which have made this therapy more tolerable. These new anthralin preparations can be used on both the body and scalp.

Anthralin is applied topically to the affected area and can be left on for a short period of time or overnight depending on the doctor's orders. Anthralin preparations are also used in combination with UVB. The NPF publishes a booklet on the use of anthralin that specifically details its use.

Vitamin D

Vitamin D_3, or calcipotriene, is the newest topical medication available for mild-moderate psoriasis. It was approved for use in the United States in 1994. It is a prescription medication that has few side effects if used as directed. It is odorless and nonstaining. Generally, it is applied to the lesions twice a day. This medication should not be used on the face or genitals because it can be irritating. It is not recommended for children or for use during pregnancy.

Vitamin D_3 is not the same as that found in commercial vitamin supplements taken orally. These commercial vitamin supplements should not be used to treat psoriasis, as ingesting large doses of over-the-counter vitamin D can lead to serious side effects.

Currently, the only available brand name of this medication is Dovonex. For more information, refer to the NPF booklet "Topical Vitamin D_3."

Other Topical Preparations

Salicylic acid is used to help remove scales and is often combined with steroids, anthralin, and tar to enhance their effectiveness. Salicylic acid is a prescription compound in higher strengths.

Oatmeal baths can be helpful in making the skin more comfortable and reducing the itching that might accompany psoriasis.

Ultraviolet Light, Type B (UVB)

UVB is a common choice for treating psoriasis. If the psoriasis is fairly extensive, physicians will generally initiate UVB treatments because it is considered to be effective and pose limited side effects. UVB has been used to treat psoriasis for many years. UVB occurs naturally in sunlight, and it is that spectrum of the sunlight which causes sunburns. Artificial UVB is used to treat many skin disorders, including psoriasis.

UVB therapy can produce a temporary clearance in most psoriasis patients. The length of remission varies among individuals. Recent studies indicate that the remission is prolonged by maintenance UVB treatments.

The UVB can be administered to a particular area of the body or the entire body surface. The UVB can be given in a physician's office or home light units can be purchased.

UVB can be used alone, with emollients like petrolatum, or with over-the-counter or prescription tar preparations. Combined UVB and tar therapy is known as the Goeckerman regimen or modified Goeckerman regimen.

The NPF publishes booklets specifically on the use of "UVB" and "Home UVB." The Goeckerman regimen is fully described in the NPF's booklet on "Tar."

PUVA (Psoralen and Ultraviolet Light, Type A)

PUVA involves the combined use of a photosensitizing medication called psoralen and a long-wave ultraviolet light, UVA. The patient takes an oral dose of the psoralen medication (available only by prescription), which makes the skin sensitive to UVA light, and a short time later, exposes their skin to UVA light. There are also ways to use the psoralen medication topically, though the topical use isn't as common as the oral use.

PUVA is effective in 85-90 percent of patients and the length of remission varies from a few weeks to a year or more. In an NPF survey of PUVA patients, 68 percent said PUVA was the first therapy to clear their psoriasis. Once a person is clear, periodic treatment may be given to maintain a clearance, or treatments may resume only when the psoriasis returns.

The NPF's booklet on PUVA provides a detailed report about the ways in which PUVA is administered.

Methotrexate (MTX)

Methotrexate is a prescription, systemic drug used in small doses to clear severe and/or disabling psoriasis. Methotrexate is taken orally or given by injection.

Methotrexate is generally recommended only if other psoriasis therapies have not been effective or if other therapies are not tolerated by the patient for some reason. It is a potent drug that can cause serious side effects.

The NPF provides more detailed information about methotrexate in a booklet entitled "Methotrexate (MTX)."

Retinoid Therapy (Tegison and Accutane)

Tegison (generic name etretinate) is a prescription medication for treating severe, recalcitrant (stubbornly resistant) psoriasis. It is indicated when patients with severe psoriasis are unresponsive to standard therapies or, for some reason, cannot use other therapies. It is generally used in combination with other psoriasis treatments such as PUVA.

Because Tegison can cause birth defects, women of childbearing potential must use effective contraception throughout treatment and for an indefinite period of time after stopping Tegison. In fact, **it is highly recommended that women DO NOT take this drug until their childbearing is absolutely completed.**

Another form of this medication called acetretin (Soriatane) is awaiting approval by the FDA. Acetretin may pose fewer risks to women of childbearing age.

Accutane is another oral prescription medication sometimes used to control psoriasis. It, too, has the potential to cause birth defects, though childbearing is acceptable once the drug is discontinued and the woman has complied with a specific waiting period.

These childbearing side effects do not apply to males and conception. The NPF booklet "Retinoid Therapy: Tegison & Accutane" outlines the side effects of retinoids for both men and women. The NPF booklet "Conception, Pregnancy & Psoriasis" sheds further light on treatments to avoid when childbearing is an issue.

A Guide to Understanding Psoriasis

Other Treatments

New treatment developments are always featured in the NPF's national newsletter the *BULLETIN*. If a treatment is prescribed for you that is not mentioned in this chapter, you may always contact the NPF about that specific treatment. The NPF has information on other less commonly used therapies, nontraditional treatments, and experimental medications as well.

Commonly-asked Questions

Can psoriasis itch?

Yes, psoriasis often causes the skin to itch, sometimes intensely. It has been estimated that about 50 percent of those with psoriasis experience itching.

Various oral antihistamines and baths are often recommended to reduce the itching. The only guaranteed way to eliminate itching is to eliminate its cause—the psoriasis itself.

Can diet affect psoriasis?

To date, no specific dietary or herbal regimen has been identified through scientific investigation that will clear or improve psoriasis. More specific information can be obtained by requesting NPF's booklet "Your Diet & Psoriasis."

Does pregnancy and nursing have an effect on psoriasis?

Psoriasis sometimes goes into remission during pregnancy; other women experience a flare during pregnancy.

Women should talk to their doctor about the safety of anti-psoriasis therapies while nursing. There has been concern reported in medical journals that steroids can be excreted in milk and can adversely affect your baby. Therefore, the use of topical steroids when nursing must be carefully supervised.

The NPF's booklet "Conception, Pregnancy & Psoriasis" provides complete information about this aspect of psoriasis.

Does weather affect psoriasis?

The lesions can be affected by the seasons. Most people who have psoriasis get worse during the winter months and improve in the summer. It is presumed this is a result of the availability of natural sunlight.

What can cause psoriasis to worsen?

Psoriasis will often appear following physical and/or emotional trauma. Drug reactions and infections can lead to an appearance or worsening of psoriasis. Drugs that have been identified as having the potential to worsen psoriasis in some cases are: antimalarial drugs; Inderal and other beta blocker medications to control high blood pressure; lithium; Quinidine (a heart medication), and prolonged use of topical and systemic steroids. More information on these drugs is provided in the NPF's booklet "Practical Information About Psoriasis."

If someone plans to spend long hours in the sun, it is recommended that a sunscreen be used on the unaffected areas of skin. Also, avoid burning as that can cause psoriasis to worsen.

Does emotional stress cause psoriasis?

There is no evidence that stress is a direct cause of psoriasis, but studies have shown that psoriasis can be aggravated by emotional stress in some individuals.

Can suntan parlors be used to treat psoriasis?

Consult a dermatologist before using the lights in a suntan parlor. There are various medications that make people sensitive to ultraviolet light and which can produce burns. Some diseases, such as lupus erythematosus, are worsened by ultraviolet light and people with those diseases should not be exposed to UVB light. UVA light used alone is not very effective against psoriasis. Ask the parlor operators what light spectrums you will be receiving. You want the most UVB available. Some states have laws banning UVB from suntan parlors.

Is someone who has psoriasis protected from job discrimination?

Depending on the type of employment and the particular state in which someone lives, there are generally state and federal laws that protect an employee from being terminated for reasons not related to job performance or job qualifications.

Can psoriasis be disabling?

Psoriasis can result in job disability. The Social Security Administration (SSA) will grant job disability because of psoriasis under certain circumstances. These circumstances, as defined by the SSA, are when the skin is:

> *"with extensive lesions, including involvement of the hands and feet, which impose a severe limitation of function and which are not responding to prescribed treatment."*

The NPF provides informal guidelines on things to consider in applying for disability.

Can someone with psoriasis serve in the military?

Psoriasis normally disqualifies an individual from military service.

Can alcohol consumption worsen psoriasis?

There does not seem to be any pattern. Studies have not discovered a link between alcohol consumption and flares of psoriasis. Individuals have observed a worsening of psoriasis with alcohol consumption; others note it does not seem to make a difference.

Can psoriasis be associated with any other disease?

To date, no other disease, with the exception of psoriatic arthritis, has been associated with psoriasis. Psoriasis, however, can appear simultaneously with any other disease.

Should scales be removed before applying topical medications?

Yes. It is important to remove the scales from psoriasis since they block the penetration of medications and ultraviolet light. The scales should be removed carefully either by hydration (use of water) or by medication that softens the skin. Hydration can be done simply by soaking in a tub of water. Softening medications include creams containing one or more of the following common ingredients: propylene glycol, glycerin, salicylic acid, lactic acid and urea.

Tips to Help Your Skin

- **Keep your skin lubricated.** Oils, creams, and petroleum jelly preparations are good moisturizers or emollients. During the winter months, low temperatures and humidity draw moisture from the skin, and can result in discomfort and itching.

- **Use a humidifier in the home.** When the air is dry from home heating, a humidifier may be helpful.

- **Take advantage of the sunshine when possible.** Sunlight will clear psoriasis for some people if obtained in sufficient doses on a regular basis. The use of oils and lubricants may enhance the effects of the natural ultraviolet light. For more information about treating psoriasis with sunlight, request the NPF's educational booklet "Sunshine & Psoriasis."

- **Bathing in hot water may help reduce scaling.** Some people report a flattening of their plaques or reduced scaling from soaking in hot water.

- **Minimize contact with soap and chemicals.** Use mild soaps or soap-free cleansers. Consult your physician or pharmacist for guidance.

- **Minimize stress.** Though NPF is not aware of any study on the benefits of exercise, some people observe that their psoriasis improves when they exercise regularly. The relaxing effects of exercise may lend to the skin's improvement. Consult a professional to develop an appropriate exercise program for you.

- **Protect against skin injuries.** This includes skin irritations like soap under a ring, tight waistbands or shaving with a dull razor. Harsh chemicals and cosmetics, such as depilatories (preparations used to remove hair from the body), can increase redness and scaling.

- **Protect yourself from infections.** Children, especially, should try to avoid exposure to throat infections which may make psoriasis worse.

- **Check in with the NPF or your physician occasionally** if you are not actively treating your psoriasis. Many people with psoriasis drop out of treatment and just learn to live with it. By staying informed, you know about new treatment options, are more likely to find something you've never tried, and/or discover a treatment that didn't work once, will work now. It is worthwhile to keep an open mind.

- **Call or write the NPF.** The NPF is a valuable resource for people who have psoriasis and their families. If you need information, a physician recommendation, or just want to compare notes with someone else who has psoriasis, don't hesitate to write or call. NPF is here for you.

Birth Defects with Two Drugs

Methotrexate and Tegison (etretinate), both of which are approved by FDA to treat severe psoriasis, can cause severe birth defects in children born to women who are or who become pregnant while taking either drug.

Warnings in the labeling of both drugs state that they should not be prescribed to women who are pregnant or who are likely to become pregnant. Couples are advised to avoid pregnancy for at least three months after the man takes methotrexate and for at least one menstrual cycle after the woman takes it.

The period during which a woman should avoid pregnancy after treatment with Tegison is not known. It is known that, in some women etretinate may still be detected in blood three years after they stopped taking the drug.

Birth defects associated with Tegison include high palate, fused bones, webbed hands and feet, and malformed skull, spinal cord, face, fingers, and toes. Tegison is a retinoid, chemically similar to vitamin A.

Both drugs also should not be used by nursing women. Despite the risks, doctors can prescribe these drugs to women of childbearing age in cases where other treatments have been unsuccessful and both the doctor and patient consider that the medical benefits of treatment outweigh the risks.

Susan Harris, 38, of Alpharetta, Ca., has had severe psoriasis since she was 3 years old. When she was hospitalized for a severe outbreak of the disease at 17, she says her dermatologist sat her down and said, "I know you're barely 18 and will probably want to have children some day, but the only thing I can think of to put you on is methotrexate."

Harris, aware that she could not become pregnant while taking the drug, agreed to try it anyway. It cleared her psoriasis almost immediately, and she has continued taking methotrexate for most of the past 20 years. Although she has tried other therapies for her psoriasis, including PUVA, Tegison, and Sandimmune (cyclosporine), methotrexate is the only treatment that has brought her sustained relief and enabled her to lead a normal life.

"If there's one thing that breaks my heart, it's not being able to have children," says Harris. "But in a way it might be a good thing because I'm not passing [psoriasis] on to my kids."

National Psoriasis Foundation

Past recipient of the American Academy of Dermatology's Excellence in Education Award.

6600 S.W. 92nd Avenue, Suite 300
Portland, OR 97223-7195
USA
(503) 244-7404
FAX (503) 245-0626

NATIONAL PSORIASIS FOUNDATION® *A Guide to Understanding Psoriasis* is published as an educational service and is not intended to replace the counsel of a physician. NPF and Omnigraphics advise that you consult a physician before initiating any treatment. The NPF and Omnigraphics do not endorse any medications, products, or treatments for psoriasis.

The NPF is a 501(c)(3) nonprofit, lay organization working to improve the quality of life of people with psoriasis. Tax-deductible donations support the NPF's public education and research programs. The NPF's annual report is available by writing or calling NPF.

Chapter 14

The Immune Factor: When Friends Become Foes

Like a trusted friend who unexpectedly betrays you, your protective immune system may suddenly become your worst enemy. When that happens, rogue killer cells may attack organs or tissues that are essential to your survival, as if they were dangerous intruders that had to be destroyed. In recent years scientists have identified this scenario, known as an autoimmune attack, as the cause of many diseases whose origins previously were unknown. Psoriasis is among the latest to be included in this category.

Psoriasis is a skin disease that in severe cases disfigures patients' bodies and makes their lives miserable.

Affected areas of the skin—often spreading out from elbows and knees—are red and inflamed and may be covered by silvery scales. It has long been known that many psoriasis patients belong to families that have a history of the disease. And in these psoriasis-prone families, certain genetic markers—known as HLA antigens—are inherited more often than in the general population. But until a group of Rockefeller University scientists published their recent study—carried out in the Rockefeller General Clinical Research Center—it was not known whether psoriasis was primarily an immune disease or an epidermal skin disease. "Prior to this work, data existed that suggested an immune system involvement" explains principal investigator Dr. James G. Krueger. "What wasn't clear was whether the immune contribution was a secondary phenomenon, a sort of amplification loop." To distinguish the roles of the scaling, nonimmune epidermal

NCRR Reporter September/October, 1995.

skin cells—called keratinocytes—and the immune cells, the scientists used an experimental drug that eliminated specific immune cells. They reasoned that if the absence of these cells improved the patients' psoriasis, immune cells—not epidermal skin cells—were probably the main culprit in causing the disease.

In earlier studies of psoriatic skin, Dr. Alice B. Gottlieb—a co-investigator in this study—detected immune cells, known as T cells, that had surface receptors for interleukin-2 (IL-2), a cellular hormone that is an important mediator of immune reactions. Since only T cells that are activated to participate in immune reactions carry the IL-2 receptor, selective removal of these cells did not endanger all T cells in the body. "Presumably in psoriasis there is an as-yet-undefined antigen that the T cells react to in an autoimmune fashion. Those reactive cells proliferate and express the IL-2 receptor," Dr. Krueger says.

To target and kill the activated T cells, the scientists used a molecule manufactured by fusing IL-2 and diphtheria toxin. Like a Trojan horse, the innocuous IL-2 part of the fusion molecule binds to T cells that have IL-2 receptors and thereby delivers its poisonous partner to the target. After binding, the fusion molecule enters the cells and the diphtheria toxin blocks their protein-synthesizing machinery killing the cells.

This compound is an example of a drug that has been engineered to do a specific job," Dr. Krueger explains. "In many ways this is a triumph for a rational approach to discovering drugs. Instead of finding the drug by chance we've designed it based on an understanding of how cells and tissues are put together and work."

The scientists tested the experimental drug in 10 patients who had had severe psoriasis for approximately 10 years. The patients were admitted to the General Clinical Research Center at Rockefeller University and remained there under close observation for one week while they received the drug in five daily intravenous doses. Subsequently they were assessed as outpatients for 23 days. Then they received an additional round of five intravenous doses of the drug followed by another 23-day assessment period.

Four of the ten patients showed "striking clinical improvement," four had moderate improvement and two had minimal improvement after two cycles of treatment with the drug. Among the improvements were most significantly thinning of the psoriatic areas, reduced keratinocyte proliferation, and reduced inflammation with fewer T cells in the epidermis. Although the researchers saw flu-like symptoms in the patients they noted no serious toxicity. Nevertheless Dr.

The Immune Factor: When Friends Become Foes

Krueger cautions that "there is a long way to go before saying that this is a drug that is safe and widely effective. These early studies suggest that the molecule is likely to be effective. And at least these low doses are reasonably well tolerated."

This small preliminary study shows that at least some cases of psoriasis are caused by a defective immune system. "There aren't any data in our study that refute the hypothesis that the disease is immune mediated," notes Dr. Krueger. He points out however that the response was mixed since not all patients responded to the drug. "I think that has to do with the fact that we're in the early stages of development with this agent. Perhaps the doses weren't sufficient."

Dr. Krueger and his colleagues are now continuing their studies with higher doses of the IL-2/diphtheria toxin drug to see if a higher proportion of the patients may respond. Because psoriasis is a uniquely human disease it cannot be studied in animal models—an approach that allows experimental studies of many other diseases. "The General Clinical Research Center is very critical for this study because it facilitates our understanding of a chronic human disease. There is simply no other way of approaching this problem," Dr. Krueger concludes.

—by Ole Henriksen, Ph.D., and Victoria L. Contie

This study was supported by the General Clinical Research Centers program of the National Center for Research Resources, the National Cancer Institute, and the National Institute of Arthritis and Musculoskeletal and Skin Diseases.

Additional Reading

Gottlieb, S. L., Gilleaudeau, P., Johnson, R., et al., Response of psoriasis to a lymphocyte-selective toxin ($DAB_{389}IL-2$) suggest a primary immune, but not keratinocyte, pathogenic basis. *Nature Medicine* 1:442-447, 1995.

Chapter 15

Nail Psoriasis: Questions and Answers

Editors' Note: *With thanks to Dr. R. Rops, Yamanouchy/Europe, Dr. E. de Jong and Prof. P.C.M. van de Kerkhof, Academic Hospital Nijmegen, the Netherlands. This article was excerpted by permission of EURO-PSO and Dr. R. Rops, from their publication Psoriasis in Europe, newsletter number 10.*

Although psoriasis is primarily a disease of the skin, it can also cause unpleasant changes in fingernails and toenails, described as nail psoriasis. A group of Dutch dermatologists from the University Hospital Nijmegen recently decided to find out more about nail psoriasis. They wanted to get a better idea of how many psoriasis patients suffer from nail problems, and to investigate the impact that nail psoriasis has on the daily lives of the patients. Interviews were held with over 1,000 psoriasis patients to find the answers to important questions, such as:

- who suffers from nail psoriasis?
- what are the major nail problems experienced?
- how should these nail problems be treated?

The investigators who undertook the survey were particularly concerned to find out how severely patients are disturbed by their nail disease.

©1995 National Psoriasis Foundation, 6600 SW 92nd Avenue, Suite 300, Portland, Oregon 97223. For subscription information, call 1-800-723-9166. Reprinted with Permission.

Who suffers from nail psoriasis?

Nail changes in psoriasis probably occur more frequently than has previously been thought, with almost 80 percent of the patients in this survey suffering from nail problems. In fact, almost every patient with psoriasis probably has some degree of nail involvement, although the symptoms may be very brief or very mild in some people. Fingernails are more frequently affected than toenails, although many patients suffer in both areas.

People who have had psoriasis for a long time are more likely to suffer from nail psoriasis than those with relatively recent symptoms, although some patients with short-lived symptoms may also suffer from nail problems. In addition, people with widespread psoriasis are more likely to get nail symptoms than those whose psoriasis only affects a small region of the body. Those patients with psoriatic arthritis or psoriasis of the scalp are also more likely to get nail psoriasis than patients without these complications.

As with the skin, flare-ups and remissions occur with nail psoriasis.

What are the major nail problems experienced?

The following terms are used to describe the nail problems most commonly experienced by psoriasis patients:

- **pitting:** shallow or deep holes in the nail.
- **deformation:** alterations in the normal shape of the nail.
- **upward lifting:** upward movement and loosening of the nail.
- **onycholysis:** separation of the nail from the nail bed.
- **discoloration:** unusual nail coloration, such as yellow-brown.

The frequency of these symptoms in the patients surveyed follows the order in which they are listed, with pitting being the most frequent problem, experienced by three-quarters of the patients. Deformation was a problem for two-thirds of the patients, while upward lifting and onycholysis were experienced by about half the patients. Discoloration was noted in one-third of the patients. A combination of the various symptoms was present in some patients, and almost one-fifth of the patients suffered from all of the five problems listed above.

Nail Psoriasis: Questions and Answers

How should nail psoriasis be treated?

There are a range of possible treatments for nail psoriasis, and treatments can be divided into categories of topical treatment (applied in a cream or lotion), systemic treatment (given by injection or by mouth) or photochemotherapy (a drug applied as cream or taken by mouth increases sensitivity to light).

- **topical treatment:** e.g. calcipotriene, corticosteroids, dithranol, tar (lotion or cream)

- **systemic treatment:** e.g. methotrexate, retinoids, fumaric acid (not available in the U.S.—NPF), cyclosporine (injection or by mouth)

- **photochemotherapy:** e.g. PUVA (applied by cream or taken by mouth)

One-third of the patients in the survey had received treatment for their nail psoriasis. However, none of these treatments is totally successful, and even after treatment, many patients do not see much improvement in their symptoms. In fact, only one-fifth of the patients in the survey judged that their therapy had led to a "marked improvement" in their nail symptoms. If improvement does occur, it may only happen very slowly, with many therapies having to be continued for 3-6 months. Also, a number of side effects are associated with existing therapies. For instance, corticosteroids can affect normal regrowth of the nail, while retinoids can cause the nails to become fragile and develop ridges. Predictably, a large number of patients who responded to the survey (over three quarters) expressed a wish to receive better treatment for their nail problems.

Editor's Note: *As demonstrated by the authors of this article, nail psoriasis is a serious problem that aggravates thousands of people. Its course is usually prolonged and unpredictable. An ideal treatment is not currently available, and systemic therapies are rarely indicated for nail psoriasis. The development of improved therapy would be welcomed by many sufferers of nail psoriasis. Meanwhile, taking good care of the nails can help maximize a good appearance.*

Chapter 16

Research into Psoriasis

Immunosuppressive Drug Alleviates Psoriasis

The first large, controlled, single-center trial of cyclosporine as a treatment for plaque-type psoriasis has established a daily dose of the drug that is safe and effective in the short term for even the severest cases of the disease. However, the safety of cyclosporine for long-term treatment of psoriasis remains to be determined, according to investigators at the University of Michigan Medical Center in Ann Arbor, where the study took place.

Psoriasis is a common skin disorder, affecting up to 2 percent of the United States population, says principal investigator Dr. Charles N. Ellis, professor and associate chairman of the department of dermatology at the University of Michigan Medical School. Most often the condition appears as inflamed, scaly plaques on the surface of the body: the result of a buildup of rapidly dividing cells in the skin's outer layer. In rarer instances psoriasis takes the form of pustules or turns the entire body surface red. Although the exact abnormality underlying psoriasis is unknown, it is thought to involve loss of control over the skin's normal immunological responses to environmental stimuli. Minor injury to the skin, infection, stress, and a variety of drugs can trigger psoriasis in susceptible individuals.

In plaque-type psoriasis the area of affected skin is usually limited to a few patches on the elbows, knees, and scalp. All but two of the patients in the Michigan study, however, had plaques covering

1991 Research Resources Reporter.

between 25 and 80 percent of their body surface. "We were selecting for the most severe cases that exist," says Dr. Ellis. "And despite the fact that these patients' psoriasis was so severe, cyclosporine was clearly effective."

Dr. Ellis and his colleagues conducted a 16-week trial of three different daily doses of cyclosporine and a placebo. Eighty-five outpatients were assigned at random to one of the four treatment groups in a double-blind design, which means that neither the patients nor the investigators knew which patient was receiving which treatment. During the second half of the trial the patients either stayed at their assigned doses or received adjusted doses (determined by an unblinded physician) to increase the drug's efficacy or to reduce side effects.

All of the patients on the placebo were switched to the lowest cyclosporine dose during the second half of the trial. By the end of 16 weeks patients in all three dosage groups had responded well to the cyclosporine, but the patients in the two higher dosage groups showed significantly greater clearing of psoriasis plaques than those in the lowest dosage group. Of the two higher doses, the lower one proved to be optimally safe and effective.

"The difference in improvement between the two higher doses is trivial, but the difference in side effects was noticeable," explains Dr. Ellis. During the first half of the trial four of the patients assigned to the highest dose had it reduced because of side effects and decreases in kidney function. "My initial bias is toward keeping the dose as low as possible," he says. "My general policy would be to start with a cyclosporine dose of 5 mg per kg of body weight, and as the disease starts to clear to taper the dose down to the lowest possible level required to maintain the desired response."

The cyclosporines are the major, biologically active metabolites of the soil fungus *Tolypocladium inflatum*, which was plucked from obscurity by a Swiss microbiologist vacationing in the Norwegian tundra more than 20 years ago. A failure as an antibiotic, cyclosporine redeemed itself in the mid-1970s when it proved to have immunosuppressive properties that were particularly suited to prevent rejection of organ transplants. "Cyclosporine has a narrow spectrum of inhibition," notes Dr. Ellis. "It is basically turning off chemical messages called cytokines that activate a subset of white blood cells, the T-helper lymphocytes, which participate in the cellular immune response." No one understands precisely how cyclosporine works in psoriasis, but the drug's success "has stimulated a lot of research into the immunological aspects of skin disorders," according to Dr. Ellis. (For more information about the role of cytokines in psoriasis see below.)

In the 4-month Michigan study patients showed no clinical signs of general immunosuppression such as development of tumors or infections. All side effects disappeared and kidney function returned to normal when the dose of cyclosporine was reduced or the drug was discontinued. However, says Dr. Ellis, psoriasis is chronic, and long remissions in severely affected patients are unusual. Therefore, longer-term therapy would be necessary in nearly all cases. A decade of experience with cyclosporine in transplant patients, who often take the drug for years, has shown an increased risk of cancer and infection, as well as irreversible kidney damage, note Dr. Ellis and co-investigator Dr. Joseph M. Messana, assistant professor of internal medicine at the University of Michigan. Nevertheless, Dr. Ellis says, for patients whose psoriasis is severe enough to keep them in the hospital half the year and who do not respond to more conventional treatments such as ultraviolet light, cyclosporine is a "godsend." "These patients are willing to accept the risk," he says.

The key to reducing the risk of adverse effects appears to be a low cyclosporine dose. According to Dr. Messana, nearly all published reports on cyclosporine treatment in both organ transplants and immunologic diseases have linked irreversible kidney damage to initial doses at least twice as high as the daily dose of 5 mg per kg of body weight recommended by the Michigan investigators. "If cyclosporine could be used at a low dose throughout treatment, without the initial high doses, perhaps some of the kidney toxicity could be avoided," he says.

In addition to studying the use of oral cyclosporine, the Michigan researchers have tried topical application of the drug. However, their results, like those of other researchers who have explored this route, were "disappointing," Dr. Ellis reports. Direct injection of cyclosporine into psoriatic plaques produced much better results, but the procedure is painful and treats only a small area at a time. "Injection might be considered for patients with one or two tough spots," Dr. Ellis suggests. Longer-term studies of the safety of systemic cyclosporine administration are also under way.

Additional Reading:

Ellis, C. N., Fradin, M. S., Messana, J. M., et al., Cyclosporine for plaque-type psoriasis. New England Journal of Medicine 324:277-284,1991.

Borel, J. F., Mechanism of action and rationale for cyclosporin A in psoriasis. British Journal of Dermatology 122: Supplement 36:5-12,1990.

Fradin, M. S., Ellis, C. N., and Voorhees, J. J., Efficacy of cyclosporin A in psoriasis: A summary of the United States' experience. British Journal of Dermatology 122: Supplement 36:21-25,1990.

Austin, H. A., Palestine, A. G., Sabnis, S. G., et al., Evolution of ciclosporin nephrotoxicity in patients treated for autoimmune uveitis. American Journal of Nephrology 9:392-402,1989

Drs. Ellis and Messana acknowledge the research contributions of Drs. Mark Fradin and John Voorhees. The research described in this article was supported by the General Clinical Research Centers Program of the National Center for Research Resources; the Babcock Dermatologic Endowment, Ann Arbor; and Sandoz Research Institute.

—by Nancy Heneson

Interleukin-6 Linked to Psoriasis

Research Resources Reporter, May 1990.

Psoriatic skin plaques from patients with psoriasis contain high levels of the cell growth factor Interleukin-6 (IL-6) and its corresponding messenger (m) RNA, according to investigators at the Rockefeller University in New York City. IL-6 stimulates rapid growth of outer-layer skin cells called keratinocytes from normal individuals, the researchers report.

"This is the first evidence that IL-6 levels are increased in active psoriatic skin plaques and the first indication that IL-6 stimulates keratinocytes to divide," says associate professor Dr. Alice B. Gottlieb. The findings could have potential therapeutic importance, Dr. Gottlieb says, since inhibiting agents can often be designed once the role and structure of a cytokine such as IL-6 are known.

Psoriasis is a chronic skin disorder that affects about four million Americans, according to the New York investigators. It is characterized by reddish papules and plaques. The disease is usually first treated with locally applied corticosteroid preparations or crude coal tar along with exposure to ultraviolet light. In severe, disabling stages, antimetabolic drugs, which also are used in cancer treatment, may be prescribed. There is no known cure for psoriasis.

IL-6 is normally secreted by fibroblasts, endothelial cells, and macrophages as well as by keratinocytes; it is an active component of the body's response to tissue injury and infection, according to the researchers. Keratinocytes predominate in the skin's epidermis, and in psoriasis patients these cells grow faster. The cell growth cycle of the keratinocytes is decreased from 28 days to 3 or 4 days, according to other investigators.

Dr. Gottlieb's associate, Dr. Rachel M. Grossman, notes that in psoriatic skin most of the keratinocytes are either in the process of dividing or preparing to divide, instead of being in the resting phase of the cell cycle that usually predominates among cell populations.

"When the growth signals, whatever they may be, initiate the psoriatic message," she says, "they push the resting basal keratinocytes into DNA synthesis and the final phase before cell division, and the proliferation keeps on going."

Dr. Grossman sees an underlying, fairly widespread immunological defect (usually not triggered) being expressed when a person develops psoriasis. "I think a large segment of the population is predisposed to psoriasis. But we never get the disease until after some other event—exposure to certain drugs or chemicals or viruses, or when an immuno-compromising event like development of AIDS takes place," she says. "A disease this common doesn't require a single pathway," comments Dr. Gottlieb, who stresses the underlying immunologic problems that are expressed in psoriasis.

"I believe the inflammation we see in psoriasis and the hyperproliferation of the keratinocytes are linked," she says. "Activation of keratinocytes can be the result of an immune response to an unknown antigen. During the course of the immune response the cells respond by secreting cytokines such as interleukins. Subsequently, the activated keratinocytes make additional cytokines that can further activate the inflammatory infiltrate—and you have a positive feedback cycle," Dr. Gottlieb explains.

"That is why psoriasis is chronic and so hard to treat," she adds.

Drs. Grossman and Gottlieb, and their associates at Rockefeller University and Yale University in New Haven, Connecticut, conducted their studies with psoriasis patients who were treated at the General Clinical Research Center at Rockefeller University Hospital. The investigators obtained psoriatic plaques from skin biopsies of 35 patients with psoriasis and normal skin from uninvolved skin of 17 of these patients and 2 healthy individuals. The researchers monitored IL-6 production in skin sections by measuring how much antibody against IL-6 the cells could bind and how much IL-6 mRNA the cells contained. Epidermal and dermal cells from most patients contained considerably more IL-6 and IL-6 mRNA than did cells from normal individuals or from normal skin of patients who had undergone therapy.

Anti-inflammatory treatment suppresses infiltration of mononuclear cells into the skin, according to Dr. Grossman, thus preventing the release of other cytokines such as Interleukin-1 (IL-1), which plays a role in the release of IL-6. She sees this phenomenon as part of the feedback mechanism that shuts down IL-6 release in patients treated by anti-inflammatory drugs. Dr. Grossman says that IL-6 is also present in other inflammatory conditions, such as at the edge of a non-healing ulcer or in an area adjacent to skin cancer.

"IL-6 correlates with disease activity," Dr. Gottlieb says. "We observed that when psoriatic plaque disappears, the IL-6 level goes down. All we can say at this point is that there is an association. We haven't proved that the plaque disappears because the IL-6 concentration is decreased," she says.

The IL-6 gene is expressed in psoriatic skin lesions, Dr. Grossman says. She further suggests that increased IL-6 levels may stimulate the production of cell growth factors and acute phase reactants such as C-reactive protein. And the combined action of these factors may, in turn, increase the IL-6 level. "It's like the-chicken-or-the-egg question. It's hard to say which comes first," she says.

Studying potential effects of therapy on the increased IL-6 levels, the investigators obtained biopsies of psoriatic skin plaques from 10 patients before and after drug therapy. Specimens from 7 of the 10 patients contained less IL-6 after treatment than before, and these changes correlated with resolution of psoriatic plaques.

In addition to studying keratinocytes from the patients, the investigators measured IL-6 concentrations in blood samples from eight of the psoriasis patients. They found that the average IL-6 level was comparable to that seen in patients with acute bacterial infections.

The Rockefeller team, in collaboration with Dr. Angela Granelli-Piperno, also at Rockefeller, is now studying the immunosuppressive drug cyclosporine as potential therapy in psoriasis. "We are measuring the interaction of psoriatic skin with nucleic add probes before and after cyclosporine treatment to see what happens to the mRNA for various cytokines as a result of cyclosporine therapy" Dr. Gottlieb explains.

"There really is no *in vivo* model that shows the mechanism of action of immunosuppression by cyclosporine." Dr. Gottlieb says. "By doing these nucleic acid studies on skin biopsies of patients with psoriasis, we expect to have the first demonstration of the mechanism of immunosuppression by cyclosporine in a human disease," she says.

Additional Reading:

Grossman, R. M., Krueser, J., Yourish, D., Granelli-Piperno, A., Murphy, D P., May, L. T., Kupper, T. S., Sehgal, P. B. and Gottlieb, A. B, Interleukin 6 is expressed in high levels in psoriatic skin and stimulates proliferation of cultured human keratinocytes. Proceedings of the National Academy of Sciences USA 86:6367-6371, 1989.

Koj, A., The role of interleukin-6 as the hepatocyte stimulating factor in the network of inflammatory cytokines. Annals of the New York Academy of Sciences 557:1-8, 1989.

Kupper, T. S., Min, K. Sehgal, P., Mizutani, H. Birchall, N., Ray, A., and May L., Production of IL-6 by keratinocytes: Implications for epidermal inflammation and immunity. Annals of the New York Academy of Sciences 557: 454-465, 1989.

Ray, A., Tatter, S. B., May L. T., and Sehgal, P. B., Activation of the human "beta$_2$-interferon/hepatocyte-stimulating factor/interleukin 6" promoter by cytokines, viruses, and second messenger agonists. Proceedings of the National Academy of Sciences USA 85:6701-6705, 1988.

—by Jane Collins

Part Three

Skin Conditions as Allergic or Immune Responses

Chapter 17

Diagnosis and Management of Atopic Dermatitis

Atopic dermatitis (AD) is a chronic, relapsing form of pruritic eczema commonly found in young children. Although the cause of this skin disorder is unknown, several studies have shown that 75 percent to 80 percent of AD patients have a personal or family history of asthma or allergic rhinitis.[1]

Incidence

Atopic dermatitis is estimated to affect 0.5 percent to 1 percent of the general worldwide population, with a prevalence of 5 percent to 10 percent in children.[2] Onset is usually from two to six months, and 85 percent of cases occur within the first five years.[3]

Management of this illness includes accurate diagnosis, identification and elimination of exacerbating factors, hydration of the skin, infection control and use of anti-inflammatory agents, such as topical corticosteroids or tar preparations.

Clinical Features

There is no single distinguishing feature of atopic dermatitis, but a constellation of clinical features that include severe pruritis, chronically relapsing course, characteristic eczematoid appearance and distribution of the skin lesions.

©1992 National Jewish Center for Immunology and Respiratory Medicine, "Medical/Scientific Update." Reprinted with permission.

There are three types of AD skin reaction: acute, subacute and chronic. Distribution of the rash varies according to the patient's age. Over 50 percent of AD cases in infants resolve by age two and do not recur. Another 25 percent of the cases resolve by adolescence, while the condition persists into adulthood in the remaining group.

Dry, cracking, itchy skin is characteristic of AD and usually leads to rubbing and scratching, which causes many clinical changes. Pruritis is the major symptom of the disease and causes the greatest morbidity. AD patients also tend to develop viral, bacterial and fungal skin infections.

Clinical Features of Atopic Dermatitis

Major Features:

- Pruritis
- Chronic or chronically relapsing dermatitis
- Facial and extensor involvement in infants and children
- Flexural eczema and lichenification in older children and adults
- Personal or family history of atopy

Minor Features:

- Early age of onset (after two months of age)
- Course influenced by environmental or emotional factors
- Xerosis
- Ichthyosis, palmar hyper-linearity, keratosis palmaris
- Dennie-Morgan infraorbital fold
- Facial pallor or erythema
- Nonspecific dermatitis of the hands or feet
- Cutaneous infections
- Anterior subcapsular cataracts

Laboratory Features

Atopic dermatitis has no specific laboratory features that can be used for diagnosis. About 80 percent of AD patients show an increased serum IgE level and positive immediate skin test to a variety of common food and inhalant allergens.[4] Blood eosinophila is a common finding.

Diagnosis and Management of Atopic Dermatitis

Routine skin pathology does not differentiate atopic dermatitis from other inflammatory dermatoses, such as contact dermatitis, but it can rule out psoriasis and other such conditions. Thus, a skin biopsy may be helpful if the dermatitis is recalcitrant to vigorous therapy.

Identifying and Eliminating Exacerbating Factors

Irritants

Triggers of atopic dermatitis in the patient's physical environment need to be identified and eliminated. Irritants differ according to the patient. They generally include chemicals, detergents, soaps, occlusive or wool clothing, heat, cold and sunburn.

If soap is used, it should have minimal defatting activity and a neutral pH. Residual laundry detergent in clothing also may be irritating, which can be remedied by changing detergents or adding a second rinse cycle. All new clothes should be washed before wearing to remove residual fabric resins

Atopic dermatitis patients may need to modify their activities and surroundings to minimize sweating, which can cause itching. Working and sleeping in surroundings of constant temperature (68 to 75 degrees F) and humidity (45 percent to 55 percent) may be more comfortable for some AD patients.

Allergens

Several studies have demonstrated that food allergens and aeroallergens can exacerbate AD in, at least, a subset of patients. The most common food culprits are egg, peanut, milk, soy, wheat and fish.[5]

A careful history and skin tests in consultation with an allergist can identify allergens present in the diet or environment. Environmental allergens, such as dust mites, animal dander and pollen, once identified, need to be avoided. If a food allergy is suspected, the most definitive detection method is the double-blind, placebo-controlled food challenge. Foods that have been demonstrated to flare atopic dermatitis in controlled challenges need to be avoided. However, when any restrictive diet is imposed, care must be taken to avoid malnutrition.

Emotional Stress

The anger, frustration and anxiety that frequently accompany atopic dermatitis can exacerbate this disorder. AD patients often respond with itching and scratching. Patients need to be reassured about the normality of their feelings, what to expect in the course of the disease and the likelihood of effective treatment and coping strategies. Educating themselves about the disease and maintaining a positive outlook are two vital patient steps for the best possible management of atopic dermatitis.

Therapeutic Approaches

Effective management of this chronic disease requires understanding of each patient's disease pattern as well as reduction of exacerbating factors mentioned above.

While there is no magic cure, certain measures can decrease skin eruptions and relieve itching. Daily skin care with appropriate topical preparations is a must. Therapy must be individualized and is dependent on whether the atopic dermatitis is in an acute or chronic stage.

Hydration

Hydration is the key to good therapy, but is often difficult to achieve. The best way is to add water to the skin and immediately apply an occlusive substance to retain the absorbed water. This can be accomplished by soaking the affected area or bathing for 15 to 20 minutes in warm water. Adding oatmeal or baking soda to the water is soothing to some patients, but doesn't increase water absorption. Bath oils are not recommended because they provide a false sense of lubrication and make the bathtub slippery.

After the bath, patients should remove excess water by gently patting with a soft towel. Then they should immediately apply the recommended occlusive substance. If the skin is not occluded within three to five minutes, evaporation will occur. It is imperative that patients and families understand that hydration and occlusive substances will help re-establish the skin's barrier function and are critical in controlling the disease.

Wet wraps and occlusion used immediately after soaking the skin can optimize hydration and topical therapy by promoting medication

Diagnosis and Management of Atopic Dermatitis

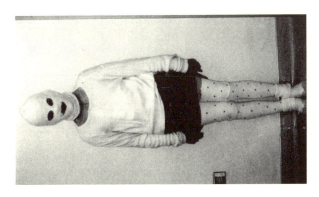

Figure 17.3. Wet dressings designed by this adolescent include the use of orthopedic stockinette on the face, long underwear on the trunk, and tube socks cut a variety of ways for the extremities.

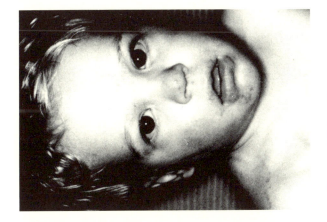

Figure 17.2. Clearing of the dermatitis results after only two weeks of appropriate hydration, topical steroids, wet dressings, and oral antibiotics.

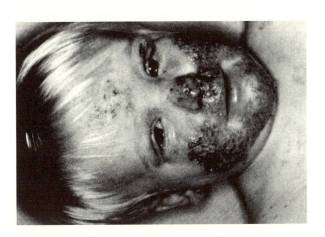

Figure 17.1. Acute dermatitis on the face of this toddler is characterized by the extensive red, oozing, crusting rash.

absorption and cooling the skin. Wraps are recommended for severely affected or persistent areas of dermatitis. Wet wraps and occlusion can be achieved by wet pajamas or long underwear and wet tube socks. A second pair of dry pajamas or sweat-suit and dry socks are worn over the wet ones. Prolonged use of wet wraps requires close supervision to prevent skin infection or maceration.

Topical Therapy

Choice of topical preparations depends on the condition of the patient's skin, the patient's tolerance for and willingness to use a given preparation and the patient's environment (dry vs. humid). Occlusives, moisturizers, corticosteroids and tar preparations can all be used topically to control atopic dermatitis. Avoid sensitizing chemicals or drugs that can cause skin eruptions.

All these preparations will be best absorbed if applied immediately after the skin has been saturated with water. When even more absorption is required, wet wraps and occlusion can be used.

Maintenance Therapy

When the skin is under optimum control, it can be maintained by bathing at least once per day and using occlusives or moisturizers. Occlusives such as petroleum jelly or Crisco are very effective in sealing in water immediately after bathing. Using occlusives without hydration is not effective because they do not contain water and only prevent evaporation from the skin. It is important to use a topical vehicle or emollient the patient likes and feels comfortable with. These should be applied as often as desired and at least three or four times a day.

Topical Steroids

Topical corticosteroids control acute flares of AD by reducing inflammation and itching. Whether a low or high potency steroid is prescribed depends on the location and severity of skin lesions. Patients should be informed of the strength of the steroid and possible side effects, of which skin thinning is the most common. Hypo-pigmentation, secondary infections, acne and permanent striae may occur. Topical steroids are available in ointments, creams, gels, sprays and lotions.

Diagnosis and Management of Atopic Dermatitis

Upon request, pharmacists can provide topical preparations in half-pound or pound quantities at lower cost.

Tar Preparations

Extracts of crude coal tar help reduce skin inflammation. Tar is not as quick acting as topical corticosteroids, but the anti-inflammatory effect lasts longer and side effects are fewer. Use of tar preparations is recommended to reduce the need for topical steroids in chronic maintenance of atopic dermatitis.

Systemic Therapy

Antibiotics and antihistamines may be necessary to treat atopic dermatitis. Use of systemic corticosteroids is rarely warranted. The "quick cure" and easy use aspects of systemic steroids sometimes make them more attractive than hydration and topical therapy to patients and parents. Unfortunately, a dramatic rebound after discontinuation is not uncommon, and serious side effects make oral steroids unwarranted in a non-life-threatening disease.

If short-term oral steroids have been used, it is important to taper the dosage when therapy is discontinued. Skin care also should be intensified, particularly with topical corticosteroids, to suppress flaring of dermatitis.

Systemic antibiotic therapy is often necessary because atopic dermatitis is characterized by chronic low-grade inflammation that often is secondarily infected. Since *Staphylococcus aureus* causes the majority of these infections, erythromycin is the first choice of therapy. However, occasionally therapeutic response is poor due to antibiotic-resistant bacteria, so dicloxacillin or clindamycin may be necessary. Long-term maintenance therapy may be indicated in patients who repeatedly develop infections.

Systemic antihistamine and antianxiety drugs may offer some relief from the highly bothersome pruritus that commonly accompanies AD, mainly through tranquilizing and sedative effects. Non-sedating antihistamines seem of little use in controlling this pruritus. Topical antihistamines and anesthetics should be avoided due to possible secondary sensitization.

Recalcitrant Disease

Hospitalization can be considered for patients resistant to therapy. In many cases, simple removal from the home environment with its potential triggers, education and assurance of therapy compliance is enough to significantly reduce dermatitis.

Ultraviolet light, under professional supervision, can be a useful adjunctive modality. However, sunburn must be avoided and the increased risk of skin cancer must be considered. In severe AD, the potential benefits usually outweigh these risks.

Because AD patients manifest immune system abnormalities, use of immuno-modulators represents one possible alternative approach as the mechanisms that cause this skin condition become more understood. Research into new therapeutic approaches to treating AD is actively being pursued at National Jewish.

Patient Education

AD patients need general disease information, detailed (verbal and written) skin care plans and updates on promising research and support groups. Strict, active compliance by patient or parent is critical to successful management.

Conclusion

Atopic dermatitis is a common chronic skin disease encountered in patients with asthma and allergic rhinitis. Each patient requires individualized therapy, and patients need to have a role in deciding their care. For the patient who appears resistant to therapy, the allergist and/or dermatologist can provide an important adjunct to the management of AD. When patient education and compliance are high, the outcome is generally rewarding, even in the most difficult AD cases.

References

1. Rajka G. Atopic Dermatitis. London, England: WB Saunders Co Ltd; 1975.
2. Hanifin J. Epidemiology of atopic dermatitis. Monogr Allergy. 1987; 21:116- 131
3. Rook A (ed). Major Problems in Dermatology: Atopic Dermatitis, Vol 3. Philadelphia, WB Saunders Co, 1975.

Diagnosis and Management of Atopic Dermatitis

4. Hoffman DR, Yamamoto FY, Geller B, Haddad Z. Specific antibodies in atopic eczema. J Allergy Clin Immunol. 1975 ;55 :256-267.

5. Sampson HA. The role of food allergy and mediator release in atopic dermatitis. J Allergy Clin Immunol. 1988; 81:635-645.

For More Information

LUNG LINE® free informational service, can save you time and act as an educational resource by helping teach patients about respiratory, allergic and immunologic diseases. Highly trained registered nurses are available to answer your patients' questions at 1-800-222-LUNG. In Denver, callers should dial 355-LUNG. LUNG LINE® nurses always encourage callers to discuss information with their physicians.

Office of Professional Communications
National Jewish Center for Immunology and Respiratory Medicine
1400 Jackson Street
Denver, CO 80206-2762

This article is drawn from extensive publications authored by Noreen H. Nicol, RN, MS, FNC, Dermatology Clinical Specialist/Nurse Practitioner at the National Jewish Center for Immunology and Respiratory Medicine, and Donald Y. M. Leung, MD, PhD, Director of Pediatric Allergy/Immunology at the National Jewish Center for Immunology and Respiratory Medicine.

Chapter 18

Atopic Dermatitis: Is it an Allergic Disease?

For many years controversy has surrounded the relation between allergy and atopic dermatitis. We critically review the evidence for the contribution of allergy, or IgE-mediated hypersensitivity reactions, to the pathogenesis of this disease. We conclude that, at present, there is scant evidence that allergy is central to the development of atopic dermatitis, although it may be an aggravating factor in a few patients. Hence there is little rationale for the routine use of allergy testing or dietary and environmental manipulation in the management of this disease. (J AM ACAD DERMATOL 1995;33:1008-18.)

Atopy, derived from a Greek word meaning "out of place," was introduced by Coca and Cooke[1] in 1923 to describe a type of inherited hypersensitivity. They defined the hypersensitive person as "one reacting with characteristic symptoms to the administration of or contact with a quantity of any substance, which, to the majority of the members of the same species of animal is innocuous." Although the mechanism of atopic hypersensitivity was unknown, it was thought to be inherited, subject to a dominant gene.

Atopic dermatitis (AD), considered one manifestation of hypersensitivity, was subsequently defined by Wise and Sulzberger[2] in 1933. In contrast to other eczematous eruptions, these authors believed the

©1995. Reproduced from the *Journal American Academy of Dermatology*, Anne R. Halbert, FACD, William L. Weston, MD, and Joseph G. Morelli, MD Denver, Colorado. "Atopic dermatitis: Is it an allergic disease?" 33.6 (1995): 1008-1018. Reprinted with permission from Mosby Year-Book.

nine cardinal features of AD included an atopic family history, antecedent infantile eczema, localization in flexural areas, gray-brown discoloration of skin, an absence of vesicles, vasomotor instability, negative patch tests but many contact irritants, many positive reactions of immediate wheal type to scratch or intradermal testing, and the presence of many reagins in the serum. In view of the latter two features, Wise and Sulzberger emphatically stated that the logical therapy for AD was the elimination of all foods and inhalants giving positive wheal reactions. They also advocated desensitization treatment with the most suspect substances. In 1935, Hill and Sulzberger[3] further emphasized the importance of food and airborne sensitivities in the development of AD, listing egg, wheat, and milk as the most common food atopens and silk and cat hair as common environmental atopens. These sensitivities were thought to be mediated by reagins frequently detected in the serum of atopic patients and subsequently identified as IgE.[4,5] Hill and Sulzberger also stated that not all substances producing positive skin test reactions or specific reagins were of clinical relevance.

During the past 60 years, controversy has surrounded the contribution of allergy, or IgE-mediated hypersensitivity, to the pathogenesis of AD. The frequently cited "evidence" in favor of allergy playing a central pathogenic role is as follows:

- Children with AD may have a strong personal history of atopy, and in 50 percent to 80 percent asthma or allergic rhinitis develops.[6,7]

- A positive family history of atopy exists in 58 percent to 68 percent of patients.[8,9]

- Total serum IgE levels are elevated in up to 80 percent of patients, and immediate skin test reactions to a variety of environmental allergens are frequent.[10,11]

- Food allergens can exacerbate skin disease in some patients with AD, and elimination of appropriate foods may ameliorate skin disease.[12]

- Epicutaneous patch testing with aeroallergens, particularly house dust mite antigens, can induce eczematous lesions in some patients with AD.[13]

Atopic Dermatitis: Is it an Allergic Disease?

Although many patients with dermatitis have an atopic constitution, this association does not necessarily mean the atopy is the cause of the dermatitis. Despite the claims already outlined, many patients with AD, particularly those with mild to moderate disease, do not have clinically relevant food or aeroallergen sensitivities. Nonspecific cutaneous hyperreactivity is thought to be the exclusive precipitating factor in this group of patients.[14] In addition, even if allergies are detected, there is still a paucity of evidence from well-planned controlled clinical trials to show that long-term benefit can be derived from dietary restriction or environmental manipulation.

A minimum set of diagnostic criteria for AD has recently been established by means of multiple logistic regression techniques.[15] Six features separate AD from other inflammatory dermatoses: a history of flexural involvement, age at onset younger than two years (omitted in children younger than four years), history of an itchy eruption, history of generalized dry skin, visible flexural dermatitis, and a personal history of asthma/hayfever (or a history of atopic disease in a first-degree relative in children younger than four years). Elevated IgE, positive skin prick tests, or radioallergosorbent tests (RASTs) to environmental allergens or a history of food intolerance are not necessary for the diagnosis of AD; indeed, these features have been shown to be neither particularly sensitive nor specific for AD.[8]

The cause of AD is still unknown, but it is believed to be a complex interplay of genetic susceptibility, immune dysregulation, and epidermal barrier dysfunction.[16] The aim of this article is to critically examine current evidence to determine the contribution of allergy to the pathogenesis of AD. With an increasing number of children being subjected to repeated allergy testing, rigid elimination diets that may be nutritionally inadequate, and anti-house-dust-mite regimens, we believe it is important to review the role of allergy and place it in perspective.

IgE and Atopy

Atopy is frequently characterized by IgE hyper-responsiveness to a range of environmental antigens.[17] When antigen binds mast cell-bound IgE, the high-affinity receptor for IgE (FcER-I) initiates events leading to the cellular release of inflammatory mediators.[18] Although this results in mucosal inflammation and hence contributes to the development of allergic rhinitis[19] and possibly some forms of asthma,[20] there is little evidence that it is central to the pathogenesis of AD.

Total serum IgE is elevated in 43 percent to 82 percent of patients with AD.[10,21] The highest levels are found in those with severe skin disease and coexisting respiratory atopy.[10,22-24] Although serum IgE has a short half-life of five to seven days, the level does not fluctuate in close association with clinical flares and remissions.[25] When severe AD is treated with systemic steroids, the clinical improvement that ensues is not accompanied by a decrease in the serum level of IgE. The IgE level returns to normal when patients with a history of severe dermatitis have been free from their disease for at least two years.[25]

The presence of serum or tissue IgE does not appear to be essential for the development of AD. In support of this, classic AD has been reported in patients with X-linked agammaglobulinemia in whom IgE was virtually absent.[26] Furthermore, when elevated IgE is present, dermatitis does not necessarily develop. Dermatitis develops only in 10 percent to 15 percent of patients with respiratory atopy and good reagin-forming capacity,[27] and it is not a complication of many other conditions with elevated IgE.

The presence of respiratory atopy in a patient with AD significantly increases the likelihood of an elevated total serum IgE level. When patients with "pure" AD are studied (i.e., those with no personal or family history of respiratory atopy), the majority do not have elevated IgE or antigen-specific sensitivities.[10,22,28-30] IgE is still correlated with disease severity in this "pure" AD group, but Uehara[28] noted only 37 percent of patients with severe "pure" AD had an elevated IgE and this elevation was only slight to moderate. In contrast, about 80 percent of patients with severe AD and a personal history of respiratory atopy have a markedly elevated IgE level.[10]

Although the genetics of IgE production are complex, recent genetic linkage studies provide some insight into the association between respiratory atopy and IgE hyper-responsiveness. These studies have identified a gene on chromosome 11q13 that is associated with respiratory atopy.[31] This gene encodes a variant of the ß subunit of the high-affinity IgE receptor (FcER-I ß) in which there is an isoleucine 181-leucine substitution within the fourth transmembrane domain of the molecule.[32] Stimulation of this variant receptor may result in increased release of proinflammatory mediators by mast cells or may enhance mast cell expression of interleukin (IL)-4, stimulating more local B lymphocyte IgE production. Of significance, linkage of atopy with this gene on 11q13 could not be shown when patients with AD were used as probands.[33] This study needs to be confirmed but does suggest caution when trying to extrapolate the pathogenesis of respiratory atopy to AD.

The Role of Food Allergy in AD

Although food hypersensitivity reactions occur in some patients with AD, the relevance of these reactions to the pathogenesis of AD is still in doubt. If food allergy does have a significant contribution, it should be possible to demonstrate that it is common in patients with AD, that challenge with the offending allergen(s) will reliably produce a flare of dermatitis, and that allergen avoidance will result in clinical improvement. In addition, prevention of food allergies should reduce the likelihood of AD developing.

Despite a large number of studies, the prevalence of food hypersensitivity in patients with AD is still not known. Immediate skin prick tests or RASTs to a range of food allergens yield one or more positive results in 51 percent to 85 percent of patients with AD,[12,23,34,35] but these tests are not useful in predicting clinically relevant reactions. Although negative skin tests virtually exclude IgE-mediated food allergy, only 25 percent to 30 percent of patients with positive skin tests will have a reaction when challenged.[35,36] In addition, skin prick tests remain strongly positive even after tolerance to foods has developed.[37]

The most reliable technique for the diagnosis of food hypersensitivity appears to be double-blind placebo-controlled food challenges (DBPCFC).[38] From the many studies utilizing this technique, 33 percent to 63 percent of patients with AD have developed a reaction when challenged.[12,34-37] However, because most of these patients were referred for management of severe dermatitis or suspected food allergies, these results do not provide a reliable estimate of food allergy prevalence. Hanifin[39] estimates 10 percent to 20 percent of patients with AD have clinically relevant food hypersensitivities although this is only a clinical impression. Guillet and Guillet,[14] using an elimination diet followed by open and blind food challenge, could not identify any food allergies in 162 patients with mild-to-moderate AD, although one or more were detectable in 96 percent of 88 patients with severe disease. These authors concluded that the detection of food allergy in a child with AD is likely to predict a prognosis of severe disease. Infants and young children appear to have a higher prevalence of food allergies, with tolerance developing to at least one third of allergens in one or two years.[40]

DBPCFC may produce cutaneous (84 percent to 96 percent), respiratory (10 percent to 52 percent), or gastrointestinal (20 percent to 42 percent) reactions.[12,34-37] These reactions develop within minutes to two hours of challenge and last only 30 to 120 minutes. A pruritic erythematous morbilliform eruption is the most common cutaneous reaction; urticaria occurs infrequently.[12,34,36,37] These eruptions are the result of IgE-mediated cutaneous mast cell activation and are accompanied by a rise in plasma histamine concentration.[41] Spontaneous basophil histamine release is increased in patients with food allergies because of the production of histamine-releasing factors from activated mononuclear cells.[42] These cytokines induce degranulation of mast cells and basophils by binding to surface-bound IgE molecules.

Much of the controversy surrounding the contribution of food allergies to AD has arisen from the inability of controlled food challenges to elicit eczematous lesions. For many years it was assumed that histamine release from repeated ingestion of food allergens produced pruritus and the scratching that ensued produced dermatitis.[43] In recent years, emphasis has been placed on the IgE-mediated late phase reaction (LPR) as the link between immediate hypersensitivity and the development of atopic eczematous skin that histologically more closely resembles a type IV delayed hypersensitivity reaction.[44] The LPR begins three to four hours after ingestion of antigen. After the expression of leukocyte adhesion molecules on post-capillary venular endothelium there is a progressive dermal accumulation of eosinophils, neutrophils, and basophils, reaching a maximum concentration at 6 to 12 hours.[45,46] By 24 to 48 hours a mononuclear cell infiltrate consisting of monocytes and T lymphocytes is present and eosinophil major basic protein deposition is detectable.[47] The T-cell infiltrate consists of Th2 cells secreting IL-3, -4, -5, and granulocyte-macrophage colony-stimulating factor.[48]

Although these findings resemble the skin lesions of AD, this IgE-mediated LPR is not accompanied by the development of clinically evident eczematous lesions. Despite systematic attempts by Sampson[49] to document delayed reactions in the large number of patients he has evaluated with DBPCFC, all positive food challenges occurred within two hours of administration of food antigen. Occasionally pruritus recurred at six to eight hours, accompanied by a nonspecific macular eruption, but this was not eczematous in type.[37,50] In contrast, delayed eczematous reactions have been reported in studies in which the suspected allergen was administered daily for several days.[51,53] Hill et al.[53] observed a delayed eczematous reaction (i.e.,

Atopic Dermatitis: Is it an Allergic Disease?

greater than 24 hours after challenge) in 17 of 135 children with suspected cow's milk allergy. Of interest, 10 of these 17 children had negative skin prick tests to cow's milk allergen extract, suggesting a non-IgE-mediated pathogenesis.

If food allergens are significantly contributing to AD, avoidance should result in clinical improvement. The detection and avoidance of relevant food allergens, however, can be a formidable task. Overall, 90 percent of children with food allergy react to only one or two foods and only six foods are responsible for 90 percent of all food allergies (egg, peanut, milk, wheat, fish, soy).[12,50] Despite this, it has been consistently shown that parents are frequently unable to correctly identify food allergens relevant to their children[12,34,53] and elimination diets conducted in the home rarely produce any benefit.[54] Many of the adverse food reactions reported by parents are caused by contact urticaria or primary irritant dermatitis.[54]

Although many studies have tried to document improvement in patients with AD after reduced exposure to food allergens, the results have been highly variable. It is frequently difficult to interpret and compare results because of differences in populations studied (different age groups and severity of dermatitis), different outcomes reported (dermatitis improved vs. cleared), and the natural history of AD, which is a chronic disease with a fluctuating course and a tendency to decrease with age.

In a study of 34 children observed for three to four years, Sampson[12] claimed the outcome was better in children with food hypersensitivity who were maintained with an elimination diet. The numbers in this study were small, however; he was comparing groups of 17, 12, and five children. In another small study with double-blind, cross-over design, Atherton et al.[55] found 14 of 20 children improved after egg and milk exclusion. Despite a similar study design, these results could not be reproduced by Neild et al.,[56] who found improvement in only 10 of 40 patients on an egg and milk exclusion diet. Results may be more impressive in infants; Casimir et al.[57] reported 31 of 64 (48 percent) cow's milk-fed infants with AD improved after avoidance of cow's milk.

More recently, several studies have been conducted in which children with severe AD have been given highly restrictive diets with gradual reintroduction of foods. Pike et al.[58] noted 24 of 66 children (36 percent) improved initially when given a "few foods" diet, but only 12 of 66 (18 percent) experienced prolonged and useful benefit. Devlin et al.[59] used a restrictive six-food diet for six weeks in 63 children with severe AD. Of the 54 who complied and completed the diet period, 21 (39 percent) did not benefit and 33 (61 percent) obtained improvement of more than 20 percent. On reintroduction of foods, 9 of these 33 patients had no reaction. Of those patients observed for 12 months or more, there was no difference in outcome between the group who responded to the diet, the group who failed to comply, and those who did not respond. It should be noted that in all these elimination studies, even when dermatitis improves it rarely completely clears.

Finally, can the prevention of food allergy in infancy modulate the incidence of atopic disease, particularly AD? Since Grulee and Sanford[60] first proposed a protective effect of breast-feeding in 1936, many studies have been performed to determine the benefits of prolonged breast-feeding, delayed introduction of solid foods, and a reduction in maternal dietary allergens in the last trimester of pregnancy and throughout lactation. Unfortunately, many of these studies have had significant methodologic flaws, making the interpretation of results difficult.[61] In addition, the results obtained have been incredibly variable. We will not provide a comprehensive review of these studies, but rather will outline a few to illustrate these inconsistent results.

In 1973, Halpern et al.[62] compared the effect of a 6-month diet of breast milk, cow's milk, or soy formula on the development of AD in 1,753 children. No significant differences in the frequency of AD were noted among the three groups. In contrast, Saarinen et al.[63] showed a reduced incidence of food allergies and eczema in 54 babies solely breast-fed for more than six months when compared with 77 babies breast-fed for only two to six months and 105 babies younger than two months of age weaned to cow's milk-based formulas. Kajosaari and Saarinen[64] and Halken et al.[65] also claimed to show a reduction in the prevalence of AD with prolonged breast-feeding and the delayed introduction of solids. In the latter study, the prevalence of AD at 18 months of life was 14 percent in 105 infants breast-fed for six months (or supplemented with a hypoallergenic formula) versus 31 percent in the control group (n=54). Gustafsson et al.,[66] however, reported finding no increase in atopic disease in children given cow's milk formulas in the first eight days of life. In this study, the cumulative incidences of atopic diseases at 7, 11, and 14 years of age were determined in a cohort of 736 children. Similarly, Kay et al.,[67] after reviewing 1,077 children in an English general practice population, did not find that breast-feeding for six months or longer affected the prevalence of AD.

Zeiger et al.,[68] in a carefully constructed randomized study, examined the effect of combined maternal and infant food allergen avoidance on the development of atopy in early infancy. The diet of the prophylactic-treated group (n=103) included maternal avoidance of cow's milk, egg, and peanut during the third trimester of pregnancy and lactation, infant use of casein hydrolysate for supplementation or weaning, and avoidance of solid foods for 6 to 24 months. At 12 months of age infants in the prophylactic group had lower cumulative and period prevalences of food allergy and AD than the control group. By 24 months of age, however, the cumulative prevalences of allergic disease were similar for the two groups and no differences in food allergy were noted.[69] Serum IgE in the two groups was comparable at 12 and 24 months, and at no age was any difference in the prevalence of respiratory atopy noted. Recently, Hide et al.[70] performed a similar study on 120 children considered to be at high risk for atopy. As with the study of Zeiger et al. the prevalence of eczema was significantly greater in the control group at 12 months of age. By two years of age, however, 8 of 58 infants in the prophylactic group and 15 of 62 infants in the control group had eczema. This was not a statistically significant difference (p=0.56).[70]

What conclusions can be drawn from these many studies of the contribution of food allergy to the pathogenesis of AD? First, food allergy affects only a minority of patients with AD, most commonly infants or those with severe disease. DBPCFCs confirm the presence of IgE-mediated food hypersensitivity reactions, but do not elicit dermatitis. Despite the histologic resemblances between the IgE-mediated LPR and AD, dermatitis has not been shown to be the clinical correlate of the LPR. Delayed eczematous reactions after repeated oral provocation have been demonstrated in some studies, but are not always IgE-mediated. When patients with known food allergies or severe AD are given supervised elimination diets there may be some initial improvement (although the dermatitis rarely clears), but few derive long-term benefit. Finally, if prolonged breast-feeding and the delayed introduction of potential allergens do protect against the development of AD, the inconsistent study results suggest the effect is small and benefits appear limited to the first year of life.

The Role of Aeroallergens in AD

Between 1918 and the 1950s, several researchers claimed inhalant allergens were important in the causation of AD. These claims were largely based on reports of small numbers of patients with ragweed pollen sensitivity who had seasonal variation in their AD and even smaller numbers of patients in whom mild eczematous eruptions in whom developed after inhalation challenge with ragweed pollen or Alternaria.[71] A pathogenic role for house dust mite was also suggested.[72]

In recent years, no well-controlled trials have studied the effect of aeroallergen inhalation on AD.[73,74] There is now evidence, however, that direct skin contact with aeroallergens may elicit a delayed-type hypersensitivity reaction and hence may contribute to cutaneous inflammation.[13,73] When patients with positive immediate skin prick tests to house dust mite (Dermatophagoides), pollens, animal epithelia, or molds are patch tested with these allergens, a proportion have an eczematous reaction at the patch test site after 24 to 72 hours. Biopsy specimens of the patch test site reveal cellular infiltrates of mononuclear cells and eosinophils, with epidermal spongiosis evident by 72 hours.[75,76]

Delayed hypersensitivity to aeroallergens is thought to be IgE-mediated with the binding of allergen to IgE-bearing epidermal Langerhans cells.[77] Allergen can bind to uncomplexed IgE attached to Langerhans cells via the high-affinity FcER-I, or preformed IgE-allergen complexes can bind to the low-affinity FcER-II/CD23.[78] Activation of FcER-l results in the release of proinflammatory mediators from the Langerhans cells (as occurs with activation of this receptor on mast cells and basophils), and activation of both FcER-I and FcER-II results in facilitated antigen presentation to CD4+ T lymphocytes in the lesional skin.[79] Many T-cell clones cultured from skin lesions of AD are aeroallergen specific, particularly to Dermatophagoides.[80] The activated T cells express a Th2 phenotype and elaborate cytokines such as IL4 and IL-5, but little interferon gamma.[80] IL4 causes increased IgE production from B cells and upregulates CD23 expression on Langerhans cells, and IL-5 is thought to contribute to local tissue damage by attracting and activating eosinophils.[77]

It should be noted that IgE-bearing Langerhans cells are not exclusive to lesional AD skin and have been identified in lesional skin of a wide range of conditions associated with elevated IgE.[81] Three types of IgE receptors occur on Langerhans cells in normal skin: FcER-I, FcER-II (CD23), and IgE-binding protein.[78,82] IgE binds to receptors in the presence of an inflammatory infiltrate83 and elevated total serum IgE.[81]

After outlining the possible mechanism of aeroallergen-induced aggravation of AD, it is now necessary to draw attention to some of the conflicting or inconsistent results that have been obtained. First, although many patients with AD have been patch tested to aeroallergens, the frequency of positive delayed hypersensitivity reactions varied greatly, from 11 percent to 100 percent.[84-89] These variable results are because of the different allergens used (e.g., different house dust mite fractions), different allergen concentrations, different application times, and varying pretreatment of skin (e.g., tape stripping, abrading, or use of normal healthy-skin). If the extremes are excluded, most studies report positive reactions in fewer than a third of patients patch tested.

In the early patch testing studies, the main criterion for patient selection was the presence of positive immediate skin tests to aeroallergens. It is now evident, however, that 30 percent to 40 percent of patients who have positive patch test reactions do not have positive skin prick tests to aeroallergens, which implies that a non-IgE-mediated pathway is involved in the development of the delayed hypersensitivity.[84,85] It has been proposed that different house dust mite fractions may induce type I and type IV allergy.[90]

Finally, although many studies claim that positive patch test reactions occur exclusively in patients with AD, several have now reported positive patch tests in patients with respiratory atopy but no history of AD.[85,87,89] For example, Seidenari et al.[85] patch tested 40 patients with rhinoconjunctivitis or asthma, but with a negative history of AD. Overall, 27.5 percent had a positive reaction and 40 percent of those with aeroallergen-specific IgE reacted. These findings need further investigation but seriously question the clinical relevance of aeroallergen-induced patch test reactions in patients with AD.

Aside from these immunologic studies, there is still a scarcity of clinical research implicating aeroallergen hypersensitivity in the pathogenesis of AD. Van Asperen and Kemp,[91] who prospectively observed 57 children up to five years of age with atopic parents, could not identify any significant differences in the incidence of IgE sensitization to inhaled allergens in children with AD and those without AD. They concluded that IgE sensitization to inhaled allergens is associated with wheeze and rhinitis in later childhood but is not associated with AD. In 1992, Guillet and Guillet[14] studied 169 patients with moderate-to-severe AD before and after a 2-month period during which relevant aeroallergens (as detected by skin prick tests and RAST) were eliminated or reduced. Sensitivity to inhaled allergens was detected and acknowledged as being clinically responsible for respiratory symptoms in 27 percent of patients, but was believed responsible for skin symptoms in only four patients. In a small controlled trial of eradication of house dust mite with natamycin and vacuum cleaning, Colloff et al.[92] found no correlation between clinical improvement and reduced mite numbers.

In contrast to these findings, a few recent studies have reported small groups of patients (n=18 to 33) in whom AD was alleviated after aeroallergen avoidance or reduced exposure to house dust mite.[57,86,93,94] Most of these studies were uncontrolled; Sanda et al.[94] included a small control group, but unfortunately neither the subjects nor the clinicians were blinded and hence a placebo effect and observer bias may have contributed to some of the symptomatic improvement reported in patients admitted to the "clean room" (a room with an air filter system reducing airborne particles). These patients did have some objective signs of improvement including a decrease in eosinophil and basophil counts and house dust mite-specific IgG. Beck and Korsgaard[95] noted an increased concentration of house dust mites in mattress dust in patients with moderate-to-severe AD but this does not prove a causal role for house dust mite.

Although there is some evidence that house dust mite hyposensitization regimens may be beneficial in children with house dust mite-provoked asthma,[96,97] Glover and Atherton[98] were unable to demonstrate significant improvement in a double-blind, controlled trial of house dust mite hyposensitization in children with AD. The numbers studied were small, however, and the duration of immunotherapy may have been insufficient. Benefit was shown in one other recent double-blind, placebo-controlled trial in which intradermal complexes containing autologous specific antibodies and *Dermatophagoides* allergens were given, but this novel technique requires further investigation.[99] It should be noted that a striking placebo effect has been observed in double-blind, controlled trials of hyposensitization.[98,99] This should be remembered when anecdotal reports of benefit or the results of uncontrolled trials are evaluated.

The Role of Infection in Ad

Two microorganisms have been implicated in the pathogenesis of AD: *Staphylococcus aureus* and *pitrosporum ovale*. We briefly examine the evidence that they contribute to the development of AD through IgE-mediated mechanisms.

Colonization of the skin with *S. aureus* is extremely common in AD, occurring in more than 90 percent of patients.[100,101] Approximately two thirds of S. aureus cultures produce one or more exotoxins although this is no greater than exotoxin production from *S. aureus* colonizing

Atopic Dermatitis: Is it an Allergic Disease?

patients without AD.[102] Two mechanisms have been proposed to explain the adverse effects of *S. aureus* on AD; i.e., IgE-mediated hypersensitivity to the organism or its exotoxins, and superantigenic stimulation of class II major histocompatibility complex (MHC) molecules and T-cell receptors.

Anti-staphylococcal IgE antibodies have been detected in a variable percentage of patients with AD studied. Nordvall et al.[103] found these antibodies in only a few patients and at low concentrations; Leung et al.[104] reported 57 percent of patients with AD had significant levels of IgE primarily directed toward exotoxins. These antibodies are more common in patients with elevated total serum IgE, and some studies show correlation with disease severity.[103,105] Anti-staphylococcal IgE antibodies are invariably detected in patients with the hyper-immunoglobulin-E syndrome.[106] These patients produce high levels of IgE antibody directed toward both the cell wall of *S. aureus*[106] and a range of exotoxins.[104]

In view of the IgE hyper-responsiveness that characterizes atopy, the development of anti-staphylococcal IgE antibodies in patients with AD does not necessarily have any clinical relevance. At present, the only evidence that IgE-mediated reactions may be a factor in exacerbating the itch of AD is the in vitro demonstration of increased basophil histamine release on exposure to anti-staphylococcal toxin IgE antibodies.[104] The *in vivo* significance of this finding is unknown.

The superantigenic activity of *S. aureus* exotoxins may be an important mechanism through which the organism exacerbates AD, although this is still in the early stages of investigation. Superantigens can bind to class II MHC molecules on epidermal Langerhans cells, macrophages, and monocytes and cause the release of proinflammatory mediators such as IL-1 and tumor necrosis factor-α.[107] In addition, through cross-linking MHC class II molecules on antigen-presenting cells and the variable domain of TCR-beta, T cells can be stimulated to proliferate and secrete a range of inflammatory cytokines.[105] *S. aureus*-derived enterotoxin B has been shown to induce a Th2 phenotype in lesional T cells, with production of IL-3, -4, and -5.[108]

P. ovale has mainly been implicated in the pathogenesis of dermatitis of the head and neck in young adults. It is particularly in these patients that anti-*Pityrosporum* IgE antibodies are found[103,100,110] and 15 percent to 65 percent have positive skin prick tests to *Pityrosporum* extracts.[110-112] Because these findings may be an epiphenomenon, much emphasis has been placed on one controlled trial in which 14 patients with head and neck dermatitis improved with ketoconazole but five patients with generalized dermatitis remained unchanged.[113] It is highly unlikely this organism plays any role in childhood dermatitis because it can only be cultured from 5 percent to 15 percent of children younger than 10 years of age,[111] and childhood AD does not favor lipophilic areas of skin.

Conclusion

The concept of AD as an allergic disease originated from the early published works of Coca and Cooke[1] and Wise and Sulzberger.[2] AD was considered the result of idiosyncratic hypersensitivity to a range of environmental atopens such as foods and inhalants. The frequent finding of positive skin prick tests and specific reagins to atopens was thought to be highly significant, and avoidance of these atopens was promoted as the most logical therapy.

Although the cause of AD is still unknown, at present there is scanty evidence that allergic mechanisms play a central pathogenetic role. Many patients with AD do have an atopic constitution, but elevated total serum IgE or antigen-specific sensitivities are not essential for the development of dermatitis and are frequently absent in those without coexisting respiratory atopy. Most patients with AD, particularly those with mild to moderate disease, do not have food allergies and do not benefit from dietary manipulation. Even when food allergies are present, total clearance of dermatitis rarely occurs with allergen avoidance, and only a small percentage of patients derive long-term benefit from supervised elimination diets. Allergen avoidance in infancy, with prolonged breast-feeding and delayed introduction of solids, may reduce the incidence of dermatitis during the first year of life but most studies show no effect on the cumulative prevalence of AD by two years of age.

The role of aeroallergens in the precipitation or exacerbation of AD is far from clear. It is now evident that direct skin contact with aeroallergens may result in an IgE-mediated, delayed hypersensitivity reaction in about one third of patients with AD. The clinical relevance of this is not known, however, because positive patch tests to aeroallergens are also found in some atopic patients with no history of dermatitis. As yet, there have been no well-conducted controlled clinical trials showing that sustained benefit can be obtained from environmental manipulation with a reduction in aeroallergen exposure. *S. aureus*, another potential environmental allergen, can undoubtedly exacerbate AD, but it is not known whether this is through an IgE-mediated pathway, superantigens, or some other mechanism.

IgE-mediated hypersensitivity reactions may at times be responsible for aggravating AD, without being central to its pathogenesis. For example, histamine release during food hypersensitivity reactions may result in a transient increase in itching without specifically producing dermatitis per se. Strauss and Kligman,[114] by inducing allergic contact dermatitis in atopic patients with allergen (atopen)-specific sensitivities, were able to show exacerbation of the contact dermatitis after inhalation challenge or topical application of the atopen. They concluded that specific atopens can provoke flares of an existing etiologically unrelated dermatitis in susceptible persons.

Finally, clarification of the influence of allergy in the pathogenesis of AD has important therapeutic implications. With our current knowledge, it appears most patients with AD do not have clinically relevant allergies. Thus there is little rationale in routinely performing allergy testing or advising dietary restriction or environmental manipulation. Rather, these patients should be encouraged to direct their energy toward optimizing their skin care regimen.

References

1. Coca AF, Cooke RA. On the classification of the phenomena of hypersensitiveness. J Immunol 1923; 8:163-82
2. Wise F, Sulzberger MB. Dermatology and syphilology [Editorial]. Chicago: Year Book, 1933:31-70.
3. Hill LW, Sulzberger MB. Evolution of atopic dermatitis. Arch Dermatol Syph 1935; 32:451-63.
4. Johansson SGO, Bennich H. Immunological studies of an atypical (myeloma) immunoglobulin. Immunology 1967; 13:381-94.
5. Ishizaka K, Ishizaka T, Holbrook MM. Identification of gamma-E antibodies as a carrier of reaginic activity. J Immunol 1967; 99:1187-98.
6. Pasternack B. The prediction of asthma in infantile eczema. J Pediatr 1965; 66:164-5.
7. Stifler WC. A twenty-one year follow-up of infantile eczema. J Pediatr 1965; 66:166-7.
8. Diepgen TL, Fartasch M. Recent epidemiological and genetic studies in atopic dermatitis. Acta Derm Venereol Suppl (Stockh) 1992; 176:13-8.
9. Rajka G. Atopic dermatitis. London: WB Saunders, 1975:47.
10. Johnson E, Irons J, Patterson R, et al. Serum IgE concentration in atopic dermatitis. J Allergy Clin Immunol 1974; 54:94-9.
11. Hoffman DR, Yamamoto FY, Sellar B, et al. Specific IgE antibodies in atopic eczema. J Allergy Clin Immunol 1975; 55:256-67.

12. Sampson HA, McCaskill CC. Food hypersensitivity and atopic dermatitis: evaluation of 113 patients. J Pediatr 1985; 107:669-75.
13. Platts-Mills TAE, Mitchell EB, Rowntree S, et al. The role of dust mite allergens in atopic dermatitis. Clin Exp Dermatol 1983; 8:233-47.
14. Guillet G, Guillet M. Natural history of sensitizations in atopic dermatitis. Arch Dermatol 1992; 128:187-92.
15. Williams HC, Burney PGJ, Hay RJ, et al. The U.K. working party's diagnostic criteria for atopic dermatitis. I: Derivation of a minimum set of discriminators for atopic dermatitis. Br J Dermatol 1994; 131:383-96.
16. Cooper KD. Atopic dermatitis: recent trends in pathogenesis and therapy. J Invest Dermatol 1994; 102:128-37.
17. Bos JD, Wierenga EA, Smitt JHS, et al. Immune dysregulation in atopic eczema. Arch Dermatol 1992; 128:1509-12.
18. Galli SJ. New concepts about the mast cell. N Engl J Med 1993; 328:257-65.
19. Hogan MB, Grammer LC, Patterson R. Rhinitis. Ann Allergy 1994; 72:293-300.
20. Platts-Mills TAE. Allergen-specific treatment for asthma: in Am Rev Respir Dis 1993; 148:553-5.
21. Juhlin L, Johansson SGO, Bennich H, et al. Immunoglobulin E in dermatoses. Arch Dermatol 1969; 100:12-5.
22. Jones HE, Inouye JC, McGerity JL, et al. Atopic disease and serum IgE. Br J Dermatol 1975; 92:17-25.
23. Ogawa M, Berger PA, McIntyre R, et al. IgE in atopic dermatitis. Arch Dermatol 1971; 103:575-80.
24. Ohman S, Johansson SGO. Immunoglobulins in atopic dermatitis. Acta Derm Venereol (Stockh) 1974; 54:193-202.
25. Johansson SGO, Juhlin L. Immunoglobulin E in healed atopic dermatitis and after treatment with corticosteroids and azathioprine. Br J Dermatol 1970,82:10-2.
26. Peterson RDA, Page ARP, Good RA. Wheal and erythema allergy in patients with agammaglobulinemia. J Allergy 1962; 33:406-11.
27. Rajka G. Atopic dermatitis. London: WB Saunders, 1975:91.
28. Uehara M. Family background of respiratory atopy: a factor of serum IgE elevation in atopic dermatitis. Acta Derm Venereol Suppl (Stockh) 1989; 144:78-82.
29. Wuthrich B, Schnyder UW. Haufigkeit genetisce asekte und prognose der neurodermatitis atopica. Allergologie 1991; 14:284-90.
30. Uehara M, Kimura C, Uenishi T. Type 1 allergy to foods in atopic dermatitis. Acta Derm Venereol Suppl (Stockh) 1992; 176:38-40.
31. Cookson WOCM, Sharp PA, Faux JA, et al. Linkage between immunoglobulin E responses underlying asthma and rhinitis and chromosome 11q. Lancet 1989; 1:1292-5.
32. Shirakawa T, Li A, Dubowitz M, et al. Association between atopy and variants of the beta subunit of the high affinity immunoglobulin E receptor. Nature Genet 1994; 7:125-30.
33. Coleman R, Trembath RC, Harper JI. Chromosome 11q13 and atopy underlying atopic eczema Lancet 1993; 341:1121-2.
34. Burks AW, Mallory SB, Williams LW, et al. Atopic dermatitis: clinical relevance of food hypersensitivity reactions. J Pediatr 1988; 113:447-51.

35. Sampson HA, Albergo R. Comparison of results of skin tests, RAST, and double-blind, placebo-controlled food challenges in children with atopic dermatitis. J Allergy Clin Immunol 1984; 74:26-33.
36. Sampson HA. Role of immediate food hypersensitivity in the pathogenesis of atopic dermatitis. J Allergy Clin Immunol 1983; 71:473-80.
37. Sampson HA. The immunopathogenic role of food hypersensitivity in atopic dermatitis, Acta Derm Venereol Suppl (Stockh) 1992; 176:34-7.
38. Anderson JA. Milestones marking the knowledge of adverse reactions to food in the decade of the 1980s. Ann Allergy 1994; 72:143-54.
39. Hanifin JM. Significance of food hypersensitivity in children with atopic dermatitis. Pediatr Dermatol 1986; 3:161-74.
40. Bock SA. The natural history of food sensitivity. J Allergy Clin Immunol 1982; 69:173-7.
41. Sampson HA, Jolie PL. Increased plasma histamine concentrations after food challenges in children with atopic dermatitis. N Engl J Med 1984; 311:372-6.
42. Sampson HA, Broadbent KR, Bernhisel-Broadbent J. Spontaneous release of histamine from basophils and histamine releasing factor in patients with atopic dermatitis and food hypersensitivity. N Engl J Med 1989; 321:228-32.
43. Engman WF, Weiss R, Engman MF. Eczema and environment. Med Clin North Am 1936; 20:651-63.
44. Gleich GJ. The late phase of the immunoglobulin-E mediated reaction: A link between anaphylaxis and common allergic disease? J Allergy Clin Immunol 1982; 70:160-9.
45. Solley GO, Gleich GJ, Jordan RE, et al. The late phase of the immediate wheal and flare skin reaction. J Clin Invest 1976; 58:408-20.
46. Leung DYM, Pober JS, Cotran RS. Expression of endothelial leukocyte adhesion molecule-1 in elicited late phase allergic reactions. J Clin Invest 1991; 87:1805-9.
47. Kapp A. The role of eosinophils in the pathogenesis of atopic dermatitis: eosinophil granule proteins as markers of disease activity. Allergy 1993; 48:1-5.
48. Kay AM, Ying S, Varney V, et al. Messenger RNA expression of the cytokine gene cluster, interleukin 3 (IL-3), IL4. IL-5 and granulocyte/macrophage CSF, in allergen-induced late phase cutaneous reactions in atopic subjects. J Exp Med 1991; 173:775-8.
49. Sampson HA. The role of "allergy" in atopic dermatitis. Clin Rev Allergy 1986; 4:125-38.
50. Sampson HA. The role of food allergy and mediator release in atopic dermatitis. J Allergy Clin Immunol 1988; 81:635-45.
51. Sloper KS, Wadsworth J, Brostoff J. Children with atopic eczema. 1: clinical response to food elimination and subsequent double blind food challenge. Q J Med 1991; 292:677-93.
52. Hammar H. Provocation with cow's milk and cereals in atopic dermatitis. Acta Derm Venereol (Stockh) 1977; 57:159-63.
53. Hill DJ, Duke AM, Hosking CS, et al. Clinical manifestations of cow's milk allergy in childhood. 11: the diagnostic value of skin tests and RAST. Clin Allergy 1988; 18:481-90.
54. Webber SA, Graham-Brown RAC, Hutchinson PE, et al. Dietary manipulation in childhood atopic dermatitis. Br J Dermatol 1989; 121:91-8.

55. Atherton DJ, Soothill JF, Sewell M, et al. A double blind controlled cross over trial of an antigen avoidance diet in atopic eczema. Lancet 1978; 1 :401-3.
56. Neild VS, Marsden RA, Bailes JA, et al. Egg and milk exclusion diets in atopic eczema. Br J Dermatol 1986; 114:117-23.
57. Casimir GJA, Duchateau J, Gossart B, et al. Atopic dermatitis: role of food and house dust mite allergens. Pediatrics 1993; 92:252-6.
58. Pike G, Carter CM, Boulton P, et al. Few food diets in the treatment of atopic eczema. Arch Dis Child 1989; 64:1691-8.
59. Devlin J, David TJ, Stanton RHJ. Six food diet for childhood atopic dermatitis. Acta Derm Venereol (Stockh) 1991; 71:204.
60. Grulee CG, Sanford HN. The influence of breast and artificial feeding on infantile eczema. J Pediatr 1936; 9:223-5.
61. Kramer MS. Does breast feeding help protect against atopic disease? Biology, methodology, and a golden jubilee of controversy. J Pediatr 1988; 112:181-90.
62. Halpern SR, Sellars WA, Johnson RB, et al. Development of childhood allergy in infants fed breast, soy, or cow milk. J Allergy Clin Immunol 1973; 51:139-51.
63. Saarinen UM, Backman G, Kajosaari M, et al. Prolonged breast feeding as prophylaxis for atopic disease. Lancet 1979; 2:163-6.
64. Kajosaari M, Saarinen UM. Prophylaxis of atopic disease by six months total solid food elimination: evaluation of 135 exclusively breast fed infants of atopic families. Acta Paediatr Scand 1983; 72:411-4.
65. Halken S, Host A, Hansen LG, et al. Effect of an allergy prevention programme on incidence of atopic symptoms in infancy: a prospective study of 159 "high risk" infants. Allergy 1992; 47:545-53.
66. Gustafsson D, Lowhagen T, Andersson K. Risk of developing atopic disease after early feeding with cow's milk based formula. Arch Dis Child 1992; 67:1008-10.
67. Kay J, Gawkrodger DJ, Mortimer MJ, et al. The prevalence of childhood atopic eczema in a general population. J AM ACAD DERMATOL 1994; 30:35-9.
68. Zeiger RS, Heller S, Mellon MH, et al. Effect of combined maternal and infant food-allergen avoidance on development of atopy in early infancy: a randomized study. J Allergy Clin Immunol 1989; 84:72-89.
69. Arshad SH, Matthews S. Gant C. et al. Effect of allergen avoidance on development of allergic disorders in infancy. Lancet 1992; 339:1493-7.
70. Hide DW, Matthews S, Matthews L, et al. Effect of allergen avoidance in infancy on allergic manifestations at age 2 years. J Allergy Clin Immunol 1994; 93:842-6.
71. Tuft L, Heck MT. Studies in atopic dermatitis. IV. Importance of seasonal inhalant allergens, especially ragweed. J Allergy 1952; 23:528-40.
72. Tuft L. Importance of inhalant allergens in atopic dermatitis. J Invest Dermatol 1949; 12:211-9.
73. Bruynzeel-Koomen CAFM, Bruynzeel PLB. A role for IgE in patch test reactions to inhalant allergens in patients with atopic dermatitis. Allergy 1988; 5(suppl):15-21.
74. Van Bever HP. Recent advances in the pathogenesis of atopic dermatitis. Eur J Pediatr 1992; 151:870-3.
75. Gondo A, Saeki N, Tokuda Y. Challenge reactions in atopic dermatitis after percutaneous entry of mite antigen. Br J Dermatol 1986; 115:485-93.

76. Bruijnzeel PLB, Kuijper PHM, Kapp A, et al. The involvement of eosinophils in the patch test reaction to aeroallergens in atopic dermatitis: its relevance for the pathogenesis of atopic dermatitis. Clin Exp Allergy 1993; 23:97-109.
77. Mudde G, Van Reijsen F, Boland G, et al. Allergen presentation by epidermal Langerhans cells from patients with atopic dermatitis is mediated by IgE. Immunology 1990; 69:335-41.
78. Bieber T. IgE-binding molecules on human Langerhans cells. Acta Derm Venereol Suppl (Stockh) 1992; 176 (suppl):54-7.
79. Van der Heijden FL, Joost van Neerven RJ, van Katwijk M, et al. Serum IgE-facilitated allergen presentation in atopic disease. J Immunol 1993; 150:3643-9.
80. Van der Heijden FL, Wierenga EA, Bos JD, et al. High frequency of IL-4 producing CD4+ allergen specific T lymphocytes in atopic dermatitis lesional skin. J Invest Dermatol 1992; 97:389-94.
81. Bieber T, Braun-Falco O. IgE-bearing Langerhans cells are not specific to atopic eczema but are found in inflammatory skin diseases. J AM ACAD DERMATOL 1991; 24:658-9.
82. Haas N, Hamann K, Grabbe J, et al. Expression of the high affinity IgE receptor on human Langerhans' cells. Acta Derm Venereol (Stockh) 1992; 72:271-2.
83. Bieber T, Dannenberg B, Prinz JC, et al. Occurrence of IgE-bearing epidermal Langerhans cells in atopic eczema: a study of the time course of the lesions and with regard to the IgE serum level. J Invest Dermatol 1989; 92:215-9.
84. Castelain M, Birnbaum J, Castelain P, et al. Patch test reactions to mite antigens: a GERDA multicentre study. Contact Dermatitis 1993; 29:246-50.
85. Seidenari S, Manzini BM, Danese P, et al. Positive patch tests to whole mite culture and purified mite extracts in patients with atopic dermatitis, asthma, and rhinitis. Ann Allergy 1992; 69:201-6.
86. Clark RAF, Adinoff AD. The relationship between positive aeroallergen patch test reactions and aeroallergen exacerbations of atopic dermatitis. Clin Immunol Immunopathol 1989; 53(suppl):S132-40.
87. Reitamo S, Visa K, Kahonen K, et al. Eczematous reactions in atopic patients caused by epicutaneous testing with inhalant allergens. Br J Dermatol 1986; 114:303-9.
88. Van Voorst Vader PC, Lier JG, Woest TE, et al. Patch tests with house dust mite antigens in atopic dermatitis patients: methodological problems. Acta Derm Venereol (Stockh) 1991; 71:301-5.
89. Mitchell EB, Chapman MD, Pope FM, et al. Basophils in allergen-induced patch test sites in atopic dermatitis. Lancet 1982; 1:127-30.
90. Sasaki K, Sugiura H, Uehara M. Lymphocyte transformation test for house dust mite in atopic dermatitis. Acta Derm Venereol Suppl (Stockh) 1992; 176:49-53.
91. Van Asperen PP, Kemp AS. The natural history of IgE sensitization and atopic disease in early childhood. Acta Paediatr Scand 1989; 78:239-45.
92. Colloff MJ, Lever RS, McSharry C. A controlled trial of house dust mite eradication using natamycin in homes of patients with atopic dermatitis: effect on clinical status and mite populations. Br J Dermatol 1989; 121:199-208.
93. Roberts DLL. House dust mite avoidance and atopic dermatitis. Br J Dermatol 1984; 110:735-6.

94. Sanda T, Yasue T, Oohashi M, et al. Effectiveness of house dust mite allergen avoidance through clean room therapy in patients with atopic dermatitis. J Allergy Clin Immunol 1992; 89:653-7.

95. Beck HI, Korsgaard J. Atopic dermatitis and house dust mites. Br J Dermatol 1989; 120:245-51.

96. Warner JO, Price JF, Soothill JF, et al. Controlled trial of hyposensitization to D. pteronyssinus in children with asthma. Lancet 1978; 2:912-5.

97. Aas K. Hyposensitization in house dust allergy asthma. Acta Paediatr Scand 1986; 60:264-8.

98. Glover MT, Atherton DJ. A double-blind controlled trial of hyposensitization to Dermatophagoides pteronyssinus in children with atopic eczema Clin Exp Allergy 1992; 22:440-6.

99. Leroy BP, Boden G, Lachapelle J-M, et al. A novel therapy for atopic dermatitis with allergen-antibody complexes: a double-blind, placebo-controlled study. J AM ACAD DERMATOL 1993; 28:232-9.

100. Leyden JE, Marples RR, Kligman AM. Staphylococcus aureus in the lesions of atopic dermatitis. Br J Dermatol 1974; 90:525-30.

101. Lever R, Hadley K, Downey D, et al. Staphylococcal colonization in atopic dermatitis and the effect of topical mupirocin therapy. Br J Dermatol 1988; 119:189-98.

102. McFadden JP, Noble WC, Camp RDR. Superantigenic exotoxin-secreting potential of staphylococci isolated from atopic eczematous skin. Br J Dermatol 1993; 128:631-2.

103. Nordvall SL, Lindgren L, Johansson SGO, et al. IgE antibodies to Pityrosporum orbiculare and Staphylococcus aureus in patients with very high serum total IgE. Clin Exp Allergy 1992; 22:756-61.

104. Leung DYM, Harbeck R, Bina P, et al. Presence of IgE antibodies to staphylococcal exotoxins on the skin of patients with atopic dermatitis. J Clin Invest 1993; 92:1374-80.

105. Neuber K, Konig W. Effects of Staphylococcus aureus cell wall products (teichoic acid, peptidoglycan) and enterotoxin B on immunoglobulin (IgE, IgA, IgG) synthesis and CD23 expression in patients with atopic dermatitis. Immunology 1992; 75:23-8.

106. Schopfer K, Baerlocher K, Price P, et al. Staphylococcal IgE antibodies, hyperimmunoglobulinaemia E and Staphylococcus aureus infections. N Engl J Med 1979; 300:835-8.

107. Leung DYM. The immunologic basis of atopic dermatitis. Clin Rev Allergy 1993;11:447-68.

108. Neuber K, Konig W. Effects of the superantigen enterotoxin B on T cells from patients with atopic dermatitis [Abstract]. Allergy 1992; 12(suppl 47):145.

109. Wessels MW, Doekes G, Van Ieperen-Van Dijk AG, et al. IgE antibodies to Pityrosporum ovale in atopic dermatitis. Br J Dermatol 1991; 125:227-32.

110. Kieffer M, Bergbrant I-M, Faergemann J, et al. Immune reactions to Pityrosporum ovale in adult patients with atopic and seborrheic dermatitis. J AM ACAD DERMATOL 1990; 22:739-42.

111. Broberg AW, Faergemann J, Johansson S, et al. Pityrosporum ovale and atopic dermatitis in children and young adults. Acta Derm Venereol (Stockh) 1992; 72:187-92.

112. Waersted A, Hjorth N. Pityrosporum orbiculare: A pathogenic factor in atopic dermatitis of the face, scalp, and neck? Acta Derm Venereol Suppl (Stockh) 1985; 114:146-8.

113. Clemmensen OJ, Hjorth N. Treatment of dermatitis of the head and neck with ketoconazole in patients with type I sensitivity to Pityrosporum orbiculare. Semin Dermatol 1983; 2:26-9.

114. Strauss JS, Kligman AM. The relationship of atopic allergy and dermatitis. Arch Dermatol 1957; 75:806-11.

—by Anne R. Halbert, FACD, William L. Weston, MD, and Joseph G. Morelli, MD Denver, Colorado.

Chapter 19

All About Contact Dermatitis

About a third of the 240,000 new occupational illness cases that occur annually involve skin diseases, according to 1988 data collected by the U.S. Bureau of Labor Statistics. The total is thought to be 10 to 50 times higher than the number of documented cases because of under-diagnosis, under-reporting, and misclassification of cutaneous disease.

Contact dermatitis is the most common occupational skin disease (OSD). The results of several studies have demonstrated that more that 90 percent of cases of OSD are contact dermatitis, and the vast majority of these cases involve a hand eruption. Hand dermatitis, also referred to as hand eczema, is a rash on the hands, characterized by scaling, redness, and itching.

Environmentally-caused skin diseases are in no way limited to the workplace. Although work-related exposures to materials such as detergents, solvents, plastics, oils, and metallic compounds are often more intense, everyday exposures to jewelry, clothing, hair products, perfumes, creams, and lotions can also result in contact dermatitis.

Causes of Contact Dermatitis

About 80 percent of cases of OSD are caused by environmental irritants, and the remaining 20 percent are caused by allergic reactions. It is exceedingly difficult to determine by examination alone which

©1993 National Jewish Center for Immunology and Respiratory Medicine. Reprinted with permission.

type of reaction a patient has. Complicating diagnosis is the fact that irritating compounds can be allergenic, and allergenic compounds can be irritating. Frequent causes of occupational allergic contact dermatitis include metallic salts, germicides, plants, rubber additives, organic dyes, plastic resins, formaldehyde, and first-aid medications.

Distinguishing between irritant and allergen-induced contact dermatitis is critical to proper management, and is best done by a physician who specializes in contact dermatitis. Irritant contact dermatitis is caused by direct toxic injury to the skin, triggering a nonspecific inflammatory response. Allergic contact dermatitis is a Type IV delayed hypersensitivity reaction. On initial exposure, an allergen is processed by epidermal Langerhans antigen-presenting cells, which then present the allergen to T-helper cells. This results in the formation of specific memory and T-effector cells. The process of sensitization takes 5 to 21 days. Re-exposure to the allergen causes the activated T-cells to proliferate, which in turn leads to the release of inflammatory mediators. The mediators attract other cells, including cytotoxic T-cells, which induce cutaneous eczematous inflammation at the site of contact, usually within 48 to 72 hours after re-exposure.

The risk of OSD increases by more than 10-fold in people who are atopic, such as those with a personal or family history of hay fever, asthma, or eczema. A history of childhood eczema is the most important risk factor for developing hand dermatitis as an adult. Women are approximately twice as vulnerable to OSD as men. Another predisposing factor is preexisting skin disease. A compromised epidermal barrier caused by stasis dermatitis or xerosis, for example, enhances the absorption of irritants and allergens and thereby increases the risk of contact dermatitis. Personal hygiene also plays a role. Inadequate washing can allow irritants or allergens to remain on the skin or clothing for prolonged periods of time; over-washing causes chapping and desiccation that compromises the skin barrier.

Environmental factors can also increase a patient's risk of OSD. Hot, humid weather leads to sweating, which can enhance the penetration of particles into the skin. Cold, dry conditions can cause chapping and desiccation.

Mathias has outlined seven criteria that are useful for determining whether contact dermatitis is occupationally related. Four of these criteria should be met to judge a patient as probably having OSD:

1. The clinical eruption is consistent with contact dermatitis.

All About Contact Dermatitis

2. The patient is exposed to irritants or allergens at work.

3. The anatomic location of the eruption is consistent with the job-related exposure.

4. The onset and time course of the eruption must be consistent with OSD.

5. Non-occupational exposures are excluded as possible sources of the dermatitis.

6. The eruption should improve when exposures to the suspected agents are eliminated. This includes exposures outside of the workplace.

7. Patch testing may reveal a likely causative agent.

Irritant or Allergen?

Although people vary widely in their susceptibility, irritants will produce a reaction in most individuals when applied in sufficient concentration for an adequate length of time. However, there is no reliable skin test for confirming an irritant reaction. Diagnosis depends on correlating an exposure history to a known irritant with the clinical appearance, distribution, and course of the dermatitis.

Irritant contact dermatitis is divided into two types: acute toxic and chronic cumulative reactions. Acute toxic reactions result from a single exposure to a strong chemical, usually appearing within minutes or hours. The skin usually heals soon after the exposure.

Chronic cumulative reactions are more common and may take weeks, months, or even years to appear. These reactions are often difficult to distinguish from chronic allergic contact dermatitis.

In contrast to irritant-induced disease, allergic contact dermatitis typically affects only a few individuals in a work place. The classic allergic response resembles poison ivy dermatitis, featuring erythema, edema, vesicle formation, and pruritus. Chronic allergic contact dermatitis and irritant reactions may both have erythema, scaling, crusting, excoriations, and lichenification. Mixed allergic and irritant reactions are also possible.

Identifying a non-occupational cause of contact dermatitis can be difficult because patients come in contact with so many materials during daily life. However, the location of the reaction often provides

Skin Disorders Sourcebook

an important clue about the cause. For example, a rash on an earlobe suggests a reaction to an earring. Dermatitis on the face may indicate that a perfume, cosmetic, or cream is the culprit. A reaction along the hair line points to a hair-care product.

Patch Testing

Patch testing is the only reliable method for diagnosing allergic contact dermatitis. The most widely used patch test is the Finn chamber method, which uses a multi-well, aluminum patch. A small amount of each allergen being tested is placed into a well, and the patch is then taped to the upper back of the patient. The patch is removed after 48 hours and an initial reading is recorded. A second reading is made a few days later. The optimal time for the second reading is 96 hours after the patch was first applied.

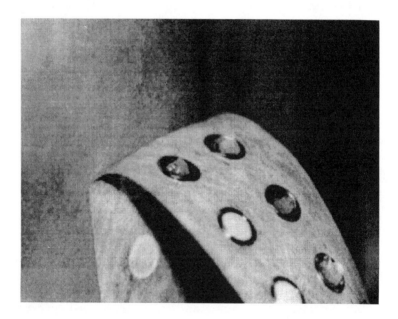

Figure 19.1. *The Finn chamber method is the most widely used patch test procedure. Small amounts of the allergen, usually in a petrolatum vehicle, are placed in the aluminum wells which are affixed to a strip of paper tape. Drops of liquid allergens are placed on filter paper discs that are placed inside the aluminum well. The upper back is the preferred testing site*

The classic, strongly positive allergic reaction to the patch test consists of erythema, edema, and closely set vesicles that persist after patch removal or may appear after two to seven days. In contrast, irritant reactions have a glazed, scalded, follicular, pustular, or bullous appearance that usually fades rapidly after patch removal. Distinguishing allergic and irritant reactions must be done carefully because the allergenic concentration of a compound may be close to the substance's irritant concentration. The patch test result must always be interpreted in the context of the patient's history and clinical presentation.

Prognosis

In general, people who develop OSD do not have a good prognosis. One study found that 75 percent of patients with OSD had either persistent or periodic dermatitis, while only 25 percent had complete clearing. Once dermatitis persists beyond the acute stage and becomes chronic it usually remains despite the best therapeutic efforts. Chronic inflammation tends to produce more permanent changes in the skin that are often difficult to resolve. For this reason, it is critical that acute contact dermatitis receives prompt evaluation and treatment.

Allergic contact dermatitis may also persist even if the primary triggering substance is eliminated because of continued exposures to other materials that contain similar, cross-reacting compounds. This possibility underscores the need for counseling the patient about the range of materials that must be avoided to resolve the allergic contact dermatitis.

Patients with contact dermatitis may also become secondarily sensitized to preservatives that are contained in the topical steroids and moisturizers that physicians use to treat contact dermatitis. Other allergens that may exacerbate dermatitis include those contained in protective gloves, waterless hand cleansers, first-aid drugs, and barrier creams.

Treatment and Prevention

The key to treatment is removing the allergen and as many irritants as possible from the patient's work and home environment. An effort should be made to replace allergens with similar, non-sensitizing agents. Patients are instructed to avoid frequent hand-washing with soap and water; mild waterless cleansers may provide an alternative. Gloves are useful to protect the hands, and many types are available.

The treatment of choice includes moisturizers and topical steroids. Topical treatments that contain the least sensitizing ingredients should be selected for high-risk patients to avoid a secondary sensitization. Systemic steroids should be reserved for acute, severe reactions, and should never be used for chronic skin eruptions.

Prevention is preferable to treatment for individuals with a history of contact dermatitis. Wet work should be avoided. Protective clothing should be used whenever possible. Selecting the right glove material is also important. A poor choice can actually exacerbate a dermatitis by allowing the allergen or irritant to penetrate the glove and be trapped against the skin.

The following two case histories exemplify the strategies used in diagnosing and managing allergic contact dermatitis:

Case 1:

A 37-year-old woman employed as a phlebotomist presented to National Jewish with a chronic hand rash. She had a history of atopic dermatitis during her childhood. Previous physicians had linked her rash to her history of eczema and current exposure to irritants. The patient had some improvement by decreasing irritant exposure, using topical steroids and moisturizers, and wearing vinyl gloves with cotton liners. However, her rash never completely resolved.

At her initial examination at National Jewish, the patient had bilateral scaly and hyper-pigmented plaques involving her central palms. Scaling also existed on her fingers. To decrease her hand washing with soap and water, the patient had been using antimicrobial wipes to clean her hands during work. Patch testing revealed that the patient reacted to parachlorometaxylenol (PCMX), the principal preservative in the wipes. A cross-reacting preservative, chlorocresol, was contained in the antiseptic soap that she occasionally used at work. After the patient discontinued her contact with PCMX and chlorocresol her hand eczema showed marked improvement.

Case 2:

A 33-year-old man presented to National Jewish with a one-year history of a rash on his hand, arm, and calf. The patient worked as a machinist, and had frequent exposure to industrial oils. Previous physicians had treated the patient with topical steroids and a moisturizing lotion.

Extensive patch testing revealed that the patient was allergic to Quaternium 15, an antimicrobial agent that was added to the oils used at the patient's work place. Quaternium 15 was also the primary preservative in the moisturizing lotion that the patient had been using.

Because Quaternium 15 is a formaldehyde-releasing preservative, we instructed the patient to avoid other formaldehyde-releasing compounds, such as Bronopol and Diazolidinyl urea. The patient's employer began using an alternative antimicrobial additive, and we switched the patient's moisturizing lotion. His rashes subsequently cleared.

References

1. Mathias CGT. Contact dermatitis and worker's compensation: criteria for establishing occupational causation and aggravation. *J Am Acad Dermatol* 1989; 20:842-48.

Additional Reading

1. Stewart LA. Occupational contact dermatitis. Immunol Aller Clin North Amer 1992; 12:831-46.
2. Hogan DJ, Dannaker CJ, Malbach HI. Contact dermatitis: prognosis, risk factors, and rehabilitation. Semin Dermatol 1990; 9:233-46.

—by Leslie Stewart, M.D.

Leslie Stewart, M.D. is Head, Division of Dermatology, Occupational and Contact Dermatitis Center, National Jewish Assistant Professor, Department of Dermatology, University of Colorado School of Medicine.

Chapter 20

The Itch of the Great Outdoors

On these hot summer days, when the realization dawns that the tiny blisters on legs or arms or wherever can only have come from a brush with poison ivy, there may be some small comfort in knowing that you are not alone. Most Americans are sensitive in some degree to this ubiquitous three-leafed plant. Only about 15 percent of the population is not affected.

Poison ivy and its cousins, poison oak and poison sumac, are responsible for more of those itchy, oozing blisters (a condition known medically as allergic contact dermatitis) than any other cause, including industrial chemicals, household products, and cosmetics. While it may be only a summer annoyance for some, for others poison ivy dermatitis can be disabling and is responsible for a considerable amount of time lost from work. Firefighters are particularly vulnerable. They not only come in contact with the plants themselves, but are exposed to smoke carrying plant particles, which when inhaled can have severe internal as well as external effects.

Despite the toll it takes in discomfort and disability, no one has come up with a way—other than avoidance—to prevent or cure this condition known simply as "poison ivy."

What causes those familiar itching blisters is a chemical called urushiol (pronounced oo r 'shee ohl). Urushiol is found in the resin, or sap, that is carried in canals within the bark, stem, leaflets, and

---

FDA Consumer, June 1986. See *Omnigraphics' Allergies Sourcebook* for a more complete discussion of poison ivy, oak, and sumac treatments, identification, avoidance and eradication.

certain flower parts of the plants. Since these canals do not connect with the plant's surface, the plant has to be broken or crushed before it can do its itchy work.

Surprising as it may seem, brushing against an intact plant will not cause a reaction. In fact, you could have a garden full of poison ivy and not get a single blister—provided, of course, the plants were undisturbed. However, what may look like an intact plant may not be, for insects chewing on the plants can cause breaks in the surface, releasing the sap.

On the other hand, you don't have to come in contact with a plant to develop dermatitis. Urushiol is sticky and can be carried on the fur of animals (they are not sensitive to it) and on garden tools, golf balls, and other objects that have come in contact with a broken plant. Touching these objects can transfer the urushiol and lead to a reaction. Once in contact with the skin, the urushiol begins to penetrate in a matter of minutes. In about 12 to 48 hours there is a visible reaction on the skin as the body marshals its forces to combat the invader. First, there is redness and swelling, followed by blisters. Itching is inevitable.

In a few days the blisters become crusted and then begin to scale. If there are no complications, such as an infection due to scratching, the dermatitis clears up in about 10 days.

One of the many myths about poison ivy dermatitis is that it can be spread from one part of the body to another, or even to other people, via the oozing material in the blisters. Not so. The blisters contain not urushiol but a fluid from the clear portion of the blood, produced as part of the body's reaction to the urushiol. This fluid cannot spread the dermatitis. The victim does the spreading before the blisters have formed, while there is still urushiol on the skin. Urushiol on the hands can be carried to other parts of the body, for instance by scratching the nose or wiping the forehead. While poison ivy dermatitis usually occurs on exposed areas of the skin, it can crop up in unlikely places, such as under clothing, thanks to this self-spreading.

Spreading the dermatitis from person to person can only occur if one person comes in contact with the urushiol on the other's body or clothing.

Sensitivity to poison ivy is not something people are born with. It develops after several encounters with the plants, sometimes over many years. Once a person has become sensitive to poison ivy, he or she is sensitive to all of the "poison" type plants. Contact with the sticky urushiol can cause almost any part of the body to break out

The Itch of the Great Outdoors

with the characteristic linear (in a line) rash. The soles of the feet and the palms of the hands are less sensitive, while areas where the skin is thinner are more sensitive to the ivy sap. The severity of the dermatitis may also depend on how big a dose of urushiol the person got. Other allergies a person may have play no part in poison ivy dermatitis.

Start Treatment Immediately

If you suspect you've gotten into poison ivy, the first thing to do is to thoroughly wash the exposed areas. Washing may not stop the initial outbreak of the rash if too much time has elapsed, but it can help prevent further spread.

Harold Baer, an FDA expert on poison ivy, advises washing with soap. The sap of the ivy and oak plants is very sticky and not very water soluble. Soap helps to break it down so that it can be removed, Baer says. Myth has it that a strong yellow soap is required. Not so, according to Baer. Any soap will do.

Clothing that has picked up the sticky sap should also be washed as soon as possible. Be sure to handle it carefully, with gloves, if necessary, to prevent any more exposure to the sap.

Considering that poison ivy has been recorded since the days of Captain John Smith, it is not surprising that a wealth of home remedies has evolved to treat this dermatitis. Not the least creative—though hardly to be recommended—are bathing in horse urine, cleaning the skin with gasoline or strychnine, and rubbing on a variety of products such as ammonia, hair spray, clear nail polish, meat tenderizer, or mouse-ear herb boiled in milk. The juice of crushed leaves of plantain, a common weed found in many yards, is favored by many hikers today. There is no scientific proof that it works.

When all is said and done, the simplest treatment is still the best. Mild cases of poison ivy may require no more than wet compresses or soaking in cool water to relieve the itching. Dilute aluminum acetate (Burrows solution), saline (salt), or sodium bicarbonate (baking soda) solutions are often recommended to dry up the oozing blisters.

Oatmeal is a drying agent as well as a cereal. You can buy an oatmeal preparation (*Aveeno*) for use in a bath or make your own by tying up about half a cupful of uncooked oatmeal in a clean cloth, such as a large handkerchief, and soaking it in water. Squeezing releases an oatmeally solution that will help dry up oozing blisters. Be warned, however, that it is messy and can make the tub extra slippery.

A variety of nonprescription drug products is also available to dry up the oozing and weeping blisters. Among the skin protectant ingredients FDA's expert advisors say are safe and effective are aluminum hydroxide gel, calamine, kaolin, zinc acetate, zinc carbonate, and zinc oxide. These ingredients were given the green light by the Advisory Review Panel on OTC Topical Analgesic, Antirheumatic, Otic, Burn, and Sunburn Prevention and Treatment Drug Products, one of 17 panels of outside experts assisting FDA in its massive review of all OTC (over-the-counter) drug products.

The same panel recommended, and FDA has concurred, that hydrocortisone preparations—hydrocortisone 0.25 and 0.5 percent and hydrocortisone acetate 0.25 and 0.5 percent—be used for the temporary relief of itching associated with poison ivy, poison oak, or poison sumac.

Other external analgesics considered by the panel and FDA as safe and effective to relieve itching associated with minor skin irritations include "caine"-type local anesthetics, such as benzocaine, lidocaine or tetracaine; alcohols, including benzyl alcohol, menthol and resorcinol; and the antihistamines diphenhydramine hydrochloride and tripelennamine hydrochloride. (Final standards for skin protectant and external analgesic drug products are under consideration by FDA.)

All these OTC drug products are intended only for the treatment of minor symptoms of poison ivy and should not be used for more than seven days. Some ingredients should not be used over large areas of the body or on raw surfaces or blistered areas and therefore would not be good for poison ivy blisters. A few ingredients are not recommended for use on young children without consulting a doctor. Always check the label of OTC drug products for specific instructions for use.

Severe poison ivy dermatitis should be treated by a doctor, who may prescribe a stronger topical steroid preparation or oral medication to be used for several days. Because side effects can be serious, such treatment is not given lightly.

Preventing poison ivy miseries should be easy—just stay away from plants. However, this is not always possible for those whose work takes them into the woods and fields where the oak and ivy grow. Unfortunately, there are no OTC products that can prevent poison ivy, oak or sumac dermatitis, according to the Advisory Review Panel on OTC Miscellaneous External Drug Products.

Another approach to preventing, or at least lessening, the consequences of poison ivy is desensitization with extracts of the plant itself. American Indians are said to have eaten poison ivy leaves for protection against the sap. This is not a practice to be recommended, however, for a nasty side effect is dermatitis at both ends of the gastrointestinal tract—the mouth and the anus. (The middle portion seems to be immune to these effects.)

Researchers at the University of California, San Francisco, are working on a potential vaccine. They claim to have found a way to neutralize the urushiol molecules, thus eliminating the itching. More testing is needed to see if the vaccine is truly safe and effective.

Because of severe reactions, injections with plant extracts (called **oleoresins**) to prevent poison ivy are not recommended, FDA noted in a proposal to establish standards for allergenic products. The proposal was based on the recommendations of the Advisory Panel on Review of Allergenic Extracts. The agency also said no injectable or oral oleoresins should be given once dermatitis has developed, because severe local or systemic reactions may occur.

There is good evidence that oral oleoresins can reduce the severity of the dermatitis—but not prevent it entirely—if the dose is strong enough and it is given for long enough before contact with the plant, said FDA. It is important that the doctor adjust the dose in response to the patient's reactions to the plant material. Sensitivity to the poison plants returns when the treatment is stopped. Currently available products in both liquid and tablet form are safe enough to remain on the market, but FDA recommended further tests to establish effectiveness.

A number of skin tests to confirm a diagnosis of poison ivy dermatitis are available. However, FDA has recommended that additional studies are needed to standardize these products.

A two-stage patch test to determine who is sensitive to poison ivy is being developed by the Forest Service of the U.S. Department of the Interior, to aid in assigning firefighters. The more sensitive people can be assigned to areas where there is less chance of exposure to the plants.

Until effective vaccines are available, the bottom line still remains—if you want to prevent poison ivy dermatitis, avoid the offending plants. Learn to recognize them in all seasons. If you're going to be in areas where they are likely to lurk, protect yourself by wearing long pants and long sleeves.

As soon as you realize that you have been in contact with poison ivy, oak or sumac, thoroughly wash all exposed areas of skin. Launder your clothes and wipe off footwear, tools and other items that may have been in contact with the sap as soon as possible.

Summertime doesn't have to be spoiled by poison ivy itches if you stay alert.

Know Thine Enemy

That old saying, "Leaflets three, let it be," is a good rule of thumb for anyone who wants to avoid the miseries of poison ivy dermatitis. The best way to identify poison ivy and poison oak is to look for the characteristic three leaves. However, there are variations depending on where the plants are growing. One or the other of these plants is found in every part of the United States except some desert areas of Nevada. They are also found in Canada and parts of Mexico, South America and the West Indies, but not in Europe. Poison ivy grows throughout the United States except in the extreme Southwest. It can be a woody, rope-like vine, a trailing shrub on the ground, or a free-standing shrub. Its leaves are green in the summer and red in the fall. Small greenish-white to cream-colored flowers appear after the leaves open in the spring. The fruit ripens into tan to yellowish berries. Eastern poison ivy leaves have smooth margins; those in the central states have notches or teeth on the leaflets. From Oklahoma to Texas, poison ivy plants have a deep, acute lobe (a so-called thumb) on—either side of the end leaflet and on the outer edge of the other two. Those from the Rio Grande basin may look like the club in a deck of playing cards.

Eastern poison oak is a low shrub found from New Jersey to eastern Texas. It grows on poor sandy soils where poison ivy generally does not. The center leaf of the three looks like an oak leaf.

Western poison oak grows on the Pacific coast from southern California to Canada in several forms: As an upright shrub it can grow into large spreading clumps six feet tall; in forests it can be a vine up to 30 feet tall. The three leaflets are irregularly lobed and resemble oak leaves.

Poison sumac is a tall rangy shrub that may reach a height of 15 feet. The bright green leaflets have no teeth on their edges, while the leaves of the nonpoisonous sumac do. The fruits are glossy pale yellow or cream colored and hang down when they are ripe. Nonpoisonous sumac fruit is red and stands erect. Poison sumac grows in damp, swampy areas, particularly east of the Mississippi River.

All of these poisonous plants are members of the Anacardiaceae family, which includes the mango, lacquer tree, and cashew nut tree. A person who is sensitive to poison ivy, oak and sumac will be sensitive to these plants as well.

The Itch of the Great Outdoors

Poison ivy, oak and sumac are most dangerous in the spring and summer, when there is plenty of sap, the urushiol content is high, and the plants are easily bruised.

Poison ivy dermatitis is generally regarded as a summer complaint, but it can be contracted in the winter when the planes are dormant, too. Cases have been reported in individuals who cut wood for the fireplace or used the vine in Christmas wreaths

If you have poison ivy in your garden and want to get rid of it, don't burn it. Plant parts can be transported in the smoke from burning plants to affect the unwary gardener. It is better to dispose of unwanted plants in sealed plastic bags or kill them with a herbicide and then bury them.

—by Annabel Hecht

Annabel Hecht is a member of FDA's public affairs staff.

Chapter 21

Living with Epidermolysis Bullosa

This chapter describes a group of genetic blistering diseases of the skin that are collectively referred to as epidermolysis bullosa or EB. It has been written for patients, their families and friends, and health professionals to explain briefly what we know about these disorders.

In addition to outlining various approaches to treatment, this chapter reviews current research in EB and related areas—research that ultimately will lead to control and possibly prevention of these distressing afflictions.

What Is Epidermolysis Bullosa?

Epidermolysis bullosa, or "EB," is a group of disorders that involve the skin and mucous membranes. The common feature of these disorders is the formation of blisters following mild injury.

According to the Dystrophic Epidermolysis Bullosa Research Association of America (DEBRA), an estimated 25,000 to 50,000 Americans have some form of EB.

Many people get blisters on their hands and feet from time to time following friction, friction that comes from the continued rubbing of skin against a hard object or surface. People with EB, however, get blisters much more easily and in much greater numbers. In severe EB, blisters seem to form without any apparent friction at all; they

---

NIH Publication No. 84-663. Prepared by the Office of Health Research reports, National Institute of Arthritis, Diabetes and Digestive and Kidney Diseases.

can even form inside the mouth, pharynx, esophagus, stomach, intestines, and respiratory and genitourinary tracts. Severe EB wounds resemble serious burns, but EB injuries keep recurring.

What Forms Does EB Take?

Although there is a non-inherited form of EB that can be acquired in adolescence or adulthood, this chapter primarily discusses inherited forms of EB, which range from mild to severe and can require major adjustments in the lifestyle of both the EB patient and his or her family.

The different types of EB are defined according to whether the blisters heal with or without scarring, the way the disease is inherited, the appearance of tissues under a microscope, and the possible underlying causes.

Each type of EB presents somewhat different symptoms and affects the patient's day-to-day living in different ways. In some instances, the right adjustments can allow the child to have a lifestyle that in many ways will not differ dramatically from that of unaffected children. In other cases, the disorder is more complex and the child's life can be seriously altered. The characteristics of the major inherited forms of EB will be described in the sections that follow.

Non-scarring Forms of EB

Epidermolysis Bullosa Simplex - Generalized

Generalized epidermolysis bullosa simplex is inherited as an autosomal dominant disease (inheritance of EB is explained later in this chapter). This form of EB has the following characteristics:

- It is usually present at birth or infancy.

- Blisters are widespread over the body's surface, occur after pressure or injury to skin, and heal without scarring.

- There may be mild involvement of mucous membranes; fingernails and toenails are sometimes involved.

- It tends to improve as the child grows older.

Epidermolysis Bullosa Simplex - Localized

Localized EB simplex also may be called Weber-Cockayne disease or recurrent bullous eruption of the hands and feet. Inheritance is autosomal dominant. This type is described as follows:

- It usually develops in childhood or adolescence, although it can occur in an infant or in adult life.

- Blisters occur almost exclusively on hands and feet and heal without permanent scarring

- There is no involvement of nails or mucous membranes.

- A greater amount of friction is needed to cause blistering than in generalized EB simplex. Some people get blisters only in hot weather.

Junctional Epidermolysis Bullosa

Junctional EB has also been called Herlitz disease, EB letalis, and junctional bullous epidermatosis. It is recessively inherited and appears in two forms, mild and severe. In junctional epidermolysis bullosa:

- Blistering is present at birth, seems to occur spontaneously, and results in large, ulcerated areas of the trunk and legs. Although the disorder is considered non-scarring, thinning and tightening of the skin does occur.

- The infant may die because of profound loss of fluid, overwhelming infection or complications resulting from blistering in the gastrointestinal, respiratory or genito-urinary tract. Some babies with junctional EB have been observed to have pyloric atresia, a closing of the opening between the stomach and the intestines that causes obstruction.

- If the baby survives the first year or so, the disease may lessen in severity.

Scarring Forms of EB

Dominant Dystrophic Epidermolysis Bullosa

This form of EB, which is an autosomal dominant condition, has the following characteristics:

- It is usually present at birth or early infancy.

- Blistering may be generalized or appear only on hands, feet, elbows, or knees; this is usually due to mechanical trauma.

- Rarely does scarring cause immobility and deformity of the hands and feet.

- There is mild involvement of the mucous membranes; nails are often thickened, malformed, or destroyed.

Another type, the albopapuloid form of dominant dystrophic EB, usually begins later in life. It is characterized by the presence of small, firm skin elevations (papules) on the trunk.

Recessive Dystrophic Epidermolysis Bullosa

This form of epidermolysis bullosa, abbreviated RDEB, is autosomal recessive. In some cases there is relatively mild blistering on hands, feet, elbows, and knees; these cases are very similar to dominant dystrophic EB. However, recessive dystrophic epidermolysis bullosa typically is characterized as follows:

- Onset is at birth or soon afterwards.

- In some cases, nearly all skin surfaces and mucous membranes (from mouth to anus) are covered by blisters. Large areas may be devoid of skin. There is widespread scarring and deformity.

- Fingers and toes may become immobile. With recurrent scarring, fingers and/or toes may fuse together.

- Hands and arms may become fixed in a flexed position with resulting contractures.

Living with Epidermolysis Bullosa

- There is difficulty swallowing; the esophagus can become scarred and interfere with passage of food into the stomach.

- Anemia and chronic malnutrition may develop; weight gain and development often are retarded.

- There is usually loss of the nails of the fingers and toes.

- Teeth may be malformed and delayed in appearing through the gums. Because routine dental care can raise blisters, many persons with RDEB have a higher than normal incidence of cavities.

- Involvement of the eyes can include eyelid inflammation with adhesions to the eyeball, as well as inflammation of the cornea or the conjunctiva (the mucous membrane covering the eyeball and the underside of the lids).

How Is Epidermolysis Bullosa Inherited?

To understand the genetics of EB, it is useful to review some general information about heredity.

The biological units of heredity are called genes. Each of us has two copies of each gene, one inherited from our mother and the other from our father. Every person has thousands of genes that interact to determine his or her traits.

Genes are strung together like beads to form thin, rod-like structures called chromosomes. Humans have 46 chromosomes in the nucleus of every cell. Each chromosome is a member of a pair, which means there are 23 pairs of chromosomes, with each member of each pair inherited from each parent. One of the 23 chromosomes from the mother is always an "X" chromosome and one from the father is either an "X," if the child is to be female, or a "Y" if male. If a gene on the X or Y chromosome causes a disorder, it is called a sex-linked disorder. If genes on the other 44 chromosomes cause a disorder, it is called an autosomal disorder, and it tends to affect males and females equally. All forms of EB are autosomally inherited.

Autosomal Dominant Inheritance

An autosomal dominant disorder is one in which the gene for the condition "dominates" and expresses itself in an individual, irrespective of the other normal gene it is paired with. A parent with an autosomal dominant form of EB has a 50:50 chance of transmitting the abnormal gene to each child. The chance is the same whether the child is a boy or a girl, and birth order does not make a difference. A child who does not inherit the gene for EB from an affected parent will not have the condition and cannot pass it on.

In some instances, neither parent has EB, but the couple has a child with an autosomal dominant form of EB. In this situation, the condition has been caused by a change, or mutation, that has occurred in the genetic material of the egg or the sperm that made the child. When a new mutation occurs, the person with it will have a 50:50 risk of passing the gene on, but his or her parents will not. They have no increased risk of having a child with EB in subsequent pregnancies.

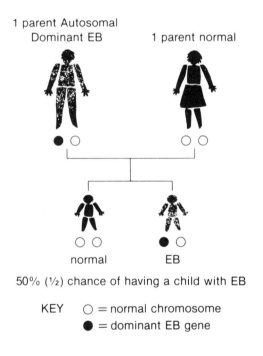

Figure 21.1. Autosomal Dominant Inheritance

Living with Epidermolysis Bullosa

Autosomal Recessive Inheritance

In the autosomal recessive forms of EB, the gene for EB must be paired with another gene for EB for the disease to be expressed in the child. If a person has one recessive EB gene paired with a normal gene, the person is a "carrier," but does not have the disorder. If a carrier marries a person whose two corresponding genes are normal, there is no chance that their children will inherit EB (although for each child there is a 50:50 chance they will carry the gene). If two carriers marry, however, there is a 25 percent chance that both may pass on the recessive EB gene to each child. Again, the sex of the child and the birth order do not matter. An individual with a recessive form of EB will have affected children only if he or she marries a carrier or another person with recessive EB.

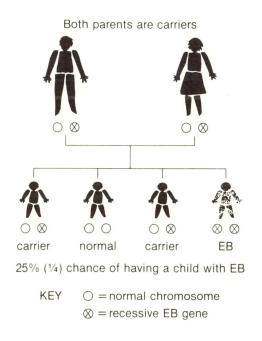

Figure 21.2. Autosomal Recessive Inheritance

It is important to recognize that the percentages given above mean odds. For example, if the first child of two carriers for recessive EB develops the disorder, the odds are still 25 percent that the next child could be born with it.

At this time, no test is available to determine whether a person is a carrier of recessive EB, although researchers are studying this important area.

Prenatal Detection and Diagnosis of EB

Although there are a number of techniques in use for "examining" the baby in the womb, only fetoscopy has been useful in research on prenatal diagnosis of junctional and recessive dystrophic EB. In fetoscopy, a delicate viewing instrument is inserted directly into the uterus to observe the fetus and take blood samples and skin biopsies. This method is experimental and is only available at a few major medical centers.

Fetoscopy should not be confused with amniocentesis, one of the most promising and best-known prenatal diagnostic techniques for certain congenital disorders. In this method, a sample of the fluid surrounding the fetus is withdrawn and analyzed. At present, EB cannot be positively diagnosed by amniocentesis; however, this technique is currently under study.

Genetic Counseling

Genetic counseling provides and interprets medical information based on expanding knowledge of human genetics. A genetic counselor will work with a couple to review their family history and explore the likelihood of recurrence of EB in subsequent children or relatives. Often the genetic counselor is a physician who will participate in the diagnosis, examine family members and provide ongoing medical care. In other instances, a geneticist (someone with an advanced degree in human genetics) may work with the child's pediatrician, dermatologist, or primary physician. The counselor, perhaps with close family advisors, such as a minister, priest or rabbi, can help a family make informed decisions about childbearing and help them cope with the impact of a genetic disorder. Genetic counselors and social workers often work together to ensure that patients and families receive all the services and benefits to which they are entitled.

How is EB Treated?

Because EB involves many systems of the body, parents and health professionals must take a "team approach" to the treatment of an EB patient. Intense and total patient care often must be provided, particularly for young and growing children. The severe forms of EB require hours of intensive nursing care that in many ways is similar to that given to burn patients. Much of this care is often provided by the parents; however, the education of all people who have contact with the patient is essential. These people may include: the primary care physician (often a pediatrician), the dermatologist, the nurse, the pediatric dentist, the specialist in gastrointestinal (digestive) diseases, the dietitian or nutritionist, the plastic surgeon, the psychologist or social worker, and the genetic counselor, as well as teachers, relatives and baby sitters, and others.

So far, research has not yet found a cure for epidermolysis bullosa or a treatment to completely control any form of EB. However, many complications can be lessened or avoided through early intervention. Many persons with milder forms have minimal symptoms and may require little or no treatment.

In all cases, treatment of EB is directed toward the symptoms and is largely supportive. This care should focus on prevention of infection, protection of the skin against trauma, attention to nutritional deficiencies and dietary complications, minimization of deformities and contractures, and the need for psychological support for the entire family.

In just the past few years, a commonly used drug has been found that can reduce blistering in the recessive dystrophic form of epidermolysis bullosa. This drug is phenytoin (Dilantin®). In some patients with RDEB, it has been shown to reduce blistering by 40 percent or more. Phenytoin and potential new EB drugs are discussed in the section on research.

The pharmaceutical industry is attempting to develop more effective dressings that will not only speed up healing, but also reduce pain and discomfort. Some of these dressings have been used successfully with burn patients and are being evaluated for use in EB.

Supportive Care

The following list of suggested methods of care has been compiled from several sources and addresses all forms of EB. Because each suggestion may not pertain to every form of EB, discretion and experimentation will guide the parents and the physician in choosing those methods that apply.

Prevention of Infection

Any raw area on the skin or mucous membranes is a potential site for infection. The best way to prevent infection is to keep the area scrupulously clean. Antibacterial soaps, antibiotic creams, wet soaks (described below), and good hand-washing techniques help to reduce the risk of infection.

Inflammation. Inflammation can be relieved through the use of "wet soaks." These are dressings made from a soft, clean handkerchief, white sheeting or diaper material that has been soaked in cool tap water, saline solution (two teaspoons of table salt per quart of water), or Burrow's solution. In the latter case, the most practical method is to dissolve prepared powders or tablets in cool tap water. The inflamed skin is covered with wet dressings for 10 to 15 minutes. This helps to dry the blisters, remove crusts, and minimize the risk of infection. This procedure can be repeated two to three times a day, or as directed by a doctor. Topical steroids are useful to reduce the inflammation, but should be used sparingly and only with a doctor's advice.

Itching. This is a common problem, and infection may occur as a result of scratching. In moderate and severe cases a mild sedative or oral antihistamine may be prescribed to help allay itching.

Skin Care and Bandaging

The purposes of good skin care and bandaging are to reduce the incidence of infection, assist healing of involved areas, and serve as a protective cushioning against friction. The best times for skin and dressing changes are following a bath, after a lesion has been cleansed, or before bedtime.

Guidelines for cleansing and bandaging for localized simplex and dystrophic EB.

1. Always wash hands before starting.

Living with Epidermolysis Bullosa

2. Release fluid in blisters by cutting a small slit on the side of the blister using a sterile scissor or scalpel blade. Many people prefer to puncture the blister in several places with a sterile needle. Do not remove the roof of the blister or the skin surrounding it.

3. To help drain the fluid and dry the blister, wet soaks can be placed over the slit or punctured blister for 10 to 15 minutes. Whenever possible, this should be repeated two or three times a day.

4. If prescribed by the doctor, an antibiotic cream may be applied.

5. In milder or localized EB, it is preferable to leave the area open to the air. If desired, a non-adherent dressing can be placed over an oozing wound. NEVER apply tape directly to the skin.

Guidelines for cleansing and bandaging generalized simplex and dystrophic EB.

1. Always wash hands before starting

2. Do not pull off any soiled dressings or clothing that may be sticking to the skin. Soak off in warm water. The physician may suggest adding an antibacterial agent to the water.

3. Release fluid in blisters using method described above. Drain the fluid.

4. Place clean gauze pads or wet soaks over the wound to drain.

5. Apply prescribed antibiotic cream to any open areas.

6. Non-adherent dressings or other dressing recommended by the doctor can be placed over the open areas. A soft, rolled type of gauze or netting can be used to secure the dressings in place. Loose ends can be secured with paper tape. NEVER apply tape directly to the skin.

Protection of the Skin

In EB, even slight friction can produce blisters, so minimal and gentle handling is absolutely necessary. A cool environment, avoidance of overheating, and skin lubrication to reduce friction can help lessen blister formation. A water or air mattress padded with foam may help reduce friction, as will a soft fleece covering or percale sheet placed over the mattress. Sheepskin is excellent for padding car seats, infant seats, or other hard surfaces. The young child with moderate or severe EB should never be picked up under the arms, but should be lifted from the bottom and carried on soft, nonirritating material.

Clothing must be made of soft, nonirritating fabric, easy to put on, and simple in design. Socks and mittens can be used to prevent the infant from rubbing his hands and feet and scratching his face. It may not be advisable to use a diaper on a baby with severe EB; instead a pad can be placed under the buttocks and the diaper area left uncovered. When a diaper is used, the area must be kept dry and clean.

Health Care Problems

The following material describes a variety of problems that can be associated with EB. It is important to bear in mind, however, that not all of these problems occur in each EB patient. Some will have none or a few; others may have nearly all of these.

Nutritional Concerns

Good nutrition is essential for all children, but may be more difficult to achieve for a child with a chronic disease such as epidermolysis bullosa.

Nutritional research on EB is in an early stage. However, knowledge gained from working with people with similar conditions, such as skin ulcers or burns, can be helpful for people with EB. Patients with skin ulcers or burns need increased protein and calories. Thus, a person with EB also may need to increase both calories and protein, depending on the severity of the disease. These extra nutritional demands on the body are due to tissue regeneration, fluid replacement and protein loss associated with blistering.

Attention to the nutrition of the child may be important from the beginning. Immediately after birth, fluid and protein loss, which may cause chemical imbalances, can be a major complication in recessive and some dominant types of EB. Unless the baby requires isolation for medical reasons, closeness of the mother and child should be encouraged and will help make early feedings successful. Oral or breast feedings can begin as soon as the sucking reflex is demonstrated, unless the doctor indicates otherwise. If the infant has difficulty sucking because of blisters in the mouth, use a preemie nipple (a soft nipple having holes large enough to permit milk to drop into the mouth), a rubber-tipped medicine dropper or a syringe. Powdered nutritional amplifiers, which can add calories and protein, are now available that can be mixed with the mother's milk, and there are formulas that have higher than average calorie and protein concentrations. Follow the physician and/or dietitian's instructions in the use of such products and in the selection of an appropriate formula.

When the child is about six months old and pureed food has been introduced, it can be helpful to add extra liquid to the pureed food to facilitate swallowing in those who have mouth blisters. Hot drinks or foods can be irritating; if so, beverages and foods should be served lukewarm, at room temperature, or cold.

Dysphagia (difficulty in swallowing) can be a major complication, as EB can cause blistering in the mouth and/or the esophagus. A parent should watch when hard-crusted foods such as toast or crackers are introduced in the child's diet to see if they provoke blistering or a problem when swallowing. Acidic foods and drinks can also be irritating when an ulcer in the mouth is active; therefore, tomatoes and citrus juices may need to be avoided. If the child can tolerate milk, whole milk can be enriched by adding an "instant breakfast" mix or flavorings. A "fortified milk" can be prepared by adding nonfat dry milk powder to whole milk. "Fortified" milk can be served plain, flavors added or used to make sauces, cream soups, hot cereals, mashed potatoes, milkshakes, custards, puddings, and cocoa; it can be used in any recipe calling for milk to add extra calories and protein. If milk is not tolerated, liquid nutritional supplements may be recommended. These can be purchased at a pharmacy upon advice of a physician and/or dietitian. Most liquid supplements can be used in recipes such as custards, puddings, and soups and are available in a variety of flavors. It is wise to interchange products and flavors to offer variety so the child will not become bored.

Even when a child with EB does not have oral blistering or swallowing problems, he or she may need supplements of high-calorie or high-protein drinks or of vitamins or minerals. The physician should be consulted as to whether a supplement is needed and, if so, the amount to be prescribed. Large doses of vitamins and minerals (megadoses) are not recommended. Caution should be exercised in terms of any diet or supplement that promises miraculous results. Such approaches are often attractive to parents of children with chronic diseases, but such alternatives to a varied, nutritious diet can result in malnutrition.

Anemia

Many children with EB become anemic due to a chronic loss of blood from blisters and open skin lesions and perhaps due to poor ingestion and absorption of blood-building substances. Specific treatment for iron deficiency anemia is often necessary. Many children have to keep taking supplemental iron even after the anemia has been corrected to prevent it from occurring again. Many commercial nutritional supplements contain iron. Use iron supplements only when recommended by the physician. An adequate intake of protein is also important.

Constipation

Many EB patients often suffer from constipation because they may rely on a semi-liquid or soft diet. A diet with foods from the various food groups (i.e., fruits and vegetables, breads and cereals, dairy products, and meat, poultry, and legumes), prepared in such a way that they can be tolerated by the child is important to prevent constipation. Those foods especially high in fiber such as vegetables, and fruits, e.g., prunes, and whole grain breads and cereals as well as an increase in fluid intake can help to control this problem.

Lactose Intolerance

Lactose Intolerance (or more properly, lactase deficiency, a condition in which enzyme production is insufficient to digest lactose, the sugar in milk products) has been observed in some children with EB. Milk can be treated with a commercial enzyme product called LactAid®, which, if added to a quart of milk, breaks down the sugar lactose and the milk can then be tolerated. Some stores also sell milk that has already been treated with the enzyme and is therefore more easily digested. In addition, in yogurt most of the lactose is broken down and thus is usually well tolerated. Lactose-free formulas and

Living with Epidermolysis Bullosa

liquid supplements are also available. Your physician and/or dietitian can help you in the selection of an appropriate product.

Minimizing Contractures and Deformity

Contractures (shortening or contraction of the skin, ligaments, and tendons) and muscle atrophy (weakening) develop as a result of disuse of a joint. The child with EB should be encouraged to be as active as possible, and physical therapy is often beneficial. Swimming is a good form of exercise for children with EB.

Fusion of Fingers and Toes (Syndactyly)

A complication of severe dystrophic epidermolysis bullosa is partial or complete side-to-side fusion of the fingers and toes caused by repealed friction, blistering and scarring. Prevention of this problem is extremely difficult, but placing custom-fitted splints between the fingers and toes may help slow down the process. These splints can be made from inexpensive heat-labile (moldable) material. Another method is to place strips of non-adherent gauze (Such as Vaseline® impregnated gauze) between the fingers.

Release of the thumb and fingers should be performed by a hand surgeon if the function of the hands has deteriorated significantly.

Eye Problems

Because many of the tissues of the eyes develop from the same fetal tissue as the skin, the eyes can be involved in EB, particularly in the dystrophic forms of EB. The cornea (the clear outer layer) and the conjunctiva (the mucous membrane covering the eyeball and the underside of the lids) can be damaged. Symptoms are pain, excessive formation of tears or discharge.

The goal of therapy for this problem is to protect the eye from irritation by increasing the amount of moisture. Eye drops can be useful as can lubrication with a specially prescribed antibiotic ointment. It may be helpful to put the ointment on the eye and patch it for a day or so.

Dental Problems

The infant or young child should begin to see the dentist (or pediatric dentist, if available) shortly after the teeth begin to emerge through the gums. Regular visits will ensure the most preventive care.

When the teeth begin to appear, they should be brushed gently with a small, soft multi-tufted toothbrush. Discourage the child eating sweets. If the water supply is not fluoridated, the dentist may suggest the use of nonirritating fluoride supplements.

Immunizations

Every child, including those with epidermolysis bullosa should receive the normal immunization shots. These include DPT (diphtheria-whooping cough-tetanus), polio, and MMR (measles, mumps, and rubella or German measles).

What Does the Future Hold for a Patient with EB?

As described earlier, EB can range from a relatively mild condition to a severely disabling, and sometimes fatal disease. Patients with milder forms may have periods of "temporary disability," but can lead a relatively normal life. In more severe forms, EB can be emotionally and physically devastating and cause the person to be disabled and deformed. Proper care and family support, however, can greatly enhance the quality of life for EB patients.

Despite the physical problems the disorder can cause, there is no impairment of intelligence.

There are many psychological problems that patients with EB must learn to cope with: the teasing of classmates, the stares from others, the jokes, the loneliness of being different. Many patients overcome these problems with the support of well-informed, caring parents and friends. As all children do, those with EB need love and acceptance.

Children's tissues become less delicate with age; many forms of EB begin to lessen to some degree as the child gets older. Patients given good, consistent, and intensive care early on have the best chances of doing well.

Support Groups

When one or more children in a family have a chronic disease that requires constant or almost around-the-clock care, the entire family is affected. Family therapy or support groups can:

- help each member of the family accept and deal with long-term chronic illness;

- help relieve guilt;

- make it easier to cope with the child's and the parents' feelings;

- make a difference because the parents' attitude can affect the way a child copes, handles his own care, and interacts socially with peers and people in general; and

- help to deal with siblings and spouses' feelings.

Support and information are also available from the Dystrophic Epidermolysis Bullosa Research Association of America, Inc. The aims and address of DEBRA are given at the end of this chapter.

What Can Research Tell Us about EB?

Researchers in epidermolysis bullosa and related areas are being supported by the Division of Arthritis, Musculoskeletal and Skin Diseases of the National Institute of Arthritis, Diabetes, and Digestive and Kidney Diseases, other components of the Federal Government's National Institutes of Health (NIH), and voluntary organizations such as DEBRA of America.

Experts have theories about how and why different forms of EB occur. Some understanding of the skin's structure can help explain these theories. The skin has two principal layers, the outermost layer known as the epidermis and the layer under the epidermis, the dermis. Between and connecting the two is the basement membrane zone.

Under a microscope, skin from patients with non-scarring forms of EB shows a splitting above the basement membrane. Skin from patients with scarring or dystrophic EB shows a split in the upper part of the dermis below the basement membrane.

During the past decade, investigators have discovered certain structures that hold the epidermis to the dermis, although no one yet knows what these structures are made of. Called anchoring fibrils, these structures are similar to the stitching that holds the leather cover of a baseball to the core. If the stitches are weak, or if there are not enough of them, or if something begins to dissolve them, the covering begins to come off.

For example, in dominant dystrophic epidermolysis bullosa, some researchers believe that the primary problem is a decreased number of anchoring fibrils. This might be caused by a change in the production of the molecules that make up the fibrils.

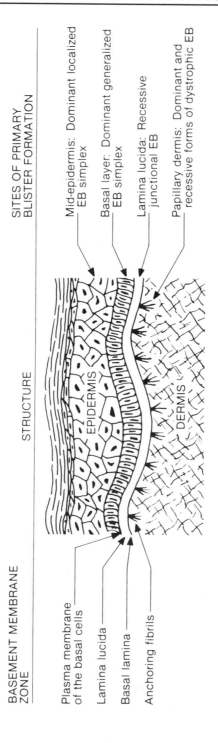

Figure 21.3. Blistering in Epidermolysis Bullosa

Living with Epidermolysis Bullosa

In recessive dystrophic epidermolysis bullosa, there are two lines of thinking as to why blisters form. Some researchers believe that EB occurs because of increased collagenase; collagenase is a natural body enzyme that controls production of collagen, the main supporting protein of the skin. Other researchers believe that there is a defect in a major structural protein, perhaps the anchoring fibrils, at the junction of the dermis and epidermis. Neither theory excludes the other, and the recessive form of EB may result from a combination of these two factors.

An NIH-supported researcher has used a new scientific technique called monoclonal antibodies to demonstrate anchoring fibrils were missing in EB skin.

In that excessive amounts of collagenase seem to be involved in some forms of EB, researchers are focusing their efforts to develop drugs that inhibit the effects of the enzyme. One example mentioned earlier is phenytoin, which was reported in 1980 to be effective against recessive dystrophic EB by NIH grantee Dr. Eugene Bauer of Washington University in St. Louis.

Other drugs that have the capacity to inhibit the enzyme collagenase are derivatives of vitamin A, known as the retinoids. It is important to note, however, that vitamin A by itself, as sold in pharmacies and elsewhere, does not have the same effects as the retinoids. High doses of vitamin A (above the Recommended Daily Allowances) can be harmful and possibly toxic.

Low concentrations of corticosteroids have also been shown to reduce collagenase activity; their effects must be tested further.

Much of science is unpredictable; there is often no way to know when and from where the answers will come. New basic research advances are constantly reshaping science and its applications. Recent developments in biology, biochemistry, pathology, immunology, and genetics are being used to study epidermolysis bullosa. The cardinal objectives are to understand the basic underlying mechanisms that lead to this distressing, disabling disease and to develop therapies directed at correcting these mechanisms.

For More Information about Epidermolysis Bullosa:

The Dystrophic Epidermolysis Bullosa Research Association of America, Inc. (DEBRA)
2936 Avenue W
Brooklyn, NY 11229
212/774-8700

DEBRA is a national nonprofit voluntary organization chartered in 1980 whose aims are: to promote and support research; to relieve physical and mental distress by giving practical advice, guidance, and support to people with EB; to assist in finding medical, social, and genetic counseling; to be an information source for health professionals; and to distribute educational material to the public.

Additional Sources of Information:

The National Center for Education in Maternal and Child Health
3520 Prospect St., N.W.
Washington, D.C. 20057
202/625-8400

This is a resource center that responds to public and professional inquiries on maternal and child health, including human genetics. Publications include a directory of clinical genetic service centers throughout the United States and a guide to Federal resources in maternal and child health. The Center is funded by the U.S. Department of Health and Human Services.

National Information Center for Handicapped Children and Youth
P.O. Box 1492
Washington, D.C. 20013
703/528-8480

The Center distributes information about services, special education programs, and laws affecting disabled children and adults. The Center is supported by the U.S. Department of Education.

Acknowledegments

Prepared by Office of Health Research Reports National Institute of Arthritis, Diabetes, and Digestive and Kidney Diseases National Institutes of Health Bethesda, MD 20205

Special thanks go to Arlene Pessar, R.N., B.S.N., Executive Director, Dystrophic Epidermolysis Bullosa Research Association of America, Inc., and to Anne Brown, R.D., M.S., Director of Dietetics, Rockefeller University Hospital, for their contributions to the text. We also acknowledge the help of members of the DEBRA Scientific Advisory Board and of a group of communications students from Rider College, Lawrenceville, New Jersey, for their thoughtful review of the manuscript. In addition, we would like to express our appreciation to several EB patients and family members for sharing with us their insights into the special problems people with EB face.

Chapter 22

Ichthyosis: An Overview

The Ichthyoses are a family of genetic skin disorders characterized by dry, thickened, scaling skin. Dermatologists estimate that there are at least twenty varieties of Ichthyosis, but the four main types are: **Ichthyosis Vulgaris, Lamellar Ichthyosis, X-linked Ichthyosis,** and **Epidermolytic Hyperkeratosis**. Some experts subdivide Lamellar Ichthyosis into two categories: **True Lamellar** and **non-bullous Congenital Ichthyosiform Erythroderma (CIE)**. There are other, even rarer, forms of Ichthyosis, too; these forms are sometimes seen with other impairments as well. A list of some of these rarer types of Ichthyosis can be found at the end of this chapter.

Most varieties of Ichthyosis affect only one person in several tens of thousands. Ichthyosis Vulgaris, sometimes called common Ichthyosis ("vulgar" means "common" in Latin), is the exception. It appears in approximately one person in every 250. The name is rarer than the disorder itself which often goes undiagnosed because people who have it often think they have simple "dry skin" and never seek treatment.

X-linked Ichthyosis is less common, usually more severe, and occurs only in males. It appears in approximately one out of every two-to-six thousand male babies. Lamellar Ichthyosis, Congenital Ichthyosiform Erythroderma and Epidermolytic Hyperkeratosis (sometimes called Bullous Congenital Ichthyosiform Erythroderma because there are blisters) are more severe still and may occur in

©1992 F.I.R.S.T. The Foundation for Ichthyosis and Related Skin Types, Inc. P.O. Box 20921, Raleigh, NC 27619-0921. Reprinted with permission.

fewer than one in 100,000 births; some estimates put the incidence at only one-to-five cases per million.

But Just What Is Ichthyosis?

In order to understand what goes wrong with the skin in the Ichthyoses, it is necessary to understand a little bit about how normal skin functions and grows.

Normal Skin Structure and Function

The skin is the largest organ in the human body, and like any other organ, it has a specific function. The skin's function is to encase and protect the entire body, regulate internal temperature, keep moisture inside and keep dirt, bacteria and other potentially harmful matter outside.

Skin is made of several layers. The top layer, called the stratum corneum, itself is made up of many very thin layers of flattened, dead cells called squames that contain keratin, a tough, thread-like protein that gives the stratum corneum strength. Between the squames there is a mixture of lipids, various fatty substances which are thought to account for the skin's impermeability to water, thus preserving the body's fluid and, conversely, preventing a flood of water into the body when we bathe or swim.

Beneath the stratum corneum is the living epidermis. As the skin constantly renews itself, cells at the bottom of the epidermis divide and move up toward the stratum corneum, maturing, making keratin, and eventually dying. The entire process takes about fourteen days. The dead, flattened cells then attach themselves at the bottom of the stratum corneum and become part of it.

Meanwhile, at the outside surface of the skin, cells are separating from each other and shedding, invisibly, thus making room for the newly-arriving cells and allowing the stratum corneum to renew itself at a constant rate. The process goes on constantly, with each new cell migrating from the living epidermis to the stratum corneum and then falling off within fourteen days. As long as the dead cells are shed from the surface at the same rate that new cells are created in the epidermis, the skin is normal and in a state of equilibrium, or "steady state."

And with Ichthyosis?

Equilibrium is not maintained when Ichthyosis occurs, and cells build up in the stratum corneum. Ichthyosis can be visualized as a

Ichthyosis: An Overview

traffic jam of skin cells, the same traffic jam that would result from cars entering a freeway in greater numbers than they are leaving it. A jam will result if an inordinate number of cars enter the highway (rush hour, for instance), or if the normal number of cars cannot get off at the proper rate because of an accident or a barrier or other obstruction in the road. In Ichthyosis, the "traffic jam" of skin cells in the stratum corneum can occur for either of these reasons: because the production of cells is too rapid or because the natural shedding process is slowed or inhibited, or both.

In Congenital Ichthyosiform Erythroderma and Epidermolytic Hyperkeratosis there is an over-production of skin cells in the epidermis. These cells reach the stratum corneum in as few as four days instead of the usual fourteen. The cells are made faster than they are shed and therefore build up in the stratum corneum.

In Ichthyosis Vulgaris, X-linked Ichthyosis, and classical Lamellar Ichthyosis, the skin cells are produced at a normal rate, but they do not separate normally at the surface of the stratum corneum and are not shed as quickly as they should be. The result, again, is a build-up of skin cells.

An increased stickiness in the stratum corneum, the cause of which is yet unknown but may be related to abnormal lipid content, may also contribute to the build-up of skin cells in some of these disorders. Now imagine those cars on the freeway with magnets on them.

In all instances of Ichthyosis the result is a thickened stratum corneum, often accompanied by an excessive loss of water (moisture) from the skin. The thickened skin gets drier and drier; it shrinks and cracks; the cracks deepen and widen, and the skin begins to look as though it is covered with scales. The process can be visualized by picturing what happens to a muddy river bed if the water dries up and the mud is exposed to the air and sun.

Ichthyotic skin does eventually shed, but only after it has built up considerably and formed into spines and/or scales. Cells of normal skin shed individually and invisibly; cells of ichthyotic skin shed in clumps, in the form of easily visible scales. The shedding of these easily visible scales is often a source of considerable annoyance and embarrassment to the person with Ichthyosis.

In classical Lamellar Ichthyosis the entire body is covered with broad, dark, plate-like scales separated by deep cracks. With Ichthyosis Vulgaris only a portion of the body may be involved, and the scale is usually fine and white. In Congenital Ichthyosiform Erythroderma the scales are also fine and white; unlike Ichthyosis Vulgaris, however, CIE covers the entire body, and the skin is often quite reddish beneath the scales. The scales of X-linked Ichthyosis are dark like those of classical Lamellar Ichthyosis, but they are usually not as large and cover only a portion of the person's body. Epidermolytic Hyperkeratosis exhibits flattened scales on some portions of the patient's body and tall, spiny scales on other parts, particularly joints and crevices; there can often be redness, blisters, and considerable fragility to bumps or abrasions.

Is It Contagious?

People with Ichthyosis are frequently asked if it is contagious. Children with Ichthyosis are often asked, "Is that catching?" The answer is "No." Ichthyosis is definitely not contagious. It is not caused by bacteria, virus, or a germ, and thus it cannot be passed from one person to another.

The term "Ichthyosis" refers to a group of disorders caused by a genetic defect which may have been spontaneous (due to a mutation of a gene) or passed on through family inheritance. It is present at conception, though in some cases the symptoms do not become apparent until sometime during the first year of a child's life; in other instances it is obvious immediately that something is wrong with the baby's skin.

(There are some acquired [non-genetic] forms of Ichthyosis but these, too, are non-contagious. They occur in a variety of conditions, including cancer, endocrine diseases, and severe nutritional deficiencies. These forms of Ichthyosis do not have their onset in infancy or early childhood as the genetic forms do.)

The genetics of Ichthyosis are discussed in much greater detail in Ichthyosis: *The Genetics of Its Inheritance*, a brochure available from the Foundation for Ichthyosis and Related Skin Types and reprinted in this sourcebook.

The Implications of Ichthyosis

The more severe forms of Ichthyosis can cause other problems: medical, social, psychological.

When the skin loses moisture, it becomes dry, tight and inelastic. This rigidity makes moving uncomfortable as it can cause the skin to crack and break open. Extreme thickening of the skin on the soles of the feet makes walking difficult for many patients, and cracking around the fingers can make even simple tasks difficult or painful.

Ichthyosis: An Overview

In some types of Ichthyosis the skin is very fragile and will rub off from even a slight abrasion. Cracks and abrasions then leave the skin open to infections.

People with very thick scaling, especially those with classical Lamellar Ichthyosis and Congenital Ichthyosiform Erythroderma, often have difficulty sweating which makes them quite vulnerable to overheating if they spend time in a hot environment, exercise too vigorously, or get a high fever. Severe scaling on the scalp may inhibit the growth of hair. Producing excess skin and fighting infections use a lot of energy and can inhibit a child's natural growth rate.

Some people with Ichthyosis, especially children with classical Lamellar Ichthyosis, have trouble closing their eyes completely because of the tightness of the skin around the eyes and eyelids. Parents report that these children "sleep with their eyes open." In some cases the skin around the eyes pulls so tightly it causes the eyelids to turn outward, exposing the red inner lid and causing continuing irritation. This condition is called ectropion, and some physicians recommend plastic surgery to correct it because if it is left untreated damage to the cornea can develop, leading to impaired vision.

Social and Psychological Implications

Ichthyosis can be a disfiguring disorder and as such has numerous social and psychological repercussions. Children are especially vulnerable to its social and psychological side effects, and it is during childhood that the disorder's physical, medical and cosmetic manifestations are most obvious.

Impaired motor ability, a possible side effect of skin tautness, affects a child's sense of competence and can leave him or her open to ridicule from peers. So does the unusual and unsightly appearance of his skin, especially if the skin on the face is involved. Other children with Ichthyosis may be spared blatant ridicule but find themselves ostracized, ignored and isolated.

Adolescence is a time of self-consciousness, self-doubt and exaggerated concern with appearance and physical attractiveness for even the healthiest and best-looking youngsters. It can be an especially painful experience for teenagers with Ichthyosis. The appearance of the skin itself can be a major hurdle to dating, and an already-poor self-image caused by a childhood of ridicule or isolation exacerbates the problem.

A child with Ichthyosis can find himself between a rock and a hard place; the cruelty of other children hurts him deeply, but the attentions of over-protective parents and other adults can impair development. Sometimes, by the time a person with Ichthyosis reaches adulthood, the skin problems have lessened somewhat, but s/he still carries the burden of its side effects on emotional development.

Some of these emotional implications spill over to other members of the family. The children with Ichthyosis may resent their normal, healthy siblings. They, in turn, may feel guilty about their health and easy relationships with peers. "Why me?" can echo within the heads of all the children. Siblings may also find themselves continually thrust into a protective role when other children taunt the affected brother or sister.

Parents of children with Ichthyosis can add a whole new dimension to the concept of guilt, blaming themselves, or worse yet, each other for the child's condition. "Did I take good enough care of myself when I was pregnant?" "Am I doing enough to track down the best and latest treatment for my child now?" "Am I doing everything possible to help him to be well adjusted?" "Am I paying enough attention to the rest of my children?" The list is endless.

These people, children or adults with Ichthyosis and the parents and other family members, can benefit a great deal from meeting and talking with other people who share their situation.

Treatments

Treatments for Ichthyosis are exactly that: treatments, not cures. As yet, there is no cure for Ichthyosis. A true cure would require changing the faulty genetic components. Current treatments for Ichthyosis are aimed at making the skin look and feel more normal. Therapy must be repeated on a regular, ongoing basis because the errant genes keep producing the defective skin.

Topical Therapy

There are two basic goals in topical treatments (treatments applied externally to the area or areas affected by the disorder). One is to keep the layer of scale from building up so the skin will not be so thick; the other is to retain moisture in the skin so it will not be so dry and rigid. If these goals are achieved, the skin will be more flexible and less susceptible to painful cracking and tightness.

Substances called keratolytics are used to loosen scale and are found in lotions or creams containing salicylic acid, urea, or alpha

Ichthyosis: An Overview

hydroxy acids such as lactic and glycolic acids. Some keratolytics such as salicylic acid can be absorbed through the skin, though, with potentially harmful side effects on the body, and some of the acids can be irritating. Patients are advised, therefore, to use these substances only under the guidance of a physician.

Treatment for scale in Ichthyosis Vulgaris, Lamellar Ichthyosis and X-linked Ichthyosis is usually longer-lasting than it is for Congenital Ichthyosiform Erythroderma and Epidermolytic Hyperkeratosis because the skin is created at a normal rate in the former variations and at a greatly increased rate with the latter. Keeping up with the scaling in Epidermolytic Hyperkeratosis and Congenital Ichthyosiform Erythroderma is rather like keeping up with a high-speed conveyor belt.

Some patients find that occluding all or parts of the body overnight with occlusion suits or plastic food wrap allows water to soak into the skin and soften it well enough for it to slough off with minimal scrubbing the next morning. Using a propylene glycol and water mixture inside the suit may hasten the process.

The second goal of topical therapy is to keep the skin moist. This means holding water in the skin. While most people feel that dry skin lacks oil, the symptoms of dry skin are actually the result of too little water. Oils and other emollients are applied simply to hold that water in the skin. Lubricants like glycerine, mineral oil, lanolin, or simple petroleum jelly attract or seal moisture in the stratum corneum, thus keeping the skin pliable and preventing cracks and breaks. Many patients hydrate the skin with a long, soaking bath or shower, then apply the lubricants to seal in that moisture.

Systemic Therapy

The use of drugs taken internally (systemic treatment) is being investigated and tested. Ichthyosis was once thought to be an allergy to foods, while some experts believed it was the result of insufficient Vitamin A.

Generally, dietary changes have produced little or no effect in treating the symptoms of this genetic disorder. Consuming an excess of Vitamin A can, in fact, be toxic and result in damage to internal organs. Children can be particularly sensitive to toxic amounts of Vitamin A.

More recently, researchers have looked to highly specialized synthetic materials to try to offset the excess scaling symptoms of Ichthyosis. One drug in particular, a derivative of synthetic Vitamin

A called **isotretinoin**, is effective in controlling scale in some patients with Ichthyosis. Unfortunately, the synthetic versions can also be toxic, especially with continued administration which is necessary in treating Ichthyosis. Potential side effects include elevated blood fats (triglycerides) which may lead to an increased risk of coronary artery disease and degenerative bone disease. Children may be at risk for premature closure of bone growth centers, which could result in stunted or asymmetric bone growth. The drug also causes severe birth defects when taken by pregnant women. Currently used to treat acute acne on a temporary, short-term basis, Vitamin A compounds have not been approved for the treatment of Ichthyosis by the Food and Drug Administration of the United States at the time of this writing.

Diagnosing Ichthyosis

Because of its rarity, Ichthyosis can be difficult to diagnose, especially for general practitioners who almost never run into it in the course of their regular work. Many people with Ichthyosis have gone to general practitioners regarding totally unrelated problems and had the doctors ask them, "Is that Ichthyosis? I studied it in medical school but I've never actually seen it." Answering these questions from doctors is one way that people with Ichthyosis can help the medical community and, therefore, each other.

Doctors investigate many factors in diagnosing Ichthyosis and then identifying the particular variety of the disorder. In determining the type of Ichthyosis, the doctor will look at the general appearance of the skin, the types of scales, the location of those scales on the body. He may also look at skin samples through the microscope to examine the microscopic patterns or appearance. The presence or absence of blisters is also significant.

The examination and family history can also be used to rule out other problems such as cryptorchidism (undescended testes) in X-linked Ichthyosis and systemic involvement as in some of the rarer syndromes.

When Did the Problem First Appear?

The appearance of the child at birth and the first visible onset of symptoms are also pertinent. Babies with classical Lamellar Ichthyosis and Congenital Ichthyosiform Erythroderma are sometimes called collodion babies because of a clear membrane which may

Ichthyosis: An Overview

cover their bodies at birth and is then shed within a few days to a few weeks. Sometimes described as having a shellacked appearance, these newborns have skin which is taut, dark and split. Often the eyelids and lips are already forced open by the tightness of the skin, and there may be contractures around the fingers. Babies with Epidermolytic Hyperkeratosis have been described as looking completely raw because all or parts of their skin can be rubbed off during the birth process, leaving the red flesh exposed. Some already have blisters when they are born.

Since Ichthyosis is a genetic disorder, it exists at conception, but in some instances the symptoms do not become apparent until sometime during the first year of life. Babies with Ichthyosis Vulgaris and X-linked Ichthyosis often appear normal when they are born, but the skin abnormalities will almost always begin to show up by their first birthday.

A Bit of Family History

As he or she would with most medical problems, the doctor diagnosing Ichthyosis will probably ask for a family history, sometimes delving back several generations looking for ancestors with scaly skin. This information can help the physician make a diagnosis based on the varying genetic patterns of the different Ichthyoses.

Prenatal Diagnosis

Some forms of Ichthyosis can be diagnosed prenatally. Amniocentesis is a procedure whereby amniotic fluid containing some fetal cells is taken from the mother's womb and analyzed. This procedure has been used to diagnose X-linked Ichthyosis. Another test, fetoscopy, has been used successfully to diagnose Harlequin Ichthyosis, Sjögren-Larson Syndrome and Epidermolytic Hyperkeratosis in an unborn child, and it may be possible also to diagnose Lamellar Ichthyosis or CIE in this manner. In fetoscopy a tiny sample of skin is removed from the fetus and examined for abnormal cells. Presently fetoscopy is performed at only a few research centers around the country.

Some Rarer Forms of Ichthyosis

Except for Ichthyosis Vulgaris, Ichthyosis is a very rare disorder. Yet there are some very specific disorders which fall under the umbrella of

Ichthyosis which are even less common than the five major types of Ichthyosis just discussed. Among these disorders are: Harlequin Fetus, Sjögren-Larson Syndrome, the Chondrodysplasia Punctata Syndromes, Chanarin-Dorfman Syndrome, Refsum Disease, Tay Syndrome, Keratitis-Ichthyosis-Deafness (K.I.D.) Syndrome, Ichthyosis Linearis Circumflexa, Multiple Sulfatase Deficiency, Peeling Skin Syndrome, Epidermal Nevus Syndrome, Pityriasis Rubra Pilaris, and Darier Disease, to name a few.

All these disorders, plus others, are considered ichthyotic disorders, and people with them are served by the organizations listed below.

The Related Skin Types

In 1986 F.I.R.S.T.'s Board of Directors formally changed this organization's name to its present one from what had formerly been the National Ichthyosis Foundation in order to better reflect the broad range of ichthyotic disorders we represent. Because so little is known about the underlying genetic and metabolic defect in all but a few forms of ichthyosis, there remains in the medical community some disagreement about clear definitions and classification of its many forms. Furthermore, obscure forms of ichthyosis may exist which are not fully delineated in the medical literature. Regardless of these difficulties, following is a relatively complete list of the family of related ichthyotic disorders.

- Acquired Ichthyosis
- Autosomal Dominant Lamellar Ichthyosis
- Chanarin-Dorfman Syndrome (neutral lipid storage disease)
- CHILD Syndrome (unilateral hemidysplasia)
- Chondrodysplasia Punctata Syndrome (Conradi-Hunermann syndrome)
- Congenital Ichthyosiform Erythroderma (CIE)
- Darier's Disease (*keratosis follicularis*)
- Epidermal Nevus Syndrome
- Epidermolytic Hyperkeratosis (EHK) (*bullous congenital ichthyosiform erythroderma*)
- Erythrokeratodermias (*E. progressiva symmetrica, E. variabilis & E. heimalis*)
- Giroux-Barbeau Syndrome
- Harlequin Ichthyosis (harlequin fetus)
- Hailey-Hailey Disease (familial pemphigus)

Ichthyosis: An Overview

- Ichthyosis Hystrix (Curth-Maklin type)
- Ichthyosis Vulgaris
- Keratosis Follicularis Spinulosa Decalvans
- KID Syndrome (keratitis-ichthyosis-deafness)
- Lamellar Ichthyosis (recessive)
- Multiple Sulfatase Deficiency
- Netherton's Syndrome (*i. linearis circumflexa*)
- Palmoplantar Keratoderma Types (various)
- Peeling Skin Syndrome
- Pityriasis Rubra Pilaris
- Recessive X-Linked Ichthyosis (steroid sulfatase deficiency)
- Refsum's Disease (phytanic acid storage type)
- Rud's Syndrome
- Sjögren-Larson Syndrome
- Tay's Syndrome (trichothiodystropy; IBIDS syndrome)

Very little reliable information is available on the prevalence, or incidence, of the ichthyoses. Following is a table of commonly accepted figures. However, these figures are only broad estimates and the margin of error is exceedingly large.

The figures are based on 1990 census data reporting a U.S. population of approximately 250 million, with an estimated 3.8 million live births.

TYPE	PREVALENCE	PER MILLION	YEARLY BIRTHS
Lamellar (recessive)	1 : 300,000	3.3	13
CIE	1 : 300,000	3.3	13
EHK	1 : 200,000	5	19
Recessive X-Linked	1 : 6,000	167	633
Darier's Disease	1 : 200,000	5	19
Harlequin Ichthyosis	1 : 500,000	2	8
Ichthyosis Vulgaris	1 : 250	4,000	15,200

Table 22.1. Prevalence of Some Prominent Forms of Ichthyosis

Sources of Help and Information

Ichthyosis is a disorder that affects not just individuals but whole families. Parents' lives are turned upside down as they try to deal with the demands of caring for a child with an illness they have probably never even heard of, let alone had to deal with, before. There is presently no cure, at any price, and reliable information about diagnosis and treatment is scarce. Medical problems are a day-to-day reality: expensive, disruptive and exhausting.

On top of the omnipresent physical problems and demands, there is the psychological aspect of the disorder on the child and on the whole family. Parents of children with Ichthyosis, and individual adults with the disorder, have often never met a single other person who shares their situation. They can feel very isolated and alone, and depression, anger and guilt often co-exist with the physical symptoms.

F.I.R.S.T., The Foundation for Ichthyosis and Related Skin Types, Inc. (formerly The National Ichthyosis Foundation, Inc.), can help. A non-profit organization consisting of patients and families, a Board of Directors, and a Medical Advisory Board, F.I.R.S.T. supports education, self-help and research activities through a national newsletter, an annual conference, and a network of regional representatives. Members get up-to-date information about Ichthyosis and a chance to meet or correspond with others in the Ichthyosis community, to give and receive information and support.

Chapter 23

Lichen Planus and Lichen Sclerosus

Lichen Planus (li' ken pla' nus)

What is lichen planus?

Lichen planus is a skin disease characterized by angular, purple bumps called papules. White spots or lacy white lines known as Wickham's striae cover the shiny, flat surfaces of the papules. In later stages of the disease, scales may form on the papules. Affected areas are itchy, or pruritic, and may become red and swollen.

The papules are usually localized and occur most often on the arms, legs, hands, and feet. The genitalia, oral mucous membranes (or mouth), nails, and scalp may also be affected. The first occurrence of lichen planus almost always affects the limbs, however.

Who gets lichen planus?

People age 30 to 60 are most often affected. Lichen planus is uncommon in both the young and the elderly. The disease does not seem to favor any race or sex.

The National Institute of Arthritis and Musculoskeletal and Skin Diseases (NIAMS) Information Release 2/92. Office of Scientific and Health Communications.

What causes lichen planus?

The cause of lichen planus is not known. However, possible causes are infection; allergy; having a family history of the disease; a defect in the body's immune system, which fights infection; or psychological factors such as fatigue and severe emotional stress. Also, certain chemicals and drugs seem to cause lichen planus.

How is lichen planus diagnosed?

Characteristic skin papules (described above) usually establish the diagnosis of lichen planus. However, a skin biopsy, an examination of a small sample of affected skin, may be necessary to confirm the diagnosis.

How is lichen planus treated?

Treatment of lichen planus addresses the symptoms, namely itching and inflammation. Mild cases are treated with one or more of the following: lotions, steroids applied topically or injected by needle directly into the papules, or antihistamines to relieve discomfort. Severe cases of lichen planus are treated with more potent steroids.

What is the duration of lichen planus?

In two-thirds of the cases, lichen planus papules disappear by themselves, without therapy, within 8 to 12 months. With therapy, lichen planus clears within 9 to 18 months, though severe cases may last for 3 to 20 years.

Where do I go for help?

Lichen planus is treated by dermatologists, skin doctors. The American Academy of Dermatology can provide referrals to dermatologists in your area. The National Institute of Arthritis and Musculoskeletal and Skin Diseases (NIAMS) does not make physician referrals and is not currently funding clinical trials, experimental treatments, for lichen planus. Other ways to locate dermatologists who treat lichen planus include: asking your family physician to provide the name of a dermatologist, calling a local or state department of health, checking the listings of dermatologists in the phone book, or

Lichen Sclerosus (li' ken sklur o' sus)

What is lichen sclerosus?

Lichen sclerosus is a skin eruption characterized by angular, pea-sized bumps, or papules, that are nearly flat. Early in the disease, the papules are soft, pink, and slightly raised. As the disease progresses, the papules flatten, turn grey to white, and become shiny and wrinkled, like a scar. Sometimes the papules may cluster to form plaques, larger patches of affected skin. In some cases, dark horn-like plugs will appear in the lesions.

The skin of the genital area and the anal area is most often affected, but lichen sclerosus may develop on any part of the body. Itching and burning usually accompany lichen sclerosus of the genital and anal areas. Bleeding, ulceration, and shrinkage of the vulva due to scarring are also typical. In very rare cases, a form of skin cancer may develop within a patch of lichen sclerosus.

The skin of the neck, chest, and abdomen are also more frequently affected by lichen sclerosus. Lesions on non-genital skin rarely itch, bleed, or ulcerate. Cancer rarely develops in non-genital lichen sclerosus.

Who gets lichen sclerosus?

Lichen sclerosus is a rare skin disease affecting considerably more women than men, particularly women between the ages 40 and 70. It occasionally occur in children, particularly in young girls, where it generally resolves spontaneously at puberty. The disease appears to be more common in whites.

What causes lichen sclerosus?

Although the cause is unknown, studies suggest that hormonal abnormalities or a defect in the body's immune system, which fights disease, may play a role in the eruption of lichen sclerosus. No preventative measures are known.

How is lichen sclerosus diagnosed?

When lichen sclerosus is well developed, the appearance of the skin—marked by characteristic skin eruptions—is very suggestive of the diagnosis. However, a skin biopsy (an examination of a small sample of affected skin) is frequently needed to establish the diagnosis of lichen sclerosus. This is particularly true for genital lesions.

How is lichen sclerosus treated?

Non-genital lichen sclerosus is generally not treated, because itching, bleeding, and erosion do not occur. Topical corticosteroids benefit lichen sclerosus of the genital area, particularly early in the disease. They relieve the symptoms and may slow the course of the disease. Testosterone ointment may also be helpful for genital lichen sclerosus. Lichen sclerosus may remit occasionally, but no evidence suggests that treatment is responsible for remission; rather, remission seems to be spontaneous.

If a skin cancer develops within a patch of lichen sclerosus, it should be treated in a manner appropriate to the size of the affected area and the extent of involvement. Surgical removal of the affected area may be necessary.

Where do I go for help?

Lichen sclerosus is treated by dermatologists (skin doctors) and by gynecologists if the female genitalia are involved. The American Academy of Dermatology can provide referrals to dermatologists in your area, and the American College of Obstetricians and Gynecologists can refer you to a gynecologist. The National Institute of Arthritis and Musculoskeletal and Skin Diseases (NIAMS) does not make physician referrals and is not currently funding clinical trials (experimental treatments) for lichen sclerosus. Other ways to locate dermatologists or gynecologists who treat lichen sclerosus include: asking your family physician to for a referral, calling a local or state department of health, checking the listings of dermatologists and gynecologists in the phone book, or contacting the departments of dermatology and gynecology at a local medical center. Libraries at university hospitals are also excellent sources of information. The *Directory of Medical Specialists*, available at most community libraries, can help you find a physician.

Chapter 24

Skin Diseases in Lupus

Skin disease is very common in lupus erythematosus. It ranks second only to arthritis in frequency of occurrence. Approximately 20 percent of people with systemic lupus erythematosus (SLE) will have ring-shaped or coin-shaped, scarring lesions as the initial symptom of their disease. In addition, it has been estimated that as many as 60-65 percent of people with SLE will develop skin rashes or lesions at some time during the course of their illness. However, with the use of oral steroids (Prednisone) and anti-malarial drugs (hydroxychloroquine, or Plaquenil), the occurrence of these skin lesions is less frequent.

The skin rashes and lesions of lupus erythematosus can be divided into those that are specific to lupus and those that can occur in other diseases as well as lupus (non-specific lesions). There are two specific lesions associated with lupus erythematosus: discoid lesions (characteristic of discoid lupus erythematosus) and coin-shaped, non-scarring lesions (characteristic of subacute cutaneous lupus erythematosus).

Discoid Lesions

The term discoid is a very confusing term which, unfortunately, is inappropriately used by many people, including physicians. The term discoid simply means coin-shaped. The scarring, coin-shaped lupus

©1995 "Skin Diseases in Lupus" and ©1994 "Photosensitivity and Lupus Erythematosus." Lupus Foundation of America, 4 Research Place, Suite 180, Rockville, MD 20850-3226. Reprinted with permission.

lesion commonly seen on areas of the skin that are exposed to light has been termed discoid lupus erythematosus. This term refers only to the description of the lupus lesion on the skin and should not be used to distinguish cutaneous lupus from systemic lupus erythematosus. A physician cannot determine whether or not a discoid lupus lesion on the skin is occurring in the presence or absence of systemic features just by examining the shape of the lesion. This can only be done by taking a complete history and physical examination and interpreting the results of appropriate blood tests.

What is the relationship between discoid and systemic lupus erythematosus? This is a common question. Lupus erythematosus should be viewed as a continuum of a spectrum of the disease. At one end of the spectrum, in its most mild form, it is characterized by coin-shaped, scarring skin lesions which we term discoid lesions. At the other end of the spectrum are those systemic lupus erythematosus patients who have no skin lesions, but have systemic features (i.e., arthritis or renal disease). People with only discoid lesions and no systemic features commonly have no auto-antibodies in their serum (i.e., antinuclear or anti-DNA tests will be negative). On the other hand, people with systemic lupus erythematosus are characterized by the presence of one or more types of auto antibodies in their blood. From personal experience and from reviewing the literature, it has been estimated that between 5 and 10 percent of patients initially presenting with only the coin-shaped lesions of discoid lupus will, with time, develop systemic features. As noted above, approximately 20 percent of people with systemic lupus erythematosus will at the time of the initial presentation of their disease have discoid lupus lesions. These data indicate that, at times, the lupus disease process is dynamic and, with time, a small percentage of those patients who only have discoid lupus lesions will eventually develop systemic disease. In addition to these coin-shaped, scarring lesions, there are several different types of discoid lupus lesions with which people should be familiar. Occasionally, the discoid lupus lesions may occur in the scalp producing a scarring, localized baldness termed alopecia. At times, these discoid lesions may appear over the central portion of the face and nose producing a characteristic butterfly rash.

This type of lupus obviously has significant cosmetic implications. The discoid lupus lesions may develop thick, scaly (hyperkeratotic) formations and are termed hyperkeratotic or hypertrophic cutaneous lupus lesions. Discoid lupus lesions may also occur in the presence of thickening (deep induration) of the layers of underlying skin. This is termed lupus profundus.

Skin Diseases in Lupus

At the present time, research indicates that discoid lupus lesions are the result of an inflammatory process in the skin in which the patient's lymphocytes (predominantly T-cells) play a major role. This is in contrast to systemic lupus erythematosus, where autoantibodies and immune complex formation are responsible for many of the clinical symptoms.

Subacute Cutaneous Lesions

The second type of specific lupus lesion was most recently described by Sontheimer and Gilliam during the late 1970s. This lesion is characterized as a non-scarring, erythematosus (red), coin-shaped lesion which is very photosensitive (gets worse when exposed to UV light). This type of lesion, which is characteristic of subacute cutaneous lupus, occurs in lupus patients who, approximately 50 percent of the time, demonstrate features of systemic lupus erythematosus. Renal disease, however, is unusual in these patients. These skin lesions also occur in people who only have clinical evidence of skin disease, and do not show any symptoms of systemic lupus. Approximately 70 percent of people with these lesions have anti-Ro (SSA) antibodies.

The subacute cutaneous lupus lesions can sometimes mimic the lesions of psoriasis or they can appear as non-scarring, coin-shaped lesions. These lesions can occur on the face in a butterfly distribution, or can cover large areas of the body. Unlike the discoid lupus lesions, these lesions do not produce permanent scarring, but can be of major cosmetic significance.

Lesions of subacute cutaneous lupus may also be seen as a feature of neonatal lupus syndrome. Infants with neonatal lupus, born of mothers with anti-Ro (SSA) antibodies, may develop a transient lupus rash that disappears by the time they reach 6 months of age. At the present time, the best evidence suggests that the anti-Ro (SSA) antibody is passed via the placenta to the fetus and plays a major role in causing the characteristic lupus skin disease.

Non-specific Lupus Lesions: Hair Loss

The non-specific lupus lesions include several forms of hair loss (alopecia) which are not related to the presence of discoid lupus lesions in the scalp. Systemic lupus patients who have been severely ill with their disease may (over a period of time) develop a transient hair loss in which large amounts of hair evolve into a resting phase and fall out. However, this is quickly replaced by new hair. In addition, a severe flare of systemic lupus erythematosus can result in defective hair growth which causes the hair to be fragile and to break easily. The hair is broken off above the surface of the scalp, especially at the edge of the scalp, giving the characteristic appearance termed "lupus hair."

Vasculitis

Systemic lupus erythematosus patients may develop inflammatory disease of the blood vessels (vasculitis). The cutaneous manifestations of vasculitis are varied. The lesions may appear as red welts involving large areas of the body. These lesions can also present as small red lines in the cuticle nail fold or on the tips of the fingers or as red bumps on the legs. In addition, these red bumps may ulcerate. At times, the blood vessels that are involved in this inflammatory process may be deep in the skin producing painful, red nodules. These are usually found on the legs.

Photosensitivity

Photosensitivity is a common feature of lupus erythematosus. The overwhelming majority of specific lupus lesions (i.e., discoid lesions and subacute cutaneous lupus lesions) occur on sun-exposed areas. In addition, approximately 40-70 percent of people with lupus will note that their disease process, including the skin disease, is aggravated by sun exposure. Furthermore, people with subacute cutaneous lupus erythematosus, especially those who have anti-Ro (SSA) antibodies demonstrate pronounced photosensitivity. It has been estimated that 90 percent of patients with systemic or discoid lupus who have anti-Ro (SSA) antibodies are photosensitive. Furthermore, a number of these patients are so photosensitive that they will burn through window glass. Window glass filters out sunlight in the sunburn spectrum and protects normal people from developing a sunburn. However, window glass will not filter ultraviolet light of longer wavelengths and these wavelengths are capable of exacerbating (making worse) the skin lesions in people with lupus with anti-Ro (SSA) antibodies.

One recent study has shown that ultraviolet light in both the sunburn and long wavelength light spectrum (those wavelengths that are not blocked by window glass) will cause lupus lesions to appear on the skin of patients with systemic lupus erythematosus, those with lesions of subacute cutaneous lupus, and those who have only scarring lupus lesions (discoid lesions) with no evidence of systemic disease. These data provide excellent evidence for the role of ultraviolet light in the development of lupus skin lesions.

There is clinical and experimental evidence that shows that ultraviolet light can also induce flares in people with systemic lupus erythematosus. The way that ultraviolet light triggers these systemic flares (or leads to the development of skin lesions) is not known. However, there is evidence that suggests that ultraviolet light is capable of leading to an increase in the number of auto-antigens to which the person is reacting.

Treatment

The treatment of skin disease in lupus erythematosus involves the use of a number of drugs as well as the use of sunscreens. Individual lupus lesions can be treated with the topical application of steroid creams, the application of a steroid impregnated tape to cover the lupus lesion, or the intralesional injection of low doses of steroid. Widespread lupus lesions are frequently treated using hydroxychloroquine (Plaquenil) alone, or in combination with a short burst of oral steroids. On very unusual occasions, unmanageable, cosmetically objectionable lupus lesions have been successfully treated with vitamin A derivatives (such as Tegison).

Sun protection can do a lot to prevent the development of lupus skin lesions. People with lupus should avoid prolonged periods of exposure to sunlight, especially between the hours of 10 a.m. and 3 p.m., when the sun is at its brightest. It is also a good idea to wear a wide-brimmed hat and avoid clothing made of thin fabric which will admit sunlight. In addition, the regular use of sunscreens with a sun protective factor rating of SPF 15 will also provide protection. In recent years, research has shown that ultraviolet light of long wavelengths, as well as ultraviolet light in the sunburn spectrum, is capable of producing lupus skin lesions. Sunscreens capable of blocking this long-wave ultraviolet light are now available. In contrast to ordinary sunscreens which generally contain para-aminobenzoic acid (PABA) esters and benzophones, these sunscreens are actually sunblocks and contain titanium oxide. (See below for a more detailed discussion of sun exposure and Lupus.)

For specific information regarding the treatment of various skin manifestations of lupus erythematosus, as well as the employment of sunscreens, consult your dermatologist, or your local chapter of the Lupus Foundation of America.

Sun Exposure and Lupus

Photosensitivity is defined as an abnormal reaction of the skin to sunlight. Forty to sixty percent of Lupus Erythematosus (LE) patients are photosensitive. Excessive sun exposure may trigger the onset of disease, may cause flares in people who have systemic lupus and aggravate cutaneous (discoid) lupus.

Photosensitivity in lupus is usually caused by the sun's ultraviolet (UV) light: UVA, UVB, and UVC. The ozone in the stratosphere filters out UVC. Window gloss filters out UVB and offers protection from the harm it can cause.

Almost all the effects of UVA and UVB are damaging. Exposure to UV causes aging, wrinkling, pre-cancerous conditions and skin cancer and should be minimized by everyone on this basis alone. Cutaneous lesions of LE can be reproduced experimentally with both UVA and UVB light. While UVB is mainly responsible for causing skin cancer and lupus, UVA also may play a role. UVA can contribute to skin cancer, premature aging and is largely responsible for drug-induced photosensitivity. Both UVB and UVA can produce tanning.

Mechanism of UV Damage

Exactly how UV light aggravates lupus is unknown. Research suggests it alters DNA and protein in the skin. The altered DNA may act as an antigen that triggers the production of autoantibodies and provokes an autoimmune response in the skin. In photosensitive persons, UV exposure causes skin cells to release substances (cytokines, prostaglandins) that trigger inflammation. The skin reacts to these substances, becomes red, inflamed and develops a rash. Photosensitivity reactions can also affect the internal organs. In people with Systemic Lupus Erythematosus (SLE), the inflammatory substances released by skin cells can be absorbed into the blood stream and carried to other parts of the body. There, they may cause inflammation in organs and lead to systemic symptoms.

Skin Diseases in Lupus

General Considerations

UV-induced lupus erythematosus is a medical and socioeconomic problem. Injury to people with LE in the work place can be a cause for Worker's Compensation and litigation. Each case must be individually studied and expert opinion obtained. There is no question that individuals who have lupus and are photosensitive should avoid excessive sun exposure. Delivering the mail, construction work, and lifeguarding are examples of occupations that may receive excessive sun exposure. In addition, there are jobs where exposure to artificial sources of UV light can aggravate LE. Welders can be exposed to UVA, UVB and UVC in their work. Other sources of UV light in the workplace include photocopying machines, slide projector lights and TV studio lights. The case for white fluorescent lights provoking LE is not well documented but may occur in rare instances. A plastic shield over fluorescent lights blocks UV "leakage."

Sometimes trauma or injury to the skin may lead to the Koebner phenomenon where the skin reacts by producing LE lesions in the area of injury. Sunburn, thermal burn, lacerations and blunt mechanical trauma all can induce LE.

Photoprotection

Many factors contribute to photoprotection which is the ability of your skin to protect itself from damaging sun rays. Skin type is an important consideration. There are six classifications of sun-reactive skin types. Skin types 1 and 2 (burn easily, tan minimally) need much more protection than types 3 and 4 (burn minimally, tan readily). Skin types 5 and 6 (burn rarely, tan profusely) do not need as much protection as other skin types. Types 5 and 6 contain larger quantities of melanin, a substance which darkens the pigment of the skin and has some sun protective properties. In Blacks, melanin has been said to have an SPF (sun protective factor) of 3 or 4. Blacks and Orientals tolerate more sun, but can also experience photosensitivity. No matter what skin type an individual may have, precautions should always be taken.

Factors affecting the intensity of UV rays must also be considered. These include: time of day, altitude, proximity to the equator and reflective surfaces. During the mid-part of the day, the sun's rays strike the earth more directly and increase UV penetration. People should minimize outdoor activities between the peak hours of 10:00 a.m. and

4:00 p.m.. Ultraviolet radiation also increases nearer the equator, in the mountains or anywhere one is physically closer to the sun. There is less atmosphere to absorb the sun's rays and extra protection is needed. Reflective surfaces such as sand, snow and concrete increase exposure to UV light. Snow skiing or sitting on a sandy beach exposes one to considerable reflected UV light. Snow or sand reflect about 50-75 percent of the UV rays. A person's UV exposure is significant even if they are sitting under an umbrella at the beach. An overcast sky does not reduce UV substantially and provides only minimal photoprotection from UV rays.

The simplest form of protection is clothing that can effectively block UV rays. Thin, loosely woven materials offer little protection because they allow UV to penetrate to the skin. The tighter the weave, the better the protection. The thickness of the clothing is more important than color. When sun exposure is unavoidable, wear a hat, a long sleeve shirt and long pants. Umbrellas can also provide protection from harmful sun exposure.

Certain drugs can increase the body/skin's photosensitivity, causing undesirable skin reactions. Photosensitizing drugs include: acne medications such as tretinoin (Retin-A), diuretics such as hydrochlorothiazide (Hydrodiuril), tranquilizers such as chlorpromazine (Thorazine), oral antibiotics such as tetracyclines, sulfa drugs, hypoglycemics such as chlorpropamide (Diabinese) and non-steroidal anti-inflammatories such as Naproxen. The treatment for drug-induced photosensitivity reactions involves stopping the drug and/or using sunscreens and avoiding UV exposure. Whenever a new drug is prescribed ask your physician if it may cause photosensitivity.

UVA and UVB can both induce cutaneous (discoid) LE. Although testing is rarely suggested, patients can be photo-tested to show how sensitive they may be to UVA and UVB light.

Sun-Protective Agents

Sun-protective agents can be sunblocks or sunscreens. Physical sunblocks are usually opaque formulas that protect by reflecting and scattering UV. They contain chemicals such as zinc oxide, titanium dioxide, and red veterinary petrolatum that block both UVA and UVB light. The most widely used UVA blocker is Oxybenzone. Sold as a white or a colored cream, sunblocks are particularly good for skiing and hiking at high altitudes. They are used very effectively on areas with extensive prior photo-damage like the nose.

Skin Diseases in Lupus

Sunscreens protect by absorbing UV light. They are available as creams, lotions or gels. The chemical content determines whether the sunscreen absorbs UVB, UVA or both. Chemicals that primarily absorb UVB include PABA (para-amino benzoic acid), and its esters, cinnamates and salicylates. Padimate, a PABA ester, is the most widely used UVB absorber. Benzophenones and anthranilates absorb both UVB and UVA. UVA protection is less well documented. Avobenzone (Parsol 1789), now available in the USA, is an excellent UVA absorber.

UVB sunscreens are rated according to their sun protective factor. An SPF of 15 protects the skin so it takes 15 times longer to produce erythema (redness) than it would without the sunscreen. SPF varies from 1-50; the most common strengths are 15, 30, and 50. The price often increases with the SPF. When purchasing a sunscreen consider the following: the SPF number, the type of UV absorbed and its ability to remain effective after application. While exercising, sweating, and swimming will decrease a sunscreen's effectiveness, there are "waterproof" or "water resistant" sunscreens. PABA and its esters are more waterproof than other sunscreens because they penetrate more deeply into the skin.

Sunscreens may produce side effects. Those which use alcohols or ethanol bases frequently are drying and may burn the eyes. The moisturizing lotions may appear greasy and aggravate acne. Other side effects include irritation and allergy. Irritation is most common in products with an alcohol base. The most common allergen is PABA, although any sunscreen can cause sensitivity. Each person must find a sunscreen, by trial and error, which is acceptable. If the problem of allergy is difficult to solve, a dermatologist can help identify specific allergens by patch testing. PABA also tends to stain cotton, nylon, and polyester which may make it unacceptable. PABA does not absorb UVA and will allow tanning.

Before applying a sunscreen, first test the product on a small area of skin to rule out sensitivity or allergy. A sunscreen should be applied after shaving and applied and allowed to dry before putting on makeup. For the greatest protection apply it half an hour to an hour before going out in the sun. On average, a sunscreen will last about five hours, but should be reapplied if heavy sweating or exposure to water occurs. The lips should be protected with either lipstick or a sunscreen with an ointment base. There are many benefits of using sunscreen: sunscreens prevent skin aging, reduce the risk of skin cancer and protect against the photosensitivity reactions associated with lupus.

Summary

People with lupus should realize that a tan is not necessarily healthy. The sun "is their enemy." A sensible lifestyle includes minimizing excessive UV exposure and using photoprotection. Outside activities should be completed before 10:00 a.m. and after 4:00 p.m. when the UV rays are less intense. People with lupus should not sunbathe or use tanning booths. Those who work outdoors may need to change occupations.

Common sense should prevail. People with lupus should be neither a "mole" nor a lifeguard. Through experience, each individual's skin type and degree of photosensitivity can be learned. Even if a person is not photosensitive, it is wise to be careful about sun exposure. By taking appropriate precautions and using common sense, individuals with lupus can achieve photoprotection.

Chapter 25

The McCune-Albright Syndrome

The McCune-Albright syndrome is named for the two physicians who described it over 50 years ago. They reported a group of children, most of them girls, with an unusual pattern of associated abnormalities: bone disease, with fractures, asymmetry and deformity of the legs, arms, and skull; endocrine disease, including early puberty with menstrual bleeding, development of breasts and pubic hair and an increased rate of growth; and skin changes, with areas of increased pigment distributed in an asymmetric and irregular pattern. Today, the term "McCune-Albright syndrome" is used to describe patients who have some or all of these bone, endocrine, and skin abnormalities. In the years since it was first identified, however, researchers have studied many additional patients, and have learned that the condition has a broad spectrum of severity. Sometimes, children are diagnosed in early infancy with obvious bone disease and markedly increased endocrine secretions from several glands; a very few of these severely affected children have died. At the opposite end of the spectrum, many children are entirely healthy, and have little or no outward evidence of bone or endocrine involvement. They may enter puberty close to the normal age, and have no unusual skin pigment at all. Because of this marked variability among patients, the components of this complicated syndrome are described separately below.

NIH Publication No. 93-3442.

Endocrine Abnormalities

Precocious Puberty

When the signs of puberty (development of breasts, testes, pubic and underarm hair, body odor, menstrual bleeding, and increased growth rate) appear before the age of eight years in a girl or nine and a half years in a boy, it is termed "precocious puberty." In the most common form of precocious puberty, there is early activation of the regions in the brain which control the maturation of the gonads (ovaries in a girl and testes in a boy). One brain center, the hypothalamus, secretes a substance called gonadotropin-releasing-hormone or "GnRH." This acts, in turn, on another part of the brain, the pituitary gland, to cause increased secretion of hormones called "gonadotropins" (LH and FSH) that travel through the bloodstream, and act on the ovaries or testes to stimulate secretion of estrogen or testosterone. Endocrinologists determine if a child with precocious puberty has early activation of the hypothalamus and pituitary by measuring the levels of LH and FSH in the blood after an injection of a synthetic preparation of GnRH.

After studying many girls with McCune-Albright syndrome, however, researchers have learned that most do not appear to have early activation of the hypothalamus and pituitary, because the levels of LH and FSH are usually low, or similar to those of prepubertal children. The precocious puberty in McCune-Albright girls is caused by estrogens which are secreted into the bloodstream by ovarian cysts, which enlarge, and then decrease in size over periods of weeks to days. The cysts can be visualized and measured by ultrasonography, in which sound waves are used to outline the dimensions of the ovaries. The cysts may become quite big, occasionally over 50 cc in volume (about the size of a golf ball). Frequently, menstrual bleeding and breast enlargement accompany the growth of a cyst. In fact, menstrual bleeding under two years of age has been the first symptom of McCune-Albright syndrome in 85 percent of patients. Although ovarian cysts and irregular menstrual bleeding may continue into adolescence and adulthood, many adult women with McCune-Albright syndrome are fertile, and can bear normal children.

The precocious puberty in McCune-Albright syndrome has been difficult to treat. After surgical removal of the cyst or of the entire affected ovary, cysts usually recur in the remaining ovary. A progesterone-like hormone called Provera can be given to suppress

The McCune-Albright Syndrome

the menstrual bleeding, but does not appear to slow the rapid rates of growth and bone development, and may have unwanted effects on adrenal functioning. The synthetic forms of GnRH (Deslorelin, Histerelin, and Lupron) which suppress LH and FSH, and are used to treat the common, gonadotropin-dependent form of precocious puberty, are not effective in most girls with McCune-Albright syndrome. An investigational form of treatment, using oral medications which block estrogen synthesis, (testolactone and fadrozole) is now being tested in girls with McCune-Albright syndrome, and has been beneficial in many patients.

Thyroid Function

Almost 50 percent of patients with McCune-Albright syndrome have thyroid gland abnormalities; these include generalized enlargement called goiter, and irregular masses called nodules and cysts. Some patients have subtle structural changes detected only by ultrasonography. Pituitary thyroid-stimulating hormone (TSH) levels are low in these patients, and thyroid hormone levels may be normal or elevated. Therapy with drugs which block thyroid hormone synthesis (Propylthiouracil or Methimazole), can be given if thyroid hormone levels are excessively high.

Growth Hormone

Excessive secretion of pituitary growth hormone has been seen in a few patients with McCune-Albright syndrome. Most of these have been diagnosed as young adults, when they developed the coarsening of facial features, enlargement of hands and feet, and arthritis characteristic of the condition termed "acromegaly." Therapy has included surgical removal of the area of the pituitary which is secreting the hormone, and use of new, synthetic analogs of the hormone somatostatin, which suppress growth hormone secretion.

Other Endocrine Abnormalities

Although rare, adrenal enlargement and excessive secretion of the adrenal hormone cortisol are seen in McCune-Albright syndrome. This may cause obesity of the face and trunk, weight gain, skin fragility and cessation of growth in childhood. These symptoms are called

"Cushing's syndrome." Treatment is removal of the affected adrenal glands, or use of drugs which block cortisol synthesis.

Some children with McCune-Albright syndrome have very low levels of phosphorus in their blood due to excessive losses of phosphate in their urine. This may cause bone changes associated with rickets, and may be treated with oral phosphates and supplemental vitamin D.

Bone Disease: Polyostotic Fibrous Dysplasia

The term "polyostotic fibrous dysplasia" means "abnormal fibrous tissue growth in many bones." However, the severity of bone disease in McCune-Albright syndrome is quite variable. In affected areas, normal bone is replaced by irregular masses of fibroblast cells. When this occurs in weight-bearing bones, such as the femur (upper leg bone), limping, deformity, and fractures may occur. In many children, the arms and/or legs are of unequal length, even in the absence of actual fracture. Regions of fibrous dysplasia are also very common in the bones that form the skull and upper jaw. If these areas begin to expand, skull and facial asymmetry may result.

Polyostotic fibrous dysplasia can often be seen in a plain, X-ray picture of the skeleton. A more sensitive method of finding lesions is a bone scan, in which a small amount of radioactivity (an isotope of technetium) is injected into a vein, taken up by the abnormal tissues, and detected by a scanner.

Some children may be minimally affected, with no asymmetry, deformity or fracture, and lesions detected only by a bone scan. In a few children, lesions are found only in the base of the skull. By repeating bone scans at intervals of one to two years, it has been shown that the bone disease in some children may become more extensive over time. Unfortunately, severe bone disease can have permanent effects upon physical appearance and mobility.

There is no known hormonal or medical treatment effective in controlling progressive polyostotic fibrous dysplasia. Surgical procedures to correct fracture and deformity include grafting, pinning, and casting. Skull and jaw changes are often corrected surgically, with great improvement in appearance.

Treatment and therapy for this bone disease are usually the most difficult aspect of caring for a child who has severe polyostotic fibrous dysplasia.

The McCune-Albright Syndrome

Skin Abnormalities

The irregular, flat areas of increased skin pigment in McCune-Albright syndrome are called "cafe-au-lait" spots because, in children with light complexions, they are the color of coffee with milk. In dark-skinned individuals, these spots may be difficult to see. Most children have the pigment from birth, and it almost never becomes more extensive. The pattern of the pigment distribution is unique, often starting or ending abruptly at the midline on the abdomen in front or at the spine in back. Some children have no cafe-au-lait pigment at all; in a few, it is confined to small areas, such as the nape of the neck or crease of the buttocks.

There are seldom any medical problems associated with the areas of cafe-au-lait pigment. Some adolescent children may want to use makeup to obscure areas of dark pigment on the face.

Recent Research

So far, researchers have not found a cure for the bone and endocrine disease in McCune-Albright syndrome. It cannot yet be diagnosed before birth and there is no way to accurately predict how severe the disease may become in an affected child. There are no reported cases of any parent being affected, and the children of women with McCune-Albright syndrome are normal. All races appear to be affected equally. Thus, we are not yet certain of the genetic origin of the defect. It is believed, however, that it may be the result of a mutation occurring early in the development of the embryo.

Recently, researchers have discovered abnormal mutations in DNA obtained from the affected ovaries, adrenals, and liver of several patients with McCune-Albright syndrome. The DNA contained the genetic code for one component, called a "G" protein, of a signalling system which is present in many cells, and which is known to be involved in endocrine cell growth and secretion. The presence of this mutation could result in uncontrolled cell function or hormone secretion. This research is continuing, and it may soon enable us to plan better methods of treatment for patients with the McCune-Albright syndrome.

Chapter 26

Pityriasis Rosea

An acute, self-limiting, inflammatory skin disease, pityriasis rosea produces a "herald" patch (which usually goes undetected) followed by a generalized eruption of papulosquamous lesions. Although this non-contagious disorder may develop at any age, it's most apt to occur in adolescents and young adults. The incidence rises in the spring and fall.

Causes

The cause of pityriasis rosea is unknown, but the brief course of the disease and virtual absence of recurrence suggest a viral agent or auto-immune disorder.

Signs and Symptoms

Pityriasis typically begins with an erythematous "herald" patch, which may appear anywhere on the body. Although this slightly raised, oval lesion is about 2 to 6 cm in diameter, approximately 25 percent of patients don't notice it. A few days to several weeks later, yellow-tan or erythematous patches with scaly edges (about 0.5 to 1 cm in diameter) erupt on the trunk and extremities, and sometimes on the face, hands and feet in adolescents. Eruption continues for seven to ten days, and the patches persist for two to six weeks. Occasionally,

© Professional Guide to Diseases, Third Edition. Reprinted with permission.

these patches are macular, vesicular, or urticarial. A characteristic of this disease is the arrangement of lesions along body cleavage lines, producing a pattern similar to that of a pine tree. Accompanying pruritus is usually mild but may be severe.

Diagnosis

Characteristic skin lesions support the diagnosis. Differential diagnosis must also rule out secondary syphilis (through serologic testing), dermatophytosis, and drug reaction.

Treatment and Special Considerations

Treatment focusses on relief of pruritus, with emollients, oatmeal baths, antihistamines, and occasionally, exposure to ultra-violet light or sunlight. Topical steroids in a hydrophilic cream base may be beneficial. Rarely, if inflammation is severe, systemic corticosteroids may be required.

- Reassure the patient that pityriasis rosea is non-contagious, that spontaneous remission usually occurs in two to six weeks, and that lesions generally don't recur.

- Urge the patient not to scratch. Advise him/her that hot baths may intensify itching. Encourage use of anti-pruritics.

Chapter 27

Scleroderma

What Is Scleroderma?

Scleroderma is an all-inclusive term to describe many clinical conditions. Collectively, these disorders are uncommon, but not necessarily rare.

The simplest definition of scleroderma is found in Schiffere's *Family Medical Encyclopedia*, i.e., "hardening of the skin," appropriately based on the roots of the word: *sclero*=hard and *derma*=skin.

This disease has been described for centuries and although some authors have been credited with earlier documentation, Curzio of Naples wrote the first definite description in 1753.

Gintrac introduced the current term, scleroderma, in 1847, after which it was recognized as a skin disorder. In the early twentieth century, reports suggested that this disease was not only confined to the skin but was a systemic disorder and could affect numerous internal organs. In 1945 Goetz introduced the term progressive systemic sclerosis (PSS). However, the term is not universally accepted as scleroderma is not always progressive nor systemic. Today many physicians prefer the term systemic sclerosis (SS), to describe the non-localized form of disease which may affect internal organs.

©1977 Revised 1981, 1984, 1987, 1992 United Scleroderma Foundation, Inc. Excerpted with permission.

What Forms of Scleroderma Exist?

For better understanding, the sclerodermatous disorders are divided into two major forms: Systemic and Localized.

Systemic Forms of Scleroderma

- Diffuse Systemic Sclerosis (SS)
- The CREST Syndrome, now referred to as limited

Localized Forms of Scleroderma

- Morphea (single or multiple plaques)
- Generalized Morphea
- Linear Scleroderma/En Coup de Sabre

Mixed Connective Tissue Disease (MCTD)

- Mixed Connective Tissue Disease (MCTD) is an "over lap" syndrome in which certain symptoms of scleroderma, lupus erythematosus, and polymyositis combine. It is not usually classified as systemic scleroderma.

Forms Defined

Systemic Scleroderma

Progressive Systemic Sclerosis (PSS) or Diffuse Systemic Sclerosis (SS). Progressive Systemic Sclerosis (PSS) or Diffuse Systemic Sclerosis (SS) indicates the form of scleroderma with more generalized skin involvement as well as body systems such as the esophagus, joints, intestines, lungs, heart and kidneys. The severity depends on the organ involved.

Scleroderma varies greatly in the severity and/or progression of disease. It can range from the widespread thickening of skin (diffuse) to a much more limited skin change (CREST).

Diffuse scleroderma is another term which describes systemic sclerosis and skin changes on many parts of the body. Tight, glossy skin can be present on the trunk and upper arms, as well as the face, chest and extremities.

Scleroderma

The Crest Syndrome or Limited Systemic Sclerosis

CREST. CREST is an acronym made up of the first letters of the five most prominent manifestations of this form of scleroderma: Calcinosis, Raynaud's phenomenon, esophageal dysfunction, Sclerodactyly and Telangiectasia.

- **Calcinosis.** Calcinosis is the accumulation of calcium salts under the skin. Many parts of the body can be affected such as fingers, arms, feet, and knees. Pain and infection may result as the calcium deposits may protrude through the skin.

- **Raynaud's Phenomenon.** Raynaud's Phenomenon is a disturbance of the circulation within small blood vessel thereby affecting the extremities, primarily the hands and feet. This is due to spasm of the vessels initiated by stimuli such as cold or stress. Normally, vessels constrict in order to conserve the warmth of the body for the internal organs. In scleroderma, the blood vessels (capillaries) are decreased in number and narrowed in size. The internal organs may also react to cold and stress with spasms of the small vessels.

    Poor circulation causes the hands to show color changes from the normal color to pallor/white to blue or purple; as the blood slowly returns, the skin may take on a red color. There may be pain, tingling, numbness, or a burning sensation. Care of the hands is very important as bumping or bruising may cause ulcerations (open sores). Raynaud's phenomenon is seen in 90-95 percent of systemic scleroderma patients.

- **Esophageal Dysfunction.** Esophageal Dysfunction is the loss of normal action of the lower esophagus. A common complaint is the return of food and acid from the stomach into the esophagus (acid reflux). This condition causes heartburn, and the returning acid can cause scarring in the esophagus making swallowing difficult. Some patients may experience complications in the digestive tract (gastrointestinal involvement), and many are seen with hiatal hernia.

- **Sclerodactyly.** Sclerodactyly is a condition in which the skin on the digits becomes hard. Fingers and toes may not bend, or they may become fixed into a flexed or less functional position.

- **Telangiectasia.** Telangiectasia is the appearance of small blood vessels near the surface of the skin. These capillaries become enlarged and visible, chiefly on the fingers, palms, lips, face and tongue. They appear as small red spots.

Localized Scleroderma

Morphea. Morphea is a form of localized scleroderma. It begins with an inflammatory stage, followed by the appearance of one or many patches or plaques. These plaques feel firm and hard, are oval in shape with an ivory/yellow center, and are surrounded by a violet colored area. They are seen more often on the trunk, but may also occur on the face and extremities. A large percentage of morphea patients improve spontaneously. Guttate Morphea is an uncommon form and is characterized by small, chalk-white spots which appear on the chest, neck, and shoulders. The violet colored line may surround all or some of the spots.

Generalized Morphea. Generalized Morphea is rare and a more serious problem. It can involve almost the entire skin but usually does not affect internal organs or have associated Raynaud's phenomenon.

Linear Scleroderma. Linear Scleroderma is a band-like thickening of skin which may be limited to one area, such as an arm or leg, but can affect two or more extremities. It generally begins in the first decade of life, and is most evident in children when an extremity fails to grow as rapidly as the uninvolved limb. The band may extend from hip to heel or shoulder to hand, and very often there is loss of deep tissue, such as muscle and bone.

En Coup De Sabre. En Coup De Sabre is a French term meaning "the strike of the sword." It is used to describe linear scleroderma when it occurs on the face or scalp. The deep scarring resembles a sabre wound.

Problems of the Internal Organs

Although the dermatologist or rheumatologist may first diagnose the scleroderma, often disease progression requires the services of other specialists, namely a gastroenterologist, pulmonary specialist, cardiologist, or urologist.

The stomach does not seem to be directly affected, but the loss of muscle motion in the small intestine or bowel may result in malabsorption (the body does not absorb nutrients from food). The food remains in the bowel too long and allows overgrowth of bacteria. Diarrhea can be a symptom of bacterial overgrowth. The patient may suffer from weight loss, anemia, and malnutrition.

The muscle of the large intestine or colon may lose the ability to "push" the wastes down. Some symptoms of this condition may be bloating and constipation.

Lung involvement can be severe or slight. Pleurisy-like symptoms may occur or shortness of breath and coughing. The lungs do contain a large reserve of tissue, but damaged tissue results in less oxygen to the blood system. The reflux action of the esophagus may cause pulmonary problems by aspirating foreign matter into the lungs.

Some heart involvement is seen in most scleroderma patients. Much of the time it is due to involvement of other organs. For instance, lung damage can put a strain on the heart. Scarring of the heart may cause heart rhythm disturbances, and, while uncommon, falling or fainting spells may occur.

While most patients do not have kidney involvement, patients should have blood pressure checked regularly. A sudden rise in blood pressure is a serious symptom. Patients with severe hypertension are hospitalized and treated with large doses of blood pressure medication.

Involvement of the liver may occur in the form of biliary cirrhosis, a serious disorder, particularly in patients with CREST syndrome. Fortunately, this is uncommon.

What Causes Scleroderma?

No one knows the answer, but there are many theories being studied which involve different systems of the body: the immune system, the vascular system, and connective tissue metabolism. All these are known to play a part in the disease mechanism.

The appearance of scleroderma in several members of a family has been cited, but the hereditary aspect has not been fully defined.

Some occupations involving vinyl chloride have produced scleroderma-like symptoms in workers, while prolonged exposure to silica dust increases the risk of development of true SD.

A drug, bleomycin, which is used for treating cancer patients, has also produced scleroderma-like symptoms. These seem to be self limiting, and disappear after the drug treatment is stopped.

Who Gets Scleroderma?

The disease is found in all countries and ethnic groups, with patients ranging from infants to the elderly. Symptoms usually appear between the ages of thirty to fifty, and childhood scleroderma is usually the localized form.

Approximately four times as many women as men develop scleroderma during early and middle age. The frequency tends to increase with age in both sexes, and in the older ages the relative ratio of women to men is less.

While seemingly rare, scleroderma is far more prevalent than muscular dystrophy, multiple sclerosis, and a host of other better known and understood diseases. Frequency in the U.S. suggests over 300,000 cases of systemic scleroderma. Denny Tuffanelli, M.D., UC San Francisco, the first chairman of USF's Medical Advisory Board states that the combined forms approximate 700,000. Many other patients have sclerodermoid lesions as part of other diseases.

Symptoms and Diagnosis

Two major problems of scleroderma are decreased circulation and increased production of connective tissue. For this reason, scleroderma may be defined as a disease complex of (1) vascular (blood vessel) changes; (2) fibrosis, an abnormal increase in the amount of collagenous connective tissue in an organ, (3) inflammation, that to varying degrees involves the skin and visceral (internal) organs, and (4) atrophy, loss of normal functioning tissue.

Scleroderma is classified as one of the collagen diseases. Collagen is the most abundant protein found in connective tissue, cartilage, skin and bone. It is the "binding" which holds the body together. It is produced by cells called fibroblasts. Usually, starting in the early twenties these cells function at a low level until they are needed to repair an injury or a surgery. In scleroderma, some factor triggers the overproduction of collagen causing thickening and hardening (fibrosis) of the skin or other organs. The small blood vessels (capillaries) are also affected and cannot supply sufficient blood to many parts of the body.

It is not known what the primary event may be. Changes may occur first in cells (fibroblasts) which cause over-production of collagen, or an inflammatory response may take place. It is possible for a combination of changes to occur.

Scleroderma

At first, scleroderma can be difficult to diagnose. There may be slowly evolving changes in the skin or malfunction of an internal organ. The relationship to any systemic disease may be unknown at this point. Arthritic-like symptoms may appear, and rheumatoid arthritis, lupus erythematosus, osteoarthritis, and bursitis are frequent misdiagnoses.

First symptoms may include such non-specific complaints as: arthritis, weight loss, fatigue, vague muscle pain, joint or bone aching, arthritis, Raynaud's phenomenon, stiffness of the hands, altered pigmentation (light/dark discolorations of the skin), unexplained swelling, thickening of the skin, or telangiectases.

Blood pressure problems are rare as a first symptom; however, there may be shortness of breath, loss of hair, swallowing difficulties, heartburn, or heart, lung, intestinal, or kidney problems.

If any one of these symptoms is an isolated complaint, scleroderma is not the first disorder that comes to mind. When two or more of these symptoms appear together, the true nature of the disease may be suspected.

The most frequent initial manifestations of SD are: (1) Raynaud's phenomenon, (2) puffy swelling of the hands (gradually replaced by thickening of the skin of the fingers), and (3) joint pain (polyarthralgia). There is no single test which proves the diagnosis. Careful history-taking and physical examination are emphasized. Certain tests, such as blood sedimentation rate, gamma globulin, latex fixation, antinuclear antibody, skin biopsies, and X-rays may be made. Some of the tests may be abnormal, but scleroderma is not necessarily the only possible diagnosis. The diagnosis is generally established on the basis of combined clinical findings. The American Rheumatism Association proposed criteria for clinically definite systemic sclerosis. (see table below)

Table 27.1. ARA Scleroderma Criteria Cooperative Study (SCCS): Preliminary clinical criteria for systemic sclerosis (Excludes localized scleroderma and pseudoslerdermatous disorders.)

1. Proximal scleroderma is the single major criterion; sensitivity was 91 percent and specificity was over 99 percent.

2. Sclerodactyly, digital pitting scars of fingertips or loss of substance of the distal finger pad, and bibasilar pulmonary fibrosis contributed further as minor criteria in the absence of proximal scleroderma.

3. One major or two or more minor criteria were found in 97 percent of definite systemic sclerosis patients, but only in 2 percent of the comparison patients with systemic lupus erythematosus, polymyositis/dermatomyositis, or Raynaud's phenomenon.

Reprinted from *Arthritis and Rheumatism Journal*. Used by permission of the American Rheumatism Association.

What Can Be Done?

Unfortunately, there is not yet any known therapy that will stop or reverse the progressive sclerosis involved in scleroderma. Many different medications and therapies have been tried; some of these have been met with initial hope and enthusiasm by both doctor and patient, but so far none led to a permanent cure of this disease.

After diagnosis, best results can be achieved when patients and their families become actively involved in the treatment. Many things can be done; and while the results may not be quick and dramatic, the patient's troubling symptoms may be alleviated. Scleroderma varies greatly from patient to patient and over time in any given person. Conditions may arise which are amenable to therapy, and this is one reason for regular visits to the doctor.

For many, this will be a chronic and possibly disabling illness although there are exceptional records of remission after five or ten years. The patient must face the fact that he is dealing with a long-term disorder. Many fundamental questions go unanswered as the disease varies from the sclerosis of a small bit of skin to overwhelming systemic reactions which can result in death.

Therapies and medications range from the prescription of creams and emollients for relief of skin problems to dialysis or large doses of hypertensive drugs for patients with acute renal (kidney) involvement.

Medications used in the treatment of scleroderma can be divided into two main groups:

- those designed to control (reduce) fibrosis of the skin and internal organ—chiefly D-penicillamine and colchicine;

- symptomatic measures, designed to relieve problems caused by damage to skin and internal organs by the fibrosis.

Scleroderma

Anti-hypertensive agents

alpha methyldopa (Aldomet)
catopril (Capoten)
phenoxybenzamine (Dibenzyline)
enalapril (Vasotec)
nifedipine (Procardia, Adalat)
lisinopril (Prinivil, Zestril)
diltiazem (Cardizem)
fosinopril (Monopril)

Anti-fibrotic agents

D-penicillamine (Cuprimine, Depen)
Colchicine

Immunosuppressive agents

azathioprine (Imuran)
chlorambucil (Leukeran)
cyclophosphamide (Cytoxan)
methotrexate

Anti-inflammatory agents

hydroxchloroquine (Plaquenil)
salicylates
potassium para-aminobenzoate (Potaba)

Hormones corticosteroids

Vasodilators (agents which enlarge blood vessels) may be prescribed for Raynaud's phenomenon. These include: nicotinic acid, prazosin (Minipress), phenoxybenzamine (Dibenzyline), nifedipine (Procardia) and other drugs in this category. Drugs such as propanolol (Inderal) and minoxidil have also been used for blood pressure control. The skin may be treated with lubricating creams, and if ulcerations become infected, antibiotics are generally used. Because circulation is impaired, some physicians are prescribing biofeedback, which teaches the patient to control circulation.

D-Penicillamine is a common therapy for people with diffuse disease, especially in the early stages.

Calcinosis is also treated with antibiotics, but many times the patient must be hospitalized and surgery may be required.

Aspirin, indomethacin (Indocin), naproxen (Naprosyn) or similar drugs are beneficial to patients with arthritic symptoms.

Corticosteroids may be helpful in myositis or arthritis, but it is not routinely effective in the treatment of scleroderma.

The esophagus and G.I. tract (gastro-intestinal) may be treated with antacids such as Maalox or Mylanta. Antibiotics and certain vitamins may be prescribed. Urecholine, Metoclopramide, omeprazole (Prilosec) and cimetidine (Tagamet) or other drugs in these categories have been helpful for G.I. complaints. Patients themselves can combat acid reflux (the return of stomach acid to the mouth and throat) by avoiding foods that provoke acid such as fats, spices, tea, coffee, and alcohol. For patients with difficulty swallowing or digesting foods, careful chewing, eating slowly and drinking carbonated water or other beverage will soften the food and help the digestive process. Several small meals a day may be necessary, and one should sit upright at least two hours after eating. Six inch blocks placed under the head of the bed give relief while sleeping.

The mouth of the scleroderma patient is often neglected. It is important to maintain good oral hygiene as gum disease is common in scleroderma. A knowledgeable dentist should be consulted on the proper way to keep teeth and gums clean.

Some patients have difficulty with excessive dryness of the mouth/eyes, and this condition (Sjögren's syndrome) should be brought to the attention of the doctor.

Although heart, lungs, and kidneys are not frequently affected, symptoms should be closely monitored by the physician. Regular blood pressure checks are advised as kidney involvement usually begins with elevated blood pressure. Captopril therapy (anti-hypertension medications) has shown dramatic results and given hope to patients with scleroderma renal crisis (SRC).

From time to time, the physician may order certain laboratory tests. Blood tests ordered could include: complete blood count (CBC); rheumatoid factor; Westergren sedimentation rate; antinuclear antibody test; CPK (a muscle enzyme) among others.

A urine specimen may be required to calculate kidney function. A 24-hour specimen means the patient must discard the urine passed at a specific time and then collect all urine passed for the next 24 hours. A container is usually provided. If there are any questions, the doctor should be contacted; because if the test is not done properly, it is of no use.

Scleroderma

The physician may wish to test the circulation of blood through small blood vessels in the skin. He does this by varying the temperature of small areas of skin and watching the color changes that occur. A nailfold test is done by placing a drop of oil on the fingernail and, through the microscope, observing the tiny blood vessels found in the fingernail bed. A pulmonary function test is made to determine breathing ability and capacity of air the lungs can inspire. The patient breathes into a machine which runs out a tracing of the breathing activity on a graph.

Different types of X-rays may be ordered, and some may need preparation. Patients may be asked not to eat for several hours before the X-ray is done, or they may have to take a special medicine which acts like a dye. This will enable the physician to visualize the esophagus, stomach, or intestines. A chest X-ray requires no preparation and allows the doctor to note any changes in the lungs.

If a biopsy is requested, a small piece of skin will be taken for examination under the microscope. The doctor will either spray the skin or inject the area to numb it. With a device that works like a hole punch, he removes the piece of skin; and a stitch may be placed in the area. Usually there is little discomfort.

Depending on the progression of the disease, more involved tests may be ordered.

Physical/Occupational Therapy

The goal of every therapist is to have the patient achieve his best quality of living.

Many physicians now recognize the importance of early referral of the scleroderma patient to a physical or occupational therapist. Stiffness and tight skin impair range of motion, and an early program of exercise may prolong activities. This can include exercises for arms, legs, neck, face, and trunk. Since the hands are often the first affected part, hand exercises are very important. Patients should not attempt to exercise without proper instruction as it is possible to injure oneself. A motion must never be forced but should be relaxed and within the pain limit. If there is lung involvement, deep breathing exercises may be prescribed. It must be emphasized that exercise does not stop the progression of the disease but is important therapy. Patients are cautioned to temper activity with rest but to make the exercise a definite part of every day. Whirlpool baths, isometrics, heat, and paraffin baths may also be a part of the prescribed program.

Energy saving is stressed as the scleroderma patient can tire easily. Shopping, cleaning, gardening, or similar tasks should be done a little at a time. Simplify everything you do; eliminate unnecessary jobs, and ask your family and friends for help.

Occupational therapy is designed to increase the level of independence and decrease the difficulty caused by scleroderma.

When there is a decrease in range of motion, the therapist will suggest various adaptive devices. For limited grasp, handles can be built up with sponge, or an elongated handle may be applied. Fork and spoon combinations and special cupholders are also available.

It is important to protect any body parts where pressure causes pain. Your therapist will advise you on specialized items to protect ulcerations on elbows, knees, or heels. Air or jell-filled cushions, or those of foam can protect joints from pressure pain.

The occupational therapist strives to make the patient as comfortable as possible and help him maintain a good self-concept in the activity of daily living (ADL).

Emotional Problems

Scleroderma, as with any chronic disease, is cause for emotional involvement. From the first frustrations of diagnosis, to the coping with a long-term illness which may alter the life-style, the patient encounters stress.

The "grief-process" is a very real part of the patient's adjustment, and each will cope in his own way. In varying degrees, each will pass through the stages of: shock, denial, anger, bargaining and finally acceptance.

After the initial shock of diagnosis, the patient may deny the illness. Fear of the unknown causes anger and "blame-placing." Bargaining (with God or other figure) may take place. Depression is often a natural reaction to chronic disease, so emotional support is a major factor in the treatment of scleroderma. With acceptance, there may be a need to adjust the life-style; and this can involve the entire family. All are affected by the emotional impact of this disease, and keeping communication open is essential. Many times the patient is accused of pretending illness and "spoiling things." It must be realized that scleroderma is a disease of many symptoms which can vary in intensity in a short time. Helping the patient adjust may require some role changing in the family. Certain tasks can be allotted differently. If problems are too difficult to resolve, family counseling by a physician or competent psychologist is recommended.

The patient's well-being depends on the entire health professional "team," and this includes the family. What is implemented by physicians and therapists can be carried out by the patient with the help of the family.

Hope and Living with Scleroderma

While there is no specific treatment for scleroderma, research and studies are being conducted at medical centers throughout the world and the outlook is bright. The Criteria studies allow physicians to diagnose scleroderma more readily and these studies are on-going.

New drugs are being researched, while some old ones are being reexamined.

Patients should endeavor to find a physician interested in scleroderma. Many frustrations can be eliminated if the physician understands the problems.

In general, every effort should be made to protect the hands, face, and ears from cold or overly active air-conditioning. Smoking is contraindicated in scleroderma, and one should even avoid being around those who are smoking. Clothing to reduce skin exposure and keep the trunk insulated (even to the point of slight perspiration) is important to maintain optimal blood flow to the skin at all times. Avoid the use of strong detergents or other skin irritants, and use creams or bath oils to help prevent dryness. Room humidifiers may also help to reduce dry skin. Have all infections treated immediately. Other "common sense" measures include eating balanced meals, avoiding excess alcohol, maintaining a sensible weight, and avoiding fatigue.

Impotence in men and sexual dysfunction in women should be discussed with a physician, and specialist help obtained when needed.

Chapter 28

Chronic Idiopathic Urticaria

Overview

Chronic idiopathic urticaria (CIU) is a troublesome condition for both the patient and the physician. Although it is not fatal, the manifestations of this perplexing disease create a great deal of physical discomfort and mental anguish for the patient. By the time many patients with CIU seek medical care, their physical discomfort is compounded by a feeling of frustration and anxiety.

In the United States, 15 percent to 20 percent of the population experience one or more episodes of urticaria in a lifetime. While many of these may be acute episodes, the incidence of chronic urticaria is nonetheless high. What distinguishes chronic from acute urticaria is, simply, the duration of the symptoms (Table 28.1).

Chronic urticaria is defined by persistence of the characteristic wheal and flare lesions for more than six weeks. In some patients, perhaps as many as half, the lesions may continue for as long as a year. The condition in a few patients may fluctuate over periods as long as 20 years, with deleterious effects on the patient's life style.

Chronic urticaria is idiopathic in approximately 95 percent of all cases. Very seldom is the physician able to find the cause of chronic urticaria. In contrast, the causes of acute urticarias are often detected because there is an immediate and identifiable causal relationship

©1994 National Jewish Center for Immunology and Respiratory Medicine. *Clinician* volume 12 number 4, August 1994. Reprinted with permission.

between the triggering event and the episode of urticaria; for example, the patient ate seafood, was stung by an insect, or was given a medication, and this was followed by an episode of urticaria. In chronic urticaria this direct connection is usually absent and the cause remains unknown.

Table 28.1. Chronic vs. Acute Urticaria

Chronic urticaria

- Wheal and flare lesions persist longer than six weeks
- In approximately 50 percent of patients, lesions continue for as long as a year
- In some patients, condition may fluctuate for as long as 20 years

Acute urticaria

- Causal relationship often evident

    1. patient ate seafood
    2. patient stung by insect
    3. patient took medication

- Immediate urticarial reaction follows

The appearance of urticarial lesions is familiar to all physicians and, indeed, to many patients (Table 28.2). Most urticarial lesions range from one to a few centimeters across, although the larger lesions should more properly be characterized as plaques, or clusters of lesions. Some smaller lesions, called papules, may range down to a few millimeters across; these are more commonly seen in cholinergic or aquagenic urticarias.

Table 28.2. Characteristics of Urticarial Lesions

- Most are transient, lasting longer than four hours
- If lesions last less than 24 hours, consider vasculitis
- In CIU, lesions may subside and be replaced by new ones
- Location of lesions rarely of clinical significance

Chronic Idiopathic Urticaria

Lesions can be transient; for example, physically induced urticarias last less than four hours, while most lesions of CIU last 6-18 hours. When individual lesions last longer than 24 hours, the possibility of underlying vasculitis must be considered. In individuals with CIU, lesions may subside but they are replaced by new lesions, not as a result of a new challenge, but as part of the continuing disease process. The location of urticarial lesions is rarely of clinical significance in chronic idiopathic urticaria except in the physical urticarias.

Histology and Pathophysiology

The lesions typical of chronic idiopathic urticaria are produced by localized vasodilation and an increase in the permeability of the dermal vasculature. These effects are due to the release of histamine and other mediators primarily from mast cell degranulation.

Dermal vasodilation peaks within three minutes of a histamine challenge and results in formation of a flare. The raised wheal, a result of increased vascular permeability, peaks in approximately eight minutes. Histamine injected subcutaneously provokes the characteristic urticarial wheal and flare reaction (Table 28.3). This reaction is reversed by administration of antihistamines.

Table 28.3. Lesions of CIU

- Produced by localized vasodilation and increased dermal vascular permeability
- Due to release of histamine and other mediators from mast cell degranulation
- Dermal vasodilation peaks within three minutes of histamine challenge and results in flare formation
- Raised wheal peaks in approximately eight minutes

Mediators of Urticarial Lesions

However, recent studies indicate that histamine is not the only active mediator liberated from mast cells that could be involved in the formation of urticarial lesions. Other factors may include prostaglandin D2, leukotrienes C, D and E, platelet activating factor, the kallikrein/kinin system, and possibly others (Table 28.4). The likelihood of pathogenic mediators other than histamine is supported by the fact that, in some cases, antihistamines relieve the pruritus in chronic idiopathic urticaria, but do not eliminate the hives.

Table 28.4. Other Factors of Urticarial Lesions

- Prostaglandin D2
- Leukotrienes C, D, E
- Platelet Activating Factor (PAF)
- Kallikrein/kinin system
- Others

Microscopic examination of the cellular infiltrate in biopsies of urticarial lesions in a recent study revealed a concentration of mast cells approximately nine times higher than that found in normal controls. In addition, a high number of other mononuclear cells were found. The distribution of these cells in a study of 12 CIU patients was: T-lymphocytes—47 percent, monocytes—22 percent, mast cells—11 percent, and 20 percent unidentifiable (Table 28.5).

The composition of the cellular infiltrate in urticarial lesions further confirms the role of histamine in chronic idiopathic urticaria. Moreover, histological studies have provided clues as to the nature of the factor or factors that trigger mast cell degranulation and release of histamine.

Table 28.5. Biopsies of Urticarial Lesions (based on study findings)

- Mast cell concentrations nine-times higher than normal controls
- Higher number of other mononuclear cells

Monocuclear cells	Percentage
T-lymphocytes	47 percent
monocytes	22 percent
mast cells	11 percent
unidentifiable	20 percent

Triggers of Histamine Release in CIU

Although in acute urticaria the immediate cause is not always known, the triggering factor is generally immunoglobulin (Ig)E. This type of reaction is not characteristic of chronic idiopathic urticaria. Chronic urticaria has no known association with atopy, and most patients do not show evidence of food-dependent reactivity. There is

Chronic Idiopathic Urticaria

also no evidence of immune complex involvement specifically. There is no evidence of IgG deposition, activation of immune complement or accumulation of neutrophils (Table 28.6).

Table 28.6. Chronic Urticaria

Does not show

- association with atopy
- evidence of food-dependent reactivity
- IgG deposition, activation of immune complement or neutrophil accumulation

Does produce

- increased levels of HRF in blister fluids

Increased levels of histamine releasing factor, or HRF, have been detected in the blister fluids of patients with CIU. These factors, members of the cytokine family, are derived from a large variety of mononuclear cells including lymphocytes. HRF derived from the mononuclear cells of allergic volunteers has also been shown to produce an immediate wheal-and-flare reaction in atopic subjects.

This blister-fluid histamine-releasing-factor activity is not due to the presence of IgE. This has been proven by demonstration that the HRF in specimens of blister-fluid is resistant to heat inactivation, ruling out IgE and immune complement as triggers of mast cell degranulation.

The cellular infiltrate in biopsies from patients with CIU is similar to that found in patients with cellular immune reactions in diseases with established immunologic etiologies, such as asthma and allergic rhinitis.

The Role of Autoimmunity in CIU

The autoimmune aspects of chronic idiopathic urticaria have been the subject of intense study in recent years. Investigators have found evidence of novel IgG autoantibodies, isolated from the peripheral blood of some CIU patients, some of which have the properties of an anti-IgE while others are directed toward the high-affinity IgE receptor on the mast cell surface inducing the release of histamine by acting directly on the alpha subunit of that receptor, even in the absence of IgE.

These autoantibodies suggest a role for autoimmunity in a significant percentage of CIU patients, perhaps 20 percent to 30 percent.

Diagnosis

Although in most cases the diagnosis of chronic idiopathic urticaria is not difficult, the clinician needs to consider a range of possibilities before initiating treatment. The most important step in the diagnosis of chronic urticaria is a thorough history and examination.

Physical Examination

A great deal can be learned from the examination. For example, many of the physical urticarias can be identified from the location and morphology of the lesions (Table 28.7). Small wheals, 1-3 mm across, with large surrounding erythematous flares suggest cholinergic or, less often, aquagenic urticarias. Lesions located on exposed areas suggest light- or cold-induced urticaria. Large lesions with involvement of deeper tissue at points where there is pressure or friction may indicate pressure urticarias. Contact urticarias are sometimes obvious because they are limited to the site of contact to a stimulus. Similarly, dermatographism is likely to produce a pattern of linear wheals at the site of scratching or friction.

Table 28.7. Morphology of Physical Urticarias

Cholinergic or aquagenic

- small wheals (1-3 mm diameter) with large surrounding erythematous flares

Light- or cold-induced

- lesions on exposed areas

Pressure

- large lesions, deeper tissue involvement where there is pressure or friction

Contact

- limited to area of contact

Chronic Idiopathic Urticaria

Dermatographism

- pattern of linear wheals

Urticaria Pigmentosa

Red-brown macules or papules on the trunk or extremities that urticate on stroking are a sign of urticaria pigmentosa or mastocytosis. Mastocytosis is systemic in about 10 percent of cases with an elevated number of mast cells not only in the skin but sometimes in bone, GI tract, liver, lymph nodes and spleen. Symptoms may include intense pruritus, headache, diarrhea, bronchospasm, rhinorrhea, flushing, hypotension, nausea, vomiting, tachycardia, dyspnea and syncope.

Duration of Lesions

The clinician should take notice of the duration of individual lesions. When these last a short time, two hours or less, a physical urticaria is the likely diagnosis. On the other hand, lesions that last longer, that is, 24 hours to 72 hours, are strongly suggestive of urticarial vasculitis (Table 28.8). Individual lesions in urticarial vasculitis may show petechiae and purpura and also display secondary changes as they resolve, particularly ecchymoses.

Table 28.8. Urticarial Vasculitis

- Lesions last 24 to 72 hours
- Lesions may show petechiae and purpura
- Lesions may show ecchymoses as they resolve

Drug Causes

Although the likelihood of establishing a cause for chronic urticaria is not great, the physician should consider the major etiologies of urticaria. Many drugs trigger histamine release from mast cells; the opiates, including codeine and morphine, do so to a very high degree (Table 28.9). Many antibiotics produce cutaneous drug reactions, penicillin in particular. However, these specific adverse reactions to drugs are more likely to result in episodes of acute urticaria and to be noted by both the patient and the attending physician.

Table 28.9. Drug Causes of Urticaria

- Opiates
- Antibiotics, especially penicillin
- Aspirin and other NSAIDS

Aspirin and other non-steroidal anti-inflammatory drugs exacerbate chronic urticaria in approximately 20 percent of cases. Patients frequently self-medicate with aspirin, sometimes inadvertently, because of the presence of aspirin in a variety of OTC remedies. Physicians should be aware of the potential of aspirin to aggravate urticarial symptoms.

Food Allergies

As with drugs, food allergies are more likely to be a cause of acute rather than chronic urticarias. If a patient is convinced that a food is the cause, an elimination diet may be undertaken (Table 28.10). A diet that includes a few "non-urticariogenic foods" and eliminates food additives, molds, and salicylates may be tried. If the cause of urticaria is a food, the patient should be virtually clear of symptoms at the end of a week. When this type of diet indicates that a food is causative, it may be followed by oral challenge tests or diet additions. In general, however, a food elimination diet is a slow and cumbersome way of arriving at a diagnosis. Skin and RAST tests are of minimal value because, although their sensitivity is high, their specificity is low.

Table 28.10. Elimination Diet in Diagnosis of CIU

- Include "non-urticariogenic foods"
- Eliminate food additives, molds, salicylates
- If food is causative, symptoms dissipate within a week
- Should be followed by oral challenge tests or diet additions
- Slow and cumbersome way of making diagnosis

Value of Laboratory Tests

Laboratory tests should be strongly linked to clues uncovered in the history and physical examination. Lesions that persist longer than 24 hours should be biopsied to be examined for vasculitis. These patients should also have erythrocyte sedimentation rate (ESR), immune complement and antinuclear antibody tests, especially if they also show some of the signs of an autoimmune disease such as arthralgia or fever. Patients with normal ESR rates are unlikely to have urticarial vasculitis.

Underlying Medical Conditions

Several underlying medical problems may produce urticaria as one of the symptoms (Table 28.11). These include the prodromal phase of hepatitis B. although this phase lasts only one or two weeks and should be considered acute rather than chronic. Other underlying medical problems may include focal and systemic infections of bacterial, viral, fungal, or parasitic origin, systemic lupus, thyroid disease, and carcinomas or lymphomas. It should be remembered, however, that although an elaborate laboratory workup may prove beneficial in arriving at a diagnosis for a few patients, in most cases these tests are not cost effective and are of minimal value since they show little that was not already strongly suggested in the initial interview.

Table 28.11. Medical Causes of CIU

- Hepatitis B
- Focal and systemic infections
  1. bacterial
  2. viral
  3. fungal
  4. parasitic

- Systemic lupus
- Thyroid disease
- Carcinomas/lymphomas

Management

Although the ideal treatment for chronic urticaria would be to identify and isolate the cause and remove it from the patient's diet or environment, in the great majority of cases this is not possible. Fortunately, the pathology of CIU is well-understood and agents are available that have the capacity of blocking or minimizing this pathology.

Antihistamines

Antihistamines, specifically the H_1 blockers, are the mainstay of therapy for chronic idiopathic urticaria. The strategy is to block the effects of histamine that has already been released by mast cell degranulation. The H_1 antagonists are best suited to carry out this blockade because H_1 receptors predominate in the vasculature over H_2 receptors by 85 percent to 15 percent.

However, should monotherapy with H_1 antihistamines produce insufficient results, adjunctive therapies with H_2 blockers, oral corticosteroids or tricyclic antidepressants may be instituted.

Antihistamines are commonly categorized either as older, sedating antihistamines, or as newer, non-sedating antihistamines.

Sedating Antihistamines

The older antihistamines, as represented by chlorpheniramine, diphenhydramine, and hydroxyzine, have a rapid onset of action. Their recommended dosing regimens are three to four times a day with an assumed duration of action lasting from four to six hours (Table 28.12).

Table 28.12. Sedating (Older) Antihistamines

- Includes chlorpheniramine, diphenhydramine, and hydroxyzine
- Rapid onset of action
- Recommended dosing regimen: T-QID
- Duration of action
  1. may be in excess of 24 hrs for chlorpheniramine and hydroxyzine
  2. allows for QD dosing

However, new information indicates that the half-life of chlorpheniramine and hydroxyzine may be in excess of 24 hours which allows for a once-daily dosing regimen.

The older antihistamines also readily pass through the blood brain barrier where this oftentimes results in sedation. Whereas this may be beneficial at night, it may be detrimental for use in the patient during the day. New studies indicate that the older antihistamines may impair judgement and functional ability even in the absence of sedation. Additionally, the older, sedating antihistamines may cause anticholinergic effects such as dry mouth, urinary retention, and

Chronic Idiopathic Urticaria

blurry vision. Other adverse effects include tinnitus, dizziness, GI disturbance, and palpitations (Table 28.13).

Some patients may also complain of undesirable stimulation of the central nervous system resulting in restlessness and insomnia.

However, it should be noted that one of the benefits of the older, sedating antihistamines, particularly in today's economic environment, is cost. Additionally, the dosing regimen of these agents may be increased to achieve greater potency. If taken on a regular basis, the patient may experience sedation for the first few days. However, the patient may become tolerant to this effect in four to five days and, in some cases, may not continue to experience side effects.

Table 28.13. Sedating (Older) Antihistamines: Adverse Effects

Pass through BBB

- results in sedation

Impair judgement and functional ability even if no sedation
Anticholinergic effects

- dry mouth
- urinary retention
- blurry vision

Other

- tinnitus
- dizziness
- GI disturbance
- palpitations
- restlessness
- insomnia

Non-sedating Antihistamines

The newer, non-sedating antihistamines do not cross the blood-brain barrier and as a consequence seldom produce sedation or CNS stimulation. The incidence of sedation and anticholinergic adverse effects when patients were given these drugs in clinical trials was equal to placebo (Table 28.14).

The most widely used non-sedating H_1 antihistamines in the United States are astemizole, terfenadine, and loratadine. These newer antihistamines have been studied in clinical trials of chronic urticaria comparing them with the older antihistamines. For example, terfenadine and loratadine were compared in separate trials to hydroxyzine. The non-sedating agents were found in both cases to be equal in efficacy to hydroxyzine. In a separate study, astemizole was shown to be significantly more effective than chlorpheniramine. Nevertheless, agents such as hydroxyzine or diphenhydramine can be used in doses exceeding those in such studies, if side effects are tolerable, with greater efficacy.

These non-sedating agents are approximately equal in effectiveness and all have active metabolites but show considerable differences as to pharmacokinetics and drug interactions.

Table 28.14. Non-Sedating (Newer) Antihistamines

Do not cross BBB

- no/minimal sedation or CNS stimulation

Anticholinergic/sedative adverse effects equal to placebo

Pharmacology of the Non-sedating Antihistamines

The parent compound of astemizole has a half-life of 24 hours. However, the active metabolite has a half-life of 7 to 11 days. The onset of action is within hours with peak activity occurring after several days. Astemizole's activity can continue for many days and the active metabolite can remain in the body for as long as four months after the last dose. This is of concern for patients who need skin testing, those who experience adverse reactions, or those of childbearing age. The steady state of astemizole and its active metabolite is reached in four to eight weeks. Due to its very long half-life, astemizole is dosed once a day. Lastly, the absorption of astemizole is decreased approximately 60 percent in the presence of food.

The parent compound of terfenadine has a half-life of six hours and its active metabolite has a half-life of 17 hours. It has an onset of action of one to two hours, with peak action being reached in three to

Chronic Idiopathic Urticaria

four hours. The duration of activity for terfenadine is equal to or greater than 12 hours. Steady state for parent and active metabolite is attained in 2 1/2 to 3 days. Terfenadine has a twice-daily dosing regimen. The absorption of terfenadine is unaffected by food.

The parent compound of loratadine has a half-life of eight hours and the metabolite has a half-life of 28 hours. The onset of action is from 1 to 3 hours, with the peak action being reached in 8 to 12 hours. This allows for a duration of activity equal to or greater than 24 hours. Steady state is reached within five days. Loratadine, like astemizole, has a once daily dosing regimen. Food hastens the absorption of loratadine, but this does not influence efficacy (Table 28.15).

Incidence of Torsades De Pointes

Astemizole and terfenadine have also been infrequently associated with a ventricular arrhythmia characterized by prolongation of the QT segment and changes of the T-wave, known as torsades de pointes. Several cases of this cardiac abnormality have been reported, sometimes associated with overdoses of the two agents, sometimes with concomitant use of other agents which are known to inhibit hepatic metabolism. Some of these cases have resulted in syncope and cardiac arrest. This reaction has not been associated with the use of loratadine.

The mechanism behind these potentially fatal adverse events may lie in the pharmacokinetic profiles of these antihistamines. Studies suggest that certain agents such as ketoconazole, itraconazole and erythromycin may inhibit the metabolism of astemizole and terfenadine resulting in higher than normal serum levels of these drugs. It is suggested that it is these high levels of the parent compound that lead to the potential for this cardiac arrhythmia.

Similarly, higher than recommended doses of astemizole and terfenadine create the same pharmacokinetic situation. For this reason both astemizole and terfenadine are contraindicated with ketoconazole, itraconazole and erythromycin.

Loratadine has not shown the same potential for this problem. In a recent study, loratadine, at four times the recommended dose, was given concomitantly with erythromycin without producing any cardiac abnormalities. However, further studies are needed for the conclusive confirmation of this finding.

	Half-Life	Onset	Peak Action	Duration	Steady State	Dosing	Food Effects
Astemizole	Parent = 24 hrs Metabolite = 7-11 days	Hrs	Days later	Up to 4 mos	4 to 8 wks	OD	Absorption decreased
Terfenadine	Parent = 6 hrs Metabolite = 17 hrs	1 to 2 hrs	3 to 4 hrs	≥ 12 hrs	2 1/2 to 3 days	BID	No effect
Loratadine	Parent = 8 hrs Metabolite = 28 hrs	1 to 3 hrs	8 to 12 hrs	≥ 24 hrs	5 days	OD	Absorption increased

Table 28.15. New Antihistamines: Pharmacology

H_2 Blockers

When maximal doses of H_1 antagonists are not sufficient to produce a complete remission, it may be necessary to add an agent that has some H_2 activity. This is particularly true when wheal formation and pruritus continue. Addition of an H_2 blocker, such as cimetidine or ranitidine, has been shown to produce a synergistic response of approximately 10 percent when given with an H_1 antagonist.

Tricyclic Antidepressants

Another approach has been to employ a tricyclic antidepressant such as doxepin. This agent is a very potent H_1 blocker and also has strong H_2 blocking ability. However, it is associated with sedation as well as the typical anticholinergic side effects including blurred vision, urine retention, and dry mouth.

Some clinicians use doxepin in combination with one of the non-sedating antihistamines, taking advantage of the sedating effects of doxepin at night and using the non-sedating antihistamine during the daylight hours. Doxepin may also be used as monotherapy in selected patients.

Corticosteroids

In severe or refractory cases of chronic idiopathic urticaria, the physician may need to consider the use of oral corticosteroids. In anaphylaxis or acute urticaria, prednisone is considered useful and appropriate. In chronic urticaria, some authorities suggest giving prednisone at low doses, 20 to 30 mg per day on alternate days until the symptoms have been reduced, and then tapering down. In chronic urticaria the benefits from using corticosteroids need to be weighed against the potential for adverse events. Daily steroids should be avoided, and regular therapy with antihistamines should be continued.

In summary, the first agents to try and stay with consistently are the H_1 antihistamines. Other agents may be added to improve the response in refractory cases, but the H_1 blockers are the mainstay of therapy.

Future Research

As more is learned about the mechanism of chronic idiopathic urticaria at the cellular level, there appears to be reason to believe that, at least in some cases, it has an important autoimmune component.

A significant percentage of patients with chronic idiopathic urticaria and/or angioedema also have thyroid autoimmunity. Approximately 3 percent to 6 percent of the general population can be expected to have thyroid autoimmunity. In a pool of 624 cases of patients with chronic idiopathic urticaria, 90 had evidence of thyroid autoimmunity; thus, the incidence of thyroid autoimmunity in this patient population was three to six times higher than would be expected in the population at large.

While treatment with l-thyroxin had no effect on most patients, a few patients in the study group demonstrated a dramatic response. Among the possible explanations which have been advanced for the association of thyroid autoimmunity with chronic idiopathic urticaria is that the presence of large numbers of activated CD4 T-lymphocytes in the perivascular tissue of CIU patients results in the production of excess quantities of lymphokines, which may be linked to thyroid autoimmunity. This information taken together with the work described earlier, which points to a cross-linking of the IgE receptor in chronic idiopathic urticaria, provides fertile ground for future research.

In the meantime, until more is known about the etiologies of CIU, clinicians are fortunate in having at their disposal a range of drugs that have the capabilities of resolving the symptoms of the great majority of patients. For the foreseeable future, the mainstay of therapy for CIU will be the H_1 class of antihistamines. Chronic idiopathic urticaria is a condition which has the potential for disrupting a patient's life and causing great stress and anxiety. The clinician has the opportunity to treat the disease effectively without causing disruption to the patient's daily life.

Suggested Readings

Mathews, KP. "Chronic Urticaria." In: Schocket, AL, ed. Clinical *Management of Urticaria and Anaphylaxis*. First Edition. New York City: Marcel Dekker, Inc. 1993; 21-68.

Elias, J. Boss; E. Kaplan, AP. "Studies of the cellular infiltrate of chronic idiopathic urticaria: prominence of T-lymphocytes, monocytes, and mast cells." *J Allergy Clin Immunol*. 1986; 78: 914-918.

Monroe, EW. "Urticaria." In: Callen, JP, ed. *Current problems in dermatology*. St. Louis: Mosby. 1993; 115-140.

Jacques, P. Lavoie A; Bedard, P. et al. "Chronic idiopathic urticaria: profiles of skin mast cell histamine release during active disease and remission." *J Allergy Clin Immunol*. 1992;89: 1139-1143.

Estelle, F.; Simons, R.; Simons, KJ. "Antihistamines [H_1- and H_2-receptor antagonists]." In: Schocket, AL, ed. *Clinical Management of Urticaria and Anaphylaxis*. First Edition. New York City: Marcel Dekker, Inc. 1993; 177-212.

Chapter 29

Vitiligo

What Is Vitiligo?

People with vitiligo develop patches of skin devoid of pigment (normal skin color). These patches (often called macules) are usually completely white and are smooth and irregular in shape. Vitiligo is not contagious. Areas of the body most often affected by vitiligo are:

- exposed areas such as the face and hands
- areas around body openings such as the mouth, nose, eyes, nipples, navel, and genital area
- bodily folds such as underarms and groin
- sites of injury such as scrapes, cuts, and burns
- hair, which may gray prematurely as a result of vitiligo
- areas surrounding moles.

Patches of vitiligo vary in size. They may be localized to the hands and face, or they may affect the entire skin surface. People with vitiligo are not albinos.

Vitiligo may begin slowly with the appearance of only a few spots, or there can be a rapid loss of pigment. Pigment loss is usually followed by periods during which skin color does not change. Cycles of pigment loss followed by periods of stability may continue indefinitely. It is rare for a patient to regain lost pigment spontaneously.

1992. National Institute of Arthritis and Musculoskeletal and Skin Diseases.

Who Gets Vitiligo?

Vitiligo is a common disorder, affecting approximately one to four percent of the population. Although people of all ages, all races, and both sexes are equally affected, the disease is especially pronounced in dark-skinned people because of the marked contrast between their normal skin color and the lighter patches of vitiligo. About half of the cases of vitiligo begin before age 20.

What Causes Vitiligo?

Vitiligo results when melanocytes (skin cells which produce melanin, a substance responsible for pigmenting the skin) are destroyed. The reason this substance is destroyed is unknown; however, there are three theories:

- Research indicates that vitiligo may occur when a patient's immune system backfires. Antibodies, cells that normally fight infection, attack the patient's healthy tissues instead. These destructive antibodies are called autoantibodies. In the case of vitiligo, autoantibodies attack and destroy melanin, causing the skin to loose pigment. This is called an autoimmune reaction.

- Another theory suggests that abnormally functioning nerve cells may injure adjacent pigment cells, causing vitiligo.

- Some researchers believe that vitiligo begins when the skin is exposed to chemicals that are toxic to pigment cells.

Vitiligo is often reported after a sunburn or at the end of summer when the skin is tan. Other cases of vitiligo are reported after physical or emotional stress. There seems to be a genetic component to vitiligo; in 30 to 40 percent of the cases, a family history of the disease or of other medical disorders associated with the disease exists.

How Is Vitiligo Diagnosed?

Vitiligo is diagnosed on the basis of characteristic macules and family history. Blood and urine samples are usually not necessary. However, if a thyroid disorder or anemia is suspected, special blood tests should be done.

How Can Vitiligo Be Treated?

Repigmentation: If there is not extensive involvement, patients can undergo therapy to regain the lost pigment. Psoralen therapy combines a substance called Psoralen with sun exposure, specifically ultraviolet A (UVA). Psoralen is found naturally in many plants, but is also produced synthetically. The patient ingests psoralen, then exposes him/herself to intense sunlight. This stimulates pigment cells to divide and fill in the areas where pigment was lost. In some cases, psoralen compounds are applied directly to the skin, but when this is done, the patient should be monitored carefully in order to avoid severe sunburn. Approximately 20 percent of people with ordinary vitiligo respond favorably to psoralen therapy. However, treatments are long and tedious. Psoralen therapy can take up to two years or 100 to 200 treatments.

Repigmentation can also be achieved by other methods. Creams containing hydrocortisone seem to help stabilize the disorder. Although tattooing is usually not recommended, some individuals who have vitiligo on their lips find tattooing useful. Masking depigmented areas with cosmetics can also help de-emphasize patches of vitiligo. In the near future, researchers hope to be able to transplant pigment cells directly into white patches of vitiligo, restoring normal skin color.

Depigmentation: If more than half of the skin surface is affected, the patient and his/her physician may choose to depigment the remaining patches of darker skin.

The drug monobenzyl ether of hydroquinone, which has a bleaching effect, is used in depigmentation therapy. Approximately 15 percent of patients are allergic to this medication. Though treatment may take months to years, the results can be excellent.

What Health Risks Are Associated with Vitiligo?

Most people with vitiligo are in good health. However, approximately 15 percent have a disorder of the thyroid gland, which may be either overactive (hyperthyroidism) or underactive (hypothyroidism). Other conditions associated with vitiligo are pernicious anemia (vitamin B_{12} deficiency), Addison's disease (decreased adrenal function), alopecia areata (hair loss), or uveitis (inflammation of the eyes).

People with vitiligo should take precautions when in the sun because patches of vitiligo do not contain melanocytes, which protect the skin from sun damage. Using sunscreen, wearing protective clothing, and avoiding the sun during peak hours (between 11 a.m. and 2 p.m., especially during the summer) will decrease the risk of sun damage, which can range from sunburn to severe blistering or skin cancer.

Where Do I Go for Help?

Vitiligo is treated by dermatologists (skin doctors). The American Academy of Dermatology can provide referrals to dermatologists in your area. The National Institute of Arthritis and Musculoskeletal and Skin Diseases (NIAMS) does not make physician referrals, although it does fund investigators who study vitiligo.

Other ways to locate dermatologists who may be treating vitiligo include: asking your family physician to provide the name of a dermatologist, calling a local or state department of health, checking the listings of dermatologists in the phone book, or contacting the department of dermatology at a local medical center. Libraries at university hospitals are also excellent sources of information. The Directory of Medical Specialists, available at most community libraries, can help you find a physician.

—Office of Scientific and Health Communication

Part Four

The Hazards of Sun Exposure

Chapter 30

Cancerous Skin Mutation from Solar Rays

Although most skin cancers appear in older people, the damage often begins decades earlier, when the sun's rays mutate a key gene in a single cell.

Human Skin includes three major cell types, all of which are susceptible to sunlight-induced cancer. Near the base of the epidermis lie round, basal cells. Closer to the surface are flattened, squamous cells. Melanocytes (cells that produce the protective pigment melanin) are interspersed in the basal layer and have numerous extensions that reach outward. Solar rays, which can penetrate well below the surface of the skin, damage segments of a cell's DNA that are particularly vulnerable to ultraviolet light. Damage to a gene called p53 appears crucial to basal cell and squamous cell skin cancers.

In 1775 the British physician Percivall Pott reported a curious prevalence of ragged sores on the scrotums of many chimney sweeps in London. Other doctors might have concluded that the men were afflicted with a venereal disease that was then rampant throughout the city. But Pott was more astute. He realized they were in fact suffering from a type of skin cancer. Pott's discovery was a medical milestone. By observing that men continually exposed to coal tar were "peculiarly liable" to this form of cancer, he documented for the first time that cancer could be caused by an external agent rather than by internal factors.

©1996 by Scientific American, Inc. as "Sunlight and Skin Cancer." All rights reserved. Reprinted with permission.

More recently, investigators have identified another link between the environment and skin cancer, but this time the agent is much more ubiquitous. It is nothing less than light from the sun. The painstaking efforts of dozens of researchers have revealed a great deal about how solar rays contribute to the development of an astonishingly high number of skin cancers every year.

In the U.S. alone, about a million new cases occur annually, rivaling the incidence of all other types of cancer combined. Skin cancer typically takes one of three forms corresponding to the three major types of skin cells: basal cells, squamous cells and melanocytes. Cancer of melanocytes, called malignant melanoma, is the most lethal variety and perhaps the most mysterious to researchers attempting to understand how these tumors are triggered. Fortunately, it is also the least common. In the U.S. there will be about 38,000 new cases of melanoma this year and approximately 7,000 deaths from the disease. The two other forms, together called non-melanoma skin cancer, account for the balance of the cases but kill a much smaller percentage of the affected population. A few thousand people are expected to die in the U.S. during 1996 from non-melanoma (almost exclusively squamous cell) skin cancer.

If caught early, most cases of non-melanoma skin cancer are easily treated in a doctor's office under local anesthesia. Such cancers can be cured by a variety of simple techniques, including scraping, burning, freezing or surgically excising the malignant tissue. Even melanoma, if diagnosed when the tumor is still less than one millimeter thick, can usually be cured by simple excision. But because skin cancer plagues members of all age groups, and because it can become disfiguring and deadly if left untreated, medical researchers have mounted an immense scientific effort over the years to unravel the mechanisms that cause this disease. Curiously, an accident of history contributed much to that quest.

An Accidental Experiment

At the time Pott was studying scrotal cancer, Georgian England had a legal system that inflicted severe punishments for petty crimes: forgery or thievery often resulted in a death sentence. But a backlash against the harshness of execution for such misdemeanors soon led to milder sentences—and thus to the overcrowding of jails. To unburden the country's prisons, the House of Commons voted to banish criminals to remote locales beginning in the 1780s. The destination of choice was a little known shore bordering the South Pacific Ocean.

Cancerous Skin Mutation from Solar Rays

Within a few decades, the east coast of Australia was populated with British and Irish men and women. Those early colonists often shared the Celtic features of fair skin and light hair, and today their descendants predominate on that southern continent.

What began as an 18th-century attempt at penal reform ultimately culminated in a de facto large-scale experiment on the links between complexion, solar radiation and skin cancer. With their fair skin continually exposed to intense sun, whites in Australia now have the highest rate of all kinds of skin cancer of any people in the world. Their British relatives, who live under cloudy northern skies, are more fortunate. They have a relatively low risk of acquiring these malignancies as do Australian Aborigines, who with much darker skin are rarely affected by sun-induced cancers of the skin.

Investigators recognized as early as 50 years ago that the Australian experience implicated strong sun and fair skin as important risk factors for skin cancer. But for decades scientists were unable to explain what the sun was actually doing to skin cells to make them become cancerous. Clarifying that mystery required more than an accidental experiment on a sun-drenched continent. It took years of study in research laboratories of molecular biologists around the world before the details of that process began to be uncovered.

When the two of us started to attack this problem in the late 1980s, two types of insults from the sun seemed equally suspect. In one category were mutations of specific genes within skin cells. A cell may reproduce excessively if a mutation either turns a normal gene into an overzealous growth promoter (an oncogene) or inactivates a gene that normally limits cell growth (a tumor suppressor gene). The other class of causes we considered at the outset included more widespread events—ones that would affect every sun-exposed cell. For example, the sun's radiation might suppress the skin's immune response (reducing its natural ability to eliminate tumor cells) or directly stimulate cell division. With such diverse explanations possible, we knew that isolating the causes of skin cancer would not be easy.

But we were guided by the knowledge that the damaging effects of sunlight can occur many years before tumors appear. Such delayed effects were most clearly demonstrated in studies undertaken by Anne Kricker, then at the University of Western Australia, Robin Marks of the Anti-Cancer Council of Victoria and their colleagues. They noted that people who had emigrated from cloudy England to sunny Australia before the age of 18 acquired the higher Australian incidence of skin cancers, but if they moved when they were older, they retained the native risk.

These findings indicated that Australian skin cancer patients must have received a critically high dose of sunlight years before the appearance of tumors (which rarely occurred before middle age). Widespread events, such as immunosuppression, last for only a few days after the injurious radiation ceases. But genetic changes persist (being passed from one generation of cells to another). Looking for genetic changes therefore seemed a more promising avenue for our research. So we began a hunt for sunlight-induced mutations that could occur early in life and set the stage for the development of skin cancer much later on.

A Signature Mutation

That search was daunting. The DNA in a human cell contains as many as 100,000 genes, and each gene typically includes thousands of nucleotides (the building blocks of DNA)—only some of which would be likely to bear traces of sun-induced damage. And even if we managed to identify mutations in skin cancer samples, how could we be sure that sunlight had caused them? Fortunately, other investigators had given us a useful clue by finding that ultraviolet B radiation—long suspected to be the carcinogenic factor in sunlight—had a characteristic signature.

After studying everything from viruses to human cells, groups of researchers from Switzerland, France, Canada and the U.S. had shown that ultraviolet light causes mutations at points on a DNA strand containing specific nucleotide bases. Bases are the variable parts of nucleotides and go by the names adenine (A), guanine (G), cytosine (C) and thymine (T). Ultraviolet light creates mutations where a so-called pyrimidine base—cytosine or thymine—lies adjacent to another pyrimidine. About two-thirds of these mutations are C-to-T substitutions, and about 10 percent of these changes occur at two adjacent Cs, with both bases changing to Ts. These features of the mutations created by ultraviolet light constitute a fingerprint of sorts, because they are made by no other agents.

We thus had a good idea of the kinds of distinctive mutations that should result from exposure to sunlight. But we needed to pinpoint which of the vast number of human genes mutated to produce a carcinogenic effect. Our best guess was that the solution lay with the handful of human genes already known to be involved in cancer.

Of the recognized oncogenes and tumor suppressor genes, we chose to examine a tumor suppressor gene called p53, which is now known to be mutated in more than half of all people's cancers. At the time, we suspected that p53 might be involved in many cases of skin cancer because of an intriguing connection between non-melanoma skin cancer and a rare affliction (epidermodysplasia verruciformis) that causes wart-like growths to appear on the skin.

Previous research had revealed that such growths contain DNA from the human papillomavirus and that when these growths are located on sun-exposed skin, they can progress to basal cell or squamous cell cancer. Peter M. Howley and his colleagues at the National Cancer Institute had further shown that one of the proteins made by the papillomavirus inactivates the p53 protein. (Genes give rise to proteins, and the p53 protein, as might be expected, is the product of the p53 gene.) So all indications were that p53 might play a special role in non-melanoma skin cancer. But we needed solid confirmation.

To find that proof, we studied squamous cell carcinomas, tumors unquestionably linked to sunlight (they occur on the face and hands, especially among whites living in the tropics). In collaboration with Jan Pontén of Uppsala University Hospital in Sweden, we discovered that more than 90 percent of the squamous cell carcinomas from a set of samples collected in the U.S. had a mutation somewhere in the p53 tumor suppressor gene. These mutations occurred at sites with adjacent pyrimidine bases, and they had the distinctive C-to-T pattern associated with ultraviolet exposure. Our research group, along with several others, later pinpointed sunlight-related p53 mutations in basal cell carcinomas as well. (Melanoma does not appear to be associated with alterations to p53. Researchers are still studying cancerous melanocytes for genes affected by sunlight.) After examining samples in our laboratory, Annemarie Ziegler found that precancerous skin also contains mutations of p53, indicating that the genetic changes occur long before tumors appear. But were these mutations truly the cause of non-melanoma skin cancer, or were they simply an irrelevant indicator of lifetime exposure to sunlight?

We could rule out this last possibility by the particular way the genetic code had been altered. The nucleotides in genes are arranged in well-defined codons-groups of three bases that specify different amino acids. The sequence of codons in a gene determines the sequence of amino acids that are strung together to construct a protein. But different codons can sometimes specify the same amino acid—as if the name of the amino acid could be spelled any of several ways. Typically the amino acid does not change when the first two bases of the codon are constant and only the third varies. Hence, if the p53 mutations found in skin cancer were just a random effect of exposure to the sun, we would expect to find changes in the third position occurring as often as in the first or second. That is, there would be plenty of examples where the codon mutated (underwent a nucleotide base substitution) without altering its corresponding amino acid. Yet studies of this gene in skin cancers from around the globe had consistently revealed mutations that modified one or more amino acids in the p53 protein. These genetic changes to p53, then, were not just a side effect of ultraviolet exposure. They were in fact causing the skin cancers.

To better understand how the p53 gene was affected in non-melanoma skin cancer, we investigated whether certain segments of the p53 gene were particularly prone to the mutation by sunlight of adjacent pyrimidine bases (that is, Cs or Ts). Biologists have found so-called mutation hot spots (places on a DNA strand where mutations tend to occur) whenever they expose living cells to carcinogens. After analyzing many tumors, we determined that the p53 gene in non-melanoma skin cancer contains about nine hot spots. In cancers unrelated to sunlight (such as colon or bladder cancer), five codons of p53 are most often mutated, three of which are among the hot spots in skin cancers. At the two hot spots found only in the other cancers, the mutating C is flanked on either side by a G or A but never by a T or another C. Lacking a pair of pyrimidine bases, equivalent sites on the DNA of skin cells are protected from mutation by ultraviolet light.

Of the hundreds of places on the p53 gene with adjacent pyrimidines, why do only a few sites act as hot spots when cells are exposed to sunlight? Several researchers have recently helped answer that question by building on a discovery made more than three decades ago at Oak Ridge National Laboratory by Richard B. Setlow and William L. Carrier. Setlow and Carrier determined that cells can reverse ultraviolet damage to their DNA by an enzymatic process called excision repair. Cells essentially snip out disrupted bases and replace them with intact ones. Working in our lab in 1992, Subrahmanyam Kunala showed that cells repair damage particularly slowly at some pyrimidine pairs. Subsequently, Gerd P. Pfeifer and his colleagues at the City of Hope Beckman Research Institute in Duarte, Calif., found that cells repair the p53 sites mutated in non-melanoma skin cancer more sluggishly than they do many other sites in the gene. Hence, it seems quite likely that the hot spots we found for skin cancer owe their existence to an inability of skin cells to mend these sites efficiently.

Cellular Proofreading

Even after we had identified the relevant p53 mutations, the story of carcinogenesis remained woefully incomplete. After all, genes do not get cancer, cells do. It was clear enough that the p53 protein must operate in normal skin cells to prevent cancer, but how? One hint was available from Michael B. Kastan of Johns Hopkins Hospital. He found that cells subjected to x-rays stepped up production of the p53 protein, which in turn prevented the cells from dividing. Peter A. Hall and David P. Lane of the University of Dundee and Jonathan L. Rees of the University of Newcastle have shown a similar effect on the p53 protein in skin cells exposed to ultraviolet radiation. Cancer researchers speculate that the p53 protein normally stops a DNA-damaged cell from reproducing until it has had time to make repairs.

Moshe Oren and his colleagues at the Weizmann Institute of Science in Israel have proposed another function for the p53 protein as well: it can prevent cancer in situations where the DNA damage is too extensive to be repaired. They find that elevated levels of the p53 protein in a cell lead to apoptosis-programmed cell death. (Such cell death is a normal part of many biological processes, including embryonic development.) In this case, "suicide" of a sun-damaged cell would prevent it from becoming cancerous by permanently erasing its genetic mistakes. Such apoptosis could be called cellular proofreading. Because the skin sheds cells routinely, we surmised that skin cells often used p53 in this way. But even before we began to test our idea, some evidence was already available to support it.

Dermatologists have recognized for a long time that when skin is sunburned, some cells come to resemble apoptotic cells. By 1994 we could show that sunburned cells contained breaks in their DNA similar to those in other apoptotic cells. The sunburned cells thus appeared to be in the process of committing cellular suicide, and we began immediately to wonder whether cells that had lost p53 could undergo such self-inflicted death.

At about the time we arrived at this investigative juncture, Tyler Jacks and his colleagues at the Massachusetts Institute of Technology had developed mice lacking the p53 gene. When Alan S. Jonason and Jeffrey A. Simon irradiated the skin of these so-called p53 knockout mice in our laboratory, they found far fewer sunburned, apoptotic cells than in normal mice exposed to the same ultraviolet radiation. Mice in which the p53 gene had been only partially inactivated had only a moderate tendency to undergo light-induced cell suicide. These results suggested that programmed cell death was important for preventing non-melanoma skin cancer and that loss of p53 could block this process.

Double Punch from Sunlight

It is now possible to envision how the failure of cellular proofreading would lead to skin cancer. Normal skin exposed to sunlight will accumulate DNA damage caused by the ultraviolet B part of the solar spectrum. Cells unable to repair their DNA in a timely fashion die through apoptosis. But if the p53 gene in a cell has mutated during a previous episode of exposure to sunlight, that cell will resist such self-destruction—even if it has been badly injured.

The situation is actually much worse. A cell on the verge of becoming cancerous is surrounded by normal cells that undergo apoptosis when damaged. The dying cells thus must be leaving some space into which the p53-mutated cell can grow. By inducing healthy cells to kill themselves off, sunlight favors the proliferation of p53-mutated cells. In effect, sunlight acts twice to cause cancer: once to mutate the p53 gene and then afterward to set up conditions for the unrestrained growth of the altered cell line. These two actions, mutation and tumor promotion, are the one-two blows of carcinogenesis. Although mutation and promotion are carried out by separate agents in other tumors, in skin cancer ultraviolet radiation appears to throw both punches.

There are undoubtedly other genes involved in the development of skin cancer as well as other effects of sunlight that researchers do not yet fully understand. For example, medical researchers know that Gorlin syndrome (a disease in which patients have multiple basal cell cancers) is caused by an inherited mutation in a different tumor suppressor gene. With further investigation, the various mechanisms of carcinogenesis will become even more clear, and scientists may find clever ways to interrupt the progression of normal skin cells to cancerous ones.

It is not beyond reason to hope that the detailed understanding researchers are gaining of non-melanoma skin cancer will yield new kinds of therapies. Perhaps drugs that restore normal function to a mutated p53 protein will allow doctors to offer their patients an effective remedy that does not involve surgery. Such a cure, perhaps administered as a simple skin cream that is absorbed by the affected cells, might be available within the next decade or two. If so, it will be of great benefit to countless aging members of the sun-loving baby-boom generation—a group to which we both admittedly belong.

—by David J. Leffell and Douglas E. Brash

The Authors

DAVID J. LEFFELL and **DOUGLAS E. BRASH** have worked together for nearly a decade to understand the role of the sun in causing skin cancer. Leffell, a professor of dermatology and surgery at the Yale School of Medicine, has brought to their research collaboration the experience gained in clinical practice. He earned his M.D. at McGill University in 1981 and trained at Cornell Medical School, Memorial Sloan-Kettering Cancer Center and the University of Michigan before taking a position on the faculty at Yale in 1988. Brash, too, is on the medical school faculty at Yale, and his credentials include a bachelor's degree in engineering physics from the University of Illinois. He shifted from engineering to the study of biophysics at Ohio State University, where he received his Ph.D. in 1979. Thereafter Brash pursued postdoctoral training in microbiology (at the Harvard School of Public Health) and pathology (at Harvard Medical School) until 1984. He spent the next five years at the National Cancer Institute before moving to Yale.

Further Reading

"A Role for Sunlight in Skin Cancer: UV-induced P53 Mutations in Squamous Cell Carcinoma." D. E. Brash, J. A. Rudolph, J. A. Simon, A. Lin, G. J. McKenna, H. P. Baden, A. J. Halper and J. Pontén in *Proceedings of the National Academy of Sciences U.S.A.*, Vol. 88, No. 22, pages 10124-10128; November 15, 1991.

"Sunburn and P53 in the Onset of Skin Cancer." A. Ziegler, A. S. Jonason, D. J. Leffell, J. A. Simon, H. W. Sharma, J. Kimmelman, L. Remington, T. Jacks and D. E. Brash in *Nature*, Vol. 372, pages 773-776; December 22-29, 1994.

Cancer Free: the Comprehensive Cancer Prevention Program. Sidney J. Winawer and Moshe Shike. Simon & Schuster, 1996.

Sunlight, Ultraviolet Radiation and the Skin. NIH Consensus Statement. Vol. 7, No. 8, pages 1-29; May 8-10, 1989. Available at http://text.nlm.nih.gov/nih/cdc/www/74txt.html.

Chapter 31

Deaths from Melanoma in the United States, 1973-1992

Approximately three fourths of all skin cancer-associated deaths are caused by melanoma. During 1973-1991, the incidence of melanoma increased approximately 4 percent each year.[1] In addition, the incidence of melanoma is increasing faster than that of any other cancer.[2] To characterize the distribution of deaths from melanoma in the United States, CDC analyzed national mortality data for 1973 through 1992. This report summarizes the results of that analysis.

Decedents for whom the underlying cause of death was melanoma (International Classification of Diseases, Adapted, Ninth Revision, codes 172.0-172.9) were identified from public-use, mortality data tapes from 1973 through 1992.[3] The denominators for rate calculations were derived from U.S. census population estimates.[4,5] Rates were directly standardized to the age distribution of the 1970 U.S. population and were analyzed by state, age group, sex, year, and race. To increase the precision of the rates presented, race was characterized as white and all other races because approximately 98 percent of deaths from melanoma occurred among whites

From 1973 through 1992, the overall percentage increase in the rate of deaths from melanoma (34.1 percent) was the third highest of all cancers; for males, the percentage increase for melanoma (47.9 percent) was the highest for all cancers.[6] During the same period, the increase in the rate of deaths from melanoma was greater for white males than for other racial and sex groups (Figure 31.1). In 1992, the rate of deaths from melanoma was 5.9 times higher for whites than

Morbidity and Mortality Weekly Report vol. 44 No. 17, May 5, 1995.

Skin Disorders Sourcebook

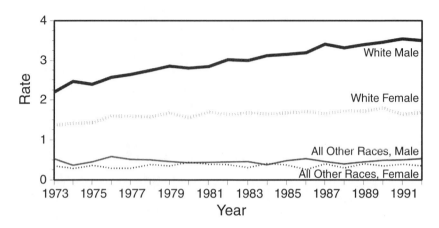

Figure 31.1. Average annual age-adjusted rate of deaths from melanoma, by race and sex—United States, 1973-1992. Per 100,000 population, adjusted to the U.S. population.

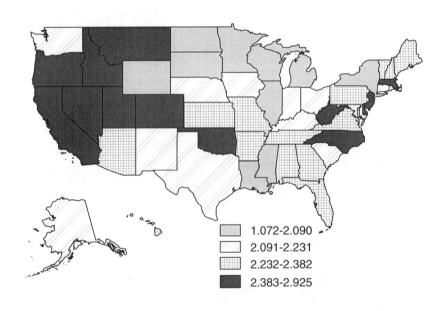

Figure 31.2. Average annual rate of deaths from melanoma, by quartile—United States, 1988-1992. Per 100,000 population, adjusted to U.S. population

Deaths from Melanoma in the United States, 1973-1992

for all other races (2.5 and 0.4 per 100,000 population, respectively), and 2.1 times higher for males than females (3.1 and 1.5, respectively).

To increase statistical precision, the rate of deaths from melanoma by state was aggregated for 1988-1992. In every state, the rate of deaths from melanoma was substantially higher for whites than for persons of all other races. For whites, the age-adjusted death rate by state ranged from 2.2 to 5.0 per 100,000 population for males and 0.8 to 2.3 for females. Most states that are in the two highest death rate quartiles are not in the lower U.S. latitudes where sun exposure is generally more intense (Figure 31.1).

During 1973-1975 and 1990-1992, death rates were highest for white men aged greater than or equal to 50 years (Figure 31.3). The death rate increased more with age for males than for females during 1990-1992.

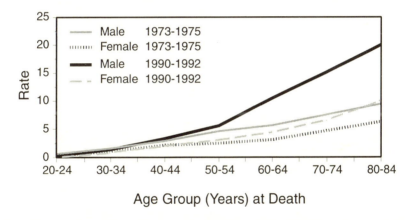

Figure 31.3. Average annual age-specific rate of deaths from melanoma among whites, by sex and time period—United States, 1973-1975 and 1990-1992. Per 100,000 population, adjusted to U.S. population

Reported by: Division of Cancer Prevention and Control, National Center for Chronic Disease Prevention and Health Promotion, CDC.

MMWR Editorial Note: The findings in this report indicate that the rate of deaths from melanoma was higher for whites than persons of all other races—a finding consistent with the more common occurrence of melanoma among persons with lightly pigmented skin[2] and an incidence among whites that is more than 10 times higher than that for blacks.[1] Based on estimates by the American Cancer Society, during 1995 an estimated 34,100 new cases of melanoma will be diagnosed and 7,200 deaths will be caused by melanoma.[1] The likelihood of survival of melanoma is substantially greater if the disease is detected early and treated.[2] Early detection of thin lesions is associated with improved prognosis and treatment outcome than is detection of thicker, later stage tumors.[2]

Risk factors[2,7,8] for melanoma related to ultraviolet radiation exposure include a history of sunburn or sun sensitivity, a tendency to freckle, the presence of lightly pigmented skin, blue eyes, and blond or red hair. Other risk factors include a family or personal history of melanoma and the presence of a large number of moles or any atypical moles. Sources for exposure to ultraviolet radiation include sunlight and artificial light (e.g., tanning booths), both of which can cause acute sunburn. The increased risk among persons who sustain intermittent, acute sunburn at an early age (i.e., less than 18 years) underscores the need for initiating prevention measures early in childhood.[9]

Adults, particularly older men in whom rates of deaths from melanoma are highest, should be encouraged to perform periodic skin self-examination or be examined by a family member[2] to monitor location, size, and color of a pigmented lesion or mole. The "ABCD approach" can be used to assess pigmented lesions and represents mole asymmetry ("A"), border irregularity ("B"), nonuniform color (i.e., pigmentation) ("C"), and diameter greater than 6 mm ("D").[1,2,8]

Recommendations for preventing melanoma should emphasize reduction of direct exposure to the sun when sunburn is most likely to occur, especially from 10:00 a.m. to 3:00 p.m.. Specific measures include wearing a broad-brimmed hat and clothes that protect sun-exposed areas, seeking shade when outdoors, using a sunscreen of sun protection factor greater than or equal to 15 that provides protection against ultraviolet radiation A and ultraviolet radiation B, and referring to the daily Ultraviolet Index rating provided by the National Weather Service and others when planning outdoor activities. The Ultraviolet Index, provided by the National Weather Service, is broadcast by television and print media in 58 U.S. cities and provides information on the intensity of the sun s rays during the solar noon hour. The index ranges from O to 10+ with greater than or equal to 10 indicating the most intense sunlight.

In 1994, CDC implemented a program to assist in achievement of the national health objectives for the year 2000 for preventing skin cancer.[10] Elements of the CDC program include funding support for state health departments to develop and implement prevention projects aimed at parents and caregivers of young children; enhancing prevention messages for the public; initiating the development of school health curriculum guidelines; enhancing Ultraviolet Index public health messages; and developing a public and professional education plan for skin cancer prevention. May is Melanoma/Skin Cancer Detection and Prevention Month.

Additional information is available from the American Academy of Dermatology, 930 North Meacham Road, Schaumburg, IL 60173-4965.

References

1. American Cancer Society. *Cancer facts and figures, 1995*. Atlanta: American Cancer Society, 1995; publication no. 5008.95.
2. Koh HK. "Cutaneous melanoma." *New England Journal of Medicine* 1991; 325:171-82.
3. NCHS. *Vital statistics mortality data, underlying cause of death, 1973-1992*. Hyattsville, Maryland: US Department of Health and Human Services, Public Health Service, CDC, 1973-1992.
4. Bureau of the Census. *1970-1989 Intercensal population estimates by race, sex, and age*. Washington, DC: US Department of Commerce, Bureau of the Census, nd.
5. Irwin R. *1990-1992 Postcensal population estimates by race, sex, and age*. Alexandria, Virginia: Demo-Detail. 1993.
6. Ries LAG, Miller BA, Hankey BF, Kosary CL, Harras A, Edwards BK, eds. *SEER cancer statistics review, 1973-1991 : tables and graphs*. Bethesda, Maryland: US Department of Health and Human Services, Public Health Service, National Institutes of Health, National Cancer Institute, 1994; publication no. (NIH)94-2789.
7. Hartman AM, Goldstein AM. "Melanoma of the skin." In: Miller BA, Ries LAG, Hankey BF, et al., eds. *SEER cancer statistics review, 1973-1990*. Bethesda, Maryland: US Department of Health and Human Services, Public Health Service, National Institutes of Health, National Cancer Institute, 1993; publication no. (NIH)93-2789.
8. Marks R, Hill D, eds. *The public health approach to melanoma control: prevention and early detection*. Geneva: International Union Against Cancer, 1992.
9. Wiley HE. "Ways to protect children from sun damage." *The Skin Cancer Foundation Journal* 1994; 12:41,98.
10. Public Health Service. *Healthy people 2000: national health promotion and disease prevention objectives*. Washington, DC: US Department of Health and Human Services, Public Health Service, 1991; DHHS publication no. (PHS)91-50213.

Chapter 32

Judging the Risks: Tips for Safer Tanning

Sunscreens

Fast Facts

- Daily exposure to the sun over a lifetime is a major cause of skin damage, including wrinkling skin cancer.
- Any tan indicates skin damage.
- Most people benefit from sunscreens with high sun protection factor (SPF) numbers such as 15 or greater.
- Even sunscreens with high SPF numbers provide less than full protection.
- The worst times to be outside are between 10:00 a.m. and 3:00 p.m.
- Keep infants under six months old out of the sun.

True or False:

- Sunscreens labeled "15" and higher do not protect you against all the sun's rays.
- A tan may protect you against some sunburn, but not against all wrinkling or skin cancer.

Facts for Consumers Federal Trade Commission, Bureau of Consumer Protection, Office of Consumer & Business Education *Sunscreens* (#FO27599), *Indoor Tanning* (FO23286) and *Protecting Kids from the Sun.*

- You can endanger your skin by using too little sunscreen or not applying it one-half hour before going out in the sun.
- Infants under six months probably should not be in the sun at all.
- Sunlight coming through a window can damage your skin.

Even if you are more careful than ever about going out in the sun nowadays, you may be surprised at the answers to the above statements. All of them are true.

While you may be used to warnings about limiting sun exposure and using sunscreens, researchers are becoming ever more cautious about how much sun is good for you. The following questions and answers may help you decide how much sun you should be exposed to and what precautions you can take to protect yourself and your family.

Is any sun exposure safe? Although sunlight is essential for human life, daily exposure to the sun over a lifetime is a major cause of skin damage, including wrinkling and skin cancer. Many of the skin changes attributed to aging are in fact signs of sun-induced skin damage. Every year, more than 700,000 people in the United States get skin cancer. It is the most common form of cancer, with rates growing 3 to 5 percent annually. Left untreated, skin cancer can be life-threatening.

Is tanning safe? Any tan indicates skin damage. Although a tan may give you some protection against sunburning, it will not fully protect you against wrinkling or skin cancer. Some people are especially vulnerable to the effects of the sun, such as fair-skinned individuals who burn easily and tan poorly or not at all. Of those who do tan well, the deeper the color of the tan, the more extensive the skin damage.

What is the best protection against the sun? Staying indoors is the best protection against getting sun-damaged skin. The hours between 10:00 a.m. and 3:00 p.m. are the worst times to be outside. To help reduce the risk of skin damage from sunlight, wear tight-weave clothing that covers the body, wear a hat, and use maximum protection sunscreens.

What kind of sunscreen protection do you need? Most people benefit from sunscreens with high sun protection factor (SPF)

Judging the Risks: Tips for Safer Tanning

numbers, such as 15 or greater. The SPF number gives you some idea how long you can remain in the sun before burning. If, for example, you would normally burn in 10 minutes without sunscreen, applying a 15-SPF sunscreen may provide you with about 150 minutes in the sun before burning. Swimming and perspiration, however, will reduce the actual SPF value for many sunscreens.

Sunscreens with SPF numbers greater than 15 may benefit those who want to minimize their exposure to the sun, especially those who are fair-skinned, live in climates close to the equator or at high altitudes, work or play outdoors, or perspire heavily. Because skin irritations may result from various sunscreen ingredients, you may want to first test a product by applying a small amount to a limited area of your skin.

Do high SPF number sunscreens fully protect you? Unfortunately, even sunscreens with high SPF numbers offer you less than full protection. Sunlight exposes you to two kinds of ultraviolet light, called UVA and UVB. Both can cause skin damage, including wrinkling and skin cancer.

Although virtually all sunscreens provide some level of protection against UVB rays, no product yet screens out all UVA rays. SPF sunscreen numbers only indicate the amount of time you can stay in the sun without burning. Even if you don't burn, the sun's rays still may be damaging your skin.

No rating system yet exists for UVA. There is no way, then, to tell how much UVA protection you are getting. Some researchers estimate that the level of protection in many products advertising UVA protection, even those with high SPF numbers, is probably equivalent to an SPF 3 or 4. So, even if you use high SPF number sunscreens, you still are vulnerable to skin damage from the sun's UVA rays.

How much sunscreen should you use? You will not get the full protection offered by the sunscreen unless you apply the recommended liberal amount on your skin. Unfortunately, many people use much less. A sunscreen with an SPF of 15 may give only half that protection if you don't use enough of it.

If you are at the beach, for example, use about an ounce of sunscreen over your whole body for one application. That means you should plan to buy about one 8-ounce container or more of sunscreen per person for each week you are at the beach.

If you frequently go swimming or perspire, use a waterproof product for the best protection. Apply the sunscreen before going outdoors and be sure to reapply it as needed—after perspiring, swimming or toweling off. Otherwise, you are not getting the protection you need from the sun's rays.

When should you use sunscreen? Skin damage does not occur only on the beach or the ski slopes. Most people who are going to be out in the sun for more than 10 minutes would benefit from daily use of sunscreen on the parts of the body exposed to the sun. Even casual exposure to sunlight—while driving a car, walking to the store, taking an outdoor lunch break—contributes to the cumulative lifetime exposure that may lead to skin damage.

Make sure you apply the sunscreen about one-half hour before going out in the sun to give your skin a chance to fully absorb it.

If you're taking medications, ask your doctor or pharmacist if these medications will sensitize your skin to the sun and aggravate sunburn or rashes. Common drugs that may do this include: certain antibiotics; birth control pills; diuretics; antihistamines; and antidepressants.

Are all sunscreens basically the same? Sunscreens contain a variety of ingredients. Although some sunscreens may provide more moisturizers, for example, those with identical SPF numbers give you equivalent sunburn protection from UVB rays. Because of the cost of buying sunscreen products year-round, you may want to shop for competitively-priced brands of sunscreen offering the level of protection you need.

How effective are sunblocks? Do not be misled by sunscreen products that claim they are sunblocks. Only opaque substances, such as zinc oxide or titanium dioxide, totally block the sunlight. These products are most practical to use on specific areas of the body most exposed to the sun, such as the nose or lips.

Are there special precautions you should take with children? Parents should see that sunscreens of SPF 15 or greater are applied routinely when children go outdoors. Because sunscreens may irritate baby skin, and babies' developing eyes are particularly vulnerable to sunlight, experts recommend that infants less than six months old should be kept out of the sun altogether.

Judging the Risks: Tips for Safer Tanning

Experts estimate that about 50 percent of an individual's sun exposure occurs by age 18. Some have suggested that schools, child care centers, and camps rearrange outdoor play times to minimize exposure to the midday sun.

Are indoor tanning devices safe? Tanning devices, like natural sunlight, emit ultraviolet rays. These UVA or UVB rays, whether from artificial or natural sources, can cause skin damage.

Indoor Tanning

Fast Facts

- Tanning is not risk-free, whether you tan in natural sunlight or in a suntan salon.
- Tanning exposes your skin to ultraviolet rays. This exposure increases your chances of skin cancer, cataracts and retinal damage, and premature skin wrinkling.
- If you tan, learn how to minimize the risks.

"Tan indoors with absolutely no harmful side effects."

"No burning, no drying, and no sun damage."

"Unlike the sun, indoor tanning will not cause skin cancer or skin aging."

You may have heard claims like these about indoor tanning and wondered whether indoor tanning devices are truly a safe alternative to outdoor tanning. But whether you tan outdoors in natural sunlight or indoors in a suntan salon, tanning is not risk-free. Overexposure can cause eye injury, premature aging and wrinkling of the skin, and increase your chances of developing skin cancer. According to the Federal Trade Commission (FTC), consumers can be harmed if advertising leads them to believe that they can get a tan without the harmful effects of the sun. The information in this chapter may help you understand how tanning devices work and why the same health risks associated with outdoor tanning are associated with indoor tanning. To help you minimize risks, including those posed by indoor tanning, a checklist is provided at the end of this section.

What the Risks Are

Whether you tan outdoors during the summer months or tan indoors exclusively, you are increasing your chances of:

- developing skin cancer later in life
- suffering cataracts and retinal damage
- developing premature skin wrinkling
- developing ultraviolet light-induced skin rashes when you eat certain foods or take some common medications, such as birth control pills or antihistamines

If you tan year 'round, you obviously will increase your skin's exposure to the dangers of ultraviolet rays. Being informed about how tanning devices work can help you spot misleading claims and avoid skin damage.

How Tanning Devices Work

The most popular device used in salons is a clamshell-like tanning bed. The customer lies down on a Plexiglas surface and relaxes as lights from above and below reach the body.

Older devices generally used light sources that emitted shortwave ultraviolet rays (UVB), often advertised as "tanning" rays, that actually caused burning. Aware of the harmful effects of UVB radiation, including the increased risk of skin cancer, salon owners began using tanning beds that emit mostly longwave (UVA) light sources, which some claimed to be safe. But the UVA rays also can be harmful to the skin because they penetrate so deeply, as explained below.

Why Certain Advertising Claims May Be False

You can make a more informed decision about indoor tanning if you learn how to spot misleading tanning claims. The following section discusses why each of four claims sometimes made about indoor tanning is misleading.

False Claim #1: *"You can achieve a deep year-round tan with gentle, comfortable, and safe UVA light."*

To understand why doctors are concerned about tanning salons, you need to understand how ultraviolet rays can affect your skin.

Judging the Risks: Tips for Safer Tanning

Shortwave ultraviolet rays called UVB can burn the outer layer of skin; longwave ultraviolet rays called UVA penetrate more deeply and can weaken the skin's inner connective tissue. Long-term exposure to the sun, to artificial sources of ultraviolet light, or to both, contributes to the risk of the three kinds of skin cancer: basal cell, an otherwise benign skin cancer that can cause scarring; squamous cell, which is usually benign but which can spread through the body if left untreated; and melanoma, one of the most fatal kinds of cancer.

False Claim #2: *"No harsh glare, so no goggles or eye shades are necessary."*

Studies show that too much exposure to ultraviolet rays, including UVA rays, can damage the retina. Over-exposure can burn the cornea, and repeated exposure over many years can change the structure of an eye lens so that it begins to cloud, forming a cataract. If left untreated, cataracts result in blindness.

The Food and Drug Administration requires tanning salons to direct all customers to wear protective eye goggles. Closing your eyes, wearing ordinary sunglasses, or using cotton wads are not strong enough measures to protect the cornea from the intensity of UV radiation in tanning devices.

Long-term exposure to natural sunlight also can result in eye damage, but, in the sun, you will be more aware that your eyelids are burning than when you tan indoors. The skin exposed to indoor UV lights remains cool to the touch. In addition, the intensity of lights used in tanning devices is much greater—and potentially more hazardous to your eyes—than the intensity of UV rays in natural sunlight.

False Claim #3: *"Tan year 'round without the harmful side effects often associated with natural sunlight."*

Exposure to tanning salon rays increases the damage caused by sunlight. This occurs because ultraviolet light actually thins the skin, making it less able to heal.

Too much exposure to ultraviolet rays also results in premature aging. A "healthy" looking tan is, in fact, damaged skin that is more likely to wrinkle and sag than skin that has not been tanned. Over time, you may notice certain undesirable changes in the way your skin looks and heals. According to some skin specialists, skin that has a dry, wrinkled, leathery appearance early in middle age is a consequence of UV exposure that occurred in youth.

False Claim #4: *"No danger in exposure or burning."*

Whether you tan indoors or outdoors, studies show the combination of ultraviolet rays and some medicines, birth control pills, cosmetics, and soaps may accelerate skin burns or produce painful adverse skin reactions, such as rashes. In addition, tanning devices may induce such common light-sensitive skin ailments as cold sores.

How to Minimize Risks: a Checklist

If you do choose to tan, either outdoors or indoors, at a salon or at home, you may want to use this checklist to help you minimize some of the associated risks:

Exposure Limits. If you do choose to tan, it is important to limit your exposure to avoid burning. If you tan with a device:

- Does the device manufacturer or the salon staff provide recommended exposure limits for your skin type?

- Is there a timer you can set on the tanning device that automatically shuts off the lights or somehow signals you regarding your exposure time?

Remember: Exposure time affects burning. Total UV dosage, whether received in a few large doses or in many smaller ones over a long period of time, can cause skin cancer and premature aging. Your age at the time of exposure also is a critical factor relative to burning. Studies suggest that children and teens are harmed more by equivalent amounts of UVB rays than are adults. The earlier you start tanning, the earlier skin injury may occur.

Eye Protection. When using a tanning device, it is important to use eye protection because UV light can harm the corneas without your being aware of any injury.

- Are safety goggles provided and is their use mandatory?
- Do the goggles fit snugly?

Judging the Risks: Tips for Safer Tanning

- Does the salon sterilize the goggles after each use to prevent the spread of eye infection?

Remember: Artificial UV light is more intense and, therefore, potentially more damaging than that found in sunlight.

Medical Histories. Whether you choose to tan indoors or outdoors, it is important to consider your medical history.

- Are you undergoing treatment for lupus or diabetes, or are you susceptible to cold sores? These conditions can be severely aggravated if you are exposed to ultraviolet radiation from tanning devices, sunlamps, or natural sunlight.

- Do you use antihistamines, tranquilizers, birth control pills, and other medications that are known to increase the likelihood of rashes, sunburns, and other allergic-type reactions when used with the sun or artificial light?

- If you tan at a salon, does it maintain such information about the medications and the treatment you are taking on a file with your medical history and does the staff update it periodically?

Remember: Check with your personal physician or other health-care provider if you have questions about possible side effects associated with tanning.

What Federal Agencies Are Doing about Deceptive Tanning Claims

The Food and Drug Administration (FDA) and the Federal Trade Commission (FTC) share responsibilities in the regulation of sunlamps and tanning devices. FDA is responsible for the labeling of the devices; the FTC is responsible for investigating false, misleading, and deceptive advertising claims. When these agencies determine that labels or advertisements are not based on valid scientific facts, they have the jurisdiction to take corrective action. The FDA also can remove the products from the salon or from the marketplace.

If you have questions or complaints about claims made in tanning device advertising, write: Correspondence Branch, Federal Trade Commission. Washington. D.C. 20580.

Protecting Kids from the Sun

Fast Facts

- Educate children about using sunscreens. Applying sunscreens regularly and liberally can greatly reduce the risk of skin damage and skin cancer later in life.

- Make sure children liberally apply sunscreen every day before going outside and after perspiring and swimming, particularly after toweling off.

- Buy sunscreens that are waterproof or water resistant and help to protect skin from the sun's UVA and UVB (ultraviolet) rays.

- When scheduling children's outdoor activities, remember the sun is strongest from 10:00 a.m. to 3:00 p.m.

Remember how much a blistering sunburn hurt as a child? Medical experts now believe that too much exposure to the sun as a child and teenager is a major cause of skin cancer and premature skin aging.

But regular sun exposure throughout the year also contributes to long-term skin damage. Tanning, for example, is a sign of skin damage. Even children with darker complexions, who have more natural protection against the sun, are at risk.

Two kinds of ultraviolet sun rays, UVA and UVB, can cause skin damage. This can range from immediate effects such as burning, photosensitive reactions (rashes), and cell and tissue damage to long-term consequences such as wrinkling and skin cancer. Experts believe that UVA also may weaken the immune system. You can help protect your child's skin from damage by taking the right steps early.

Use Sunscreens

Using sunscreens is important. Many dermatologists believe children and teenagers who regularly use sunscreens can significantly reduce the risk of skin damage, including skin cancer, later in life. To help protect children:

- Use waterproof or water-resistant sunscreens that help to protect skin from both UVA and UVB rays and have SPF (sun protection factor) numbers of at least 15.

Judging the Risks: Tips for Safer Tanning

- Apply sunscreen liberally (at least one large handful for a body) about 30 minutes before going outside. No matter what sunscreen product is used, be sure it is reapplied after swimming or perspiring heavily.

- Talk with camp counselors and others with child care responsibilities about reapplying sunscreens. Toweling off after swimming, for example, will remove even waterproof sunscreens.

Know that no sunscreen totally blocks the sun's rays. Even children wearing high SPF sunscreens get some exposure to ultraviolet rays.

Other Important Information

To help protect children from the sun, you may want to keep in mind the following:

- When scheduling children's outdoor activities, remember the sun is strongest from 10:00 a.m. to 3:00 p.m.

- Dress children for maximum protection against the sun. Hats with brims and tight-weave long-sleeved shirts and pants offer the best protection.

- Sunglasses can help protect children's eyes. Select sunglasses that help to screen out both UVA and UVB rays. UV rays may contribute to the development of cataracts. Sunglasses that are close-fitting to the face and with larger lenses also can give more protection.

- Teenagers who work outside in such jobs as lifeguards, gardeners, or construction workers may be at special risk for skin damage. They need adequate protection before going out in the sun.

- Discourage teenagers from going to tanning parlors. Tanning devices can damage the skin and eyes as much as direct sunlight.

- Keep babies younger than six months out of the sun. Know that sunscreens may irritate baby skin, and an infant's developing eyes are especially vulnerable to sunlight.

What You Should Know about Skin Cancer

Medical experts believe that the sun causes most skin cancer, which is the most common form of cancer in this country. More younger people now are being diagnosed with it. Two types of skin cancer, basal cell and squamous cell, will develop this year in more than three-quarters of a million Americans. If detected early, these cancers are usually treatable. The third kind of cancer, melanoma, is more deadly, and its incidence is increasing faster than any other form of cancer. Early detection is crucial for successful treatment. Several factors are associated with increased risk of developing skin cancer. These include having:

- Several blistering sunburns as a child or teenager.
- A family history of skin cancer.
- Light-colored skin, hair, and eyes.
- Difficulty tanning or frequent sunburns.
- Moles that: are irregular in shape or color; change in size, shape, or color; or itch or bleed.

For More Information

Be sure to check with your family doctor or dermatologist if you have questions or concerns about skin cancer or skin damage. For free FTC brochures like Best Sellers (which lists more than 140 brochures on many consumer topics) contact: Public Reference, Federal Trade Commission, Washington, DC 20580/ 202-326-2222/ TDD: 202-326-2502.

Chapter 33

Actinic Keratosis: What You Should Know about this Common Pre-Cancer

What is it?

You have surely seen an actinic keratosis. The name may be unfamiliar, but the appearance is commonplace. Anyone who spends time in the sun runs a high risk of developing one or more.

An actinic keratosis, also known as a solar keratosis, is a scaly or crusty bump that arises on the skin surface. The base may be light or dark, tan, pink, red, or a combination of these . . . or the same color as your skin. The scale or crust is horny, dry, and rough, and is often recognized by touch rather than sight. Occasionally it itches or produces a pricking or tender sensation.

The skin abnormality or lesion develops slowly to reach a size that is most often from an eighth to a quarter of an inch. It may disappear only to reappear later. You will often see several actinic keratoses at a time.

A keratosis is most likely to appear on the face, ears, bald scalp, neck, backs of hands and forearms, and lips. It tends to lie flat against the skin of the head and neck and be elevated on arms and hands.

Why is it dangerous?

Actinic keratosis can be the first step in the development of skin cancer, and, therefore, is a precursor of cancer or a precancer.

©1993 The Skin Cancer Foundation. Box 561, New York, NY 10156. Reprinted with Permission.

It is estimated that up to 10 percent of active lesions, which are redder and more tender than the rest, will take the next step and progress to squamous cell carcinomas. They are usually not life-threatening, provided they are detected and treated in the early stages. However, if this is not done, they can grow large and invade the surrounding tissues and, on rare occasions, metastasize or spread to the internal organs.

The most aggressive form of keratosis, actinic cheilitis, appears on the lips and can evolve into squamous cell carcinoma. When this happens, roughly one-fifth of these carcinomas metastasize.

The presence of actinic keratoses indicates that sun damage has occurred and that any kind of skin cancer—not just squamous cell carcinoma—can develop.

What does it look like?

Common forms of actinic keratoses are described here in the locations where they most often develop. Examine your skin to find any lesions that look like these. If you spot them, consult your doctor promptly.

- Thickened, red, scaly patches on back of hand.
- Small red bumps and small tan crusts on forehead or bald scalp.
- Fissures filled with blood or covered with horny scale on lip.
- Multiple, crusted lesions on ears ranging in color from red to brown.

What is the cause?

Sun exposure is the cause of almost all actinic keratoses. Sun damage to the skin accumulates over time, so that even a brief exposure adds to the lifetime total.

The likelihood of developing keratoses is highest in regions close to the equator. However, regardless of climate, everyone is exposed to the sun. Ultraviolet rays bounce off sand, snow, and other reflective surfaces; about 80 percent can pass through clouds.

Who is at greatest risk?

People who have fair skin, blonde or red hair, blue, green, or gray eyes are at the greatest risk. Because their skin has less protective

Actinic Keratosis: What You Should Know

pigment, they are the most susceptible to sunburn. Even those who are darker-skinned can develop keratoses if they expose themselves to the sun without protection. African-Americans, however, rarely have these lesions.

Individuals who are immunosuppressed as a result of cancer chemotherapy, AIDS, or organ transplantation, are also at higher risk.

How common is it?

One in six people will develop an actinic keratosis in the course of a lifetime, according to the best estimates.

Older people are more likely than younger ones to have actinic keratoses, because cumulative sun exposure increases with the years. A survey of older Americans found keratoses in more than half of the men and more than a third of the women aged 65 to 74 who had a high degree of lifetime sun exposure. Some experts believe the majority of people who live to the age of 80 have keratoses.

Because more than half of an average person's lifetime sun exposure occurs before the age of 20, keratoses appear even in people in their early twenties who have spent too much time in the sun with little or no protection.

How is it treated?

There are a number of effective treatments for eradicating actinic keratoses. Not all keratoses need to be removed. The decision on whether and how to treat is based on the nature of the lesion, your age, and your health.

Curettage and Electrodesiccation is the most commonly used treatment. The physician scrapes the lesion and takes a biopsy specimen to be tested for malignancy. Bleeding is controlled by electrocautery-heat produced by an electric needle.

Shave Removal utilizes a scalpel to shave the keratosis and obtain a specimen for testing. The base of the lesion is destroyed, and the bleeding is stopped by cauterization.

Cryosurgery freezes off the lesions through application of liquid nitrogen with a special spray device or cotton-tipped applicator. It does not require anesthesia and produces no bleeding, but white spots sometimes result.

Dermabrasion removes the upper layers of the skin by sanding or using a fine wire brush operating at 20-25,000 revolutions per minute. Redness and soreness usually disappear after a few days.

Topical Medications: Two medicated creams are effective in removing keratoses, particularly when lesions are numerous. The medication is applied by the patient twice daily, with progress checked by a physician. 5-Fluorouracil (5-FU) cream is used for three to five weeks. Treatment leaves the affected area temporarily reddened and may cause some discomfort resulting from skin breakdown. Masoprocol cream, 10 percent, the newest topical treatment, is applied for 28 days. Redness and flaking are the most common side effects; most reactions are usually reported as mild to moderate.

Chemical Peeling makes use of trichloroacetic acid or phenol applied while the patient is under light sedation. The top layers of the skin slough off and are usually replaced within seven days by growth of new epidermis.

Laser Surgery focuses the beam from a carbon dioxide laser onto the lesion. This treatment is rarely used, but can be effective, particularly for keratoses on the lips.

The best way to prevent actinic keratosis is to protect yourself from the sun.

- Limit the amount of time you spend in the sun. Avoid the peak hours from 10:00 a.m. to 3:00 p.m.

- Seek the shade.

- Cover up with protective clothing, including a broad-brimmed hat.

- Wear a sunscreen with a sun protection factor (SPF) of 15 or greater.

- Avoid tanning parlors and artificial tanning devices.

- Keep newborns out of the sun. Sunscreens can be used on babies over the age of six months.

Actinic Keratosis: What You Should Know

- Teach your children good sun-protective practices.

- Perform regular skin self-examination and consult a physician if you see or feel a suspicious area.

Actinic keratosis is skin cancer's warning signal. Heed that signal.

Medical Reviewers:
Rex A. Amonette, M.D.,
David J. Leffell, M.D.,
Perry Robins, M.D.

Chapter 34

Understanding Xeroderma Pigmentosum

What is xeroderma pigmentosum?

Xeroderma pigmentosum (pronounced **zer • o • der • ma pig • men • toe • sum**), XP, is a very rare inherited disease that causes extreme sensitivity to the sun's ultraviolet rays. Unless XP patients are protected from sunlight, their skin and eyes may be severely damaged. This damage may lead to cancers of the skin and eye. XP has been identified in people of every ethnic group all over the world.

What are the signs of XP?

Many people with XP will get an unusually severe sunburn after a short sun exposure. The sunburn will last much longer than expected, perhaps for several weeks. This type of sunburn will usually occur during a child's first sun exposure, and it may be a clue to the diagnosis of XP. However, some people with XP will not get a sunburn more easily than others, and the disease will be undetected until unusual skin changes appear with time.

Most XP patients will develop many freckles at an early age. Continued sun exposure will lead to further changes in the skin, including irregular dark spots, thin skin, excessive dryness, rough-surfaced growths (solar keratoses), and skin cancers. These skin changes will resemble those of elderly people who have spent many years in the

---

NIH Publication No. 94-0178P. Clinical Center Communications, National Institutes of Health, 1988.

sun. In people with XP, these changes caused by sun damage often begin in infancy, and almost always before age 20.

The eyes of a person with XP are often painfully sensitive to the sun, and may easily become irritated, "bloodshot," and clouded. Noncancerous and cancerous growths on the eyes may occur.

Skin Cancers

A series of skin changes leads to the formation of skin cancers. The first skin cancer may develop before a person is 10 years old, and many other skin cancers may continue to form in the future. All three common types of skin cancer (basal cell carcinoma, squamous cell carcinoma, and melanoma) occur much more often in people with XP. Basal cell and squamous cell carcinomas usually do not spread to internal organs, but they do destroy the local skin and underlying tissues. Melanoma can be fatal if it is not removed before it has spread to internal organs.

Other Medical Problems

In addition to skin and eye changes, about 20 percent of XP patients may have one or more nerve-related problems including the following: deafness, poor coordination, spastic muscles, or mental retardation. A few people with XP will have all of these problems, and some also may be very short and may not develop normal sexual characteristics. Some people with XP will develop only mild neurological symptoms in late childhood or adolescence. Whenever neurological problems do occur, however, they usually tend to worsen over time.

What causes xeroderma pigmentosum?

Two factors combine to cause the abnormalities in XP. First, a person inherits from both his or her parents an unusual sensitivity to the damaging effects of ultraviolet light. Second, exposure to the sun, which contains ultraviolet light, leads to changes in the skin and eyes.

DNA Damage and Repair

DNA (deoxyribonucleic acid) within our genes contains all the coded information needed to direct cell functions. Ultraviolet light damages the DNA in cells and disrupts normal cell functioning.

Understanding Xeroderma Pigmentosum

Damaged DNA is mended by the "DNA repair system." But the DNA repair systems of people with XP do not function properly. As a result, unrepaired DNA damage builds up and causes cancerous cell changes or cell death.

XP may be diagnosed by measuring the DNA repair defect in the laboratory.

The Role of Heredity in XP

XP is a "recessive" condition. This means that a person must have two XP genes (one from each parent) to develop the disease. Both parents of a person with XP are "carriers" of the XP trait because each parent has one XP gene and one normal gene. Neither parent has symptoms of XP. But when two XP carriers have a child there is a one in four chance that the child will inherit the XP gene from each parent and be born with the genetic abnormality. At present, there is no test which shows whether or not a person carries the XP trait.

The Role of Sun Exposure and the Development of Neurological Problems

Researchers do not believe that sun exposure affects the development of neurological problems in XP patients. The sun's rays are absorbed by the skin and do not penetrate the brain or other internal organs. No matter how small his or her sun exposure, a person with XP who is genetically prone to develop neurological symptoms will do so. While the cause of the neurological problems is unclear, it appears that people with the most severe reductions in their DNA repair ability are the most likely to have such problems.

Other Damaging Agents

Laboratory tests indicate that sunlight is the major DNA damaging agent to the cells of XP patients. However, tobacco smoke and some drugs (psoralens) can also cause DNA damage. People with XP should avoid exposure to tobacco smoke and should not use tobacco products.

Are there different types of XP?

There are 10 genetic types of XP. These types have been identified in research laboratories by studying cultured skin cells from XP patients. Each type is characterized by a different genetic change of the DNA repair system. Nine of the ten types show reduced activity in a DNA repair system. The tenth form shows reduced activity in another DNA repair system. This last type of XP is referred to as the "variant" form while the other nine types are known as groups A, B, C, D, E, F, G, H, and I.

Can XP be treated?

There is no cure for XP, but much can be done to prevent and treat some of the problems caused by the disease:

- protection from ultraviolet light
- frequent skin examinations
- prompt removal of cancerous tissue.

Protection from Ultraviolet Light

As soon as the diagnosis of XP is suspected, a patient should be completely protected from ultraviolet rays. This will greatly reduce the frequency and severity of skin and eye problems (including cancers). There are two types of ultraviolet light: short wavelength and long wavelength. The main source of harmful, short wavelength ultraviolet light is sunlight. These ultraviolet rays are also found in the light given off by "germicidal" lamps and by artificial sunlamps (including those found in "tanning booths"). The small amount of long wavelength ultraviolet light from regular light bulbs or from sunlight that has passed through window glass is not known to be harmful to people with XP.

To limit a person's exposure to harmful ultraviolet rays, outdoor activity should be restricted to nighttime. If daytime exposure is unavoidable, it should be limited to the very early morning or very late afternoon hours. When XP patients are indoors or in an automobile, the windows should always be closed because glass absorbs some of the harmful ultraviolet rays.

Children with XP should not play outdoors during the day unless they are under ultraviolet light-blocking shelters and away from reflective surfaces such as snow, sand, or water. Clouds do not block out harmful rays. Special arrangements for children with XP should be made at school to ensure that they are not exposed to sunlight from an open window, that they are not exposed to any unfiltered

Understanding Xeroderma Pigmentosum

fluorescent light, and that they are not permitted outside for gym, recess, fire drills, or other activities.

When XP patients are outdoors in daylight, they should wear long sleeves, long pants, and wide-brimmed hats. Two layers of clothing offer more protection than one layer. Eyeglasses or sunglasses that completely block ultraviolet light should be worn. Glasses with sideshields can be used to protect the eyelids and skin around the eyes. Long hair styles help protect the neck and ears.

Any areas of skin which are not covered by clothing or hair should be protected with an opaque sunblocking agent such as zinc oxide, titanium dioxide, or sunblocking make-up. Sunscreens are partially protective. Sunscreens may be used if they have a sun protection factor of 15 or higher. These should be applied at least 30 minutes before going out in the sun. A sunscreen may be used indoors to protect against unrecognized sources of ultraviolet light.

Frequent Skin Examinations

Patients should be examined often by a family member who has been taught to recognize the signs of skin cancer. Any suspicious spot or growth should be immediately reported to the patient's doctor. Examinations should include the eyes, scalp, ears, mouth, tongue, nostrils, and all other areas of the skin, even those that do not have sun exposure (for example, the buttocks).

Examination by a dermatologist (a doctor specializing in skin disorders) should take place at least every three to six months. The dermatologist can help detect skin cancers before they have grown or spread to internal organs. A small piece of suspicious skin growths may be removed (biopsied) and examined for cancer.

Prompt Removal of Cancerous Tissue

Skin cancer treatment for XP patients is similar to that for anyone with skin cancer. Treatment may include removal of the cancer by freezing, use of an electric needle, or surgery. Depending on the size, type, and location of the cancer, a small cancerous growth can usually be treated in a doctor's office. Large tumors may require extensive surgery and skin grafting. X-ray treatment can be used safely in XP patients. Precancerous growths, such as solar keratoses, may be frozen with liquid nitrogen.

Some XP patients who have had many skin cancers have prevented new cancers by taking an oral drug called isotretinoin, a derivative of vitamin A. However, this medicine has severe side effects that prevent its use in all but the most severe cases.

Treatment of Eye Problems

Artificial tears or soft contact lenses may provide relief for abnormally dry or irritated eyes. If the corneas of the eyes become so clouded that the patient cannot see, a corneal transplant may be considered to restore vision.

Treatment of Neurological Abnormalities

While nothing can prevent or stop the development of neurological abnormalities, it is important to be aware of such problems. Early testing and treatment for potential neurological problems may lessen the unfortunate results of undetected abnormalities. For example, detection of hearing loss and subsequent use of a hearing aid may lessen difficulties in communication and in school. XP patients should have a neurological examination (including a hearing test) once a year through age 20.

What are the lifespans of people with XP?

Many people with XP will die at an early age from skin cancer if they are untreated and unprotected from sunlight. However, if a person is diagnosed early, has no severe neurological problems, is protected from ultraviolet light, and followed carefully for early cancer detection, a normal lifespan may result. The lifespans of most people with XP will fall between these extremes. A reduced lifespan is to be expected, but there are great differences among XP patients.

If the parents of a child with XP have another child, will that child also have XP?

There is a one-in-four chance that any child of the same parents of an XP patient will also have XP. XP among affected children in the same family is usually of similar severity. For example, if the first child with XP has severe neurological problems, the next affected child may have similar problems.

Understanding Xeroderma Pigmentosum

Prenatal diagnosis of XP has been done in research laboratories, but it is not a routine test. Parents of a child with XP should seek genetic counseling before considering having another child.

Can a person with XP have children?

Most people with XP have normal sexual development and functioning, and they are able to have children. The advisability of an XP patient becoming a parent would be affected by the patient's own ability to care for a family.

The probability of a person with XP having a child with XP is very small. This would occur only if the other parent also has XP or is a carrier for the XP trait. The likelihood of a person with XP choosing a partner who carries the XP trait is very small unless the two people are related by blood. If there is any doubt about the blood relationship between two partners, family trees should be made covering several generations.

Is there any research being done on XP?

Research laboratories in the United States and throughout the world are learning about XP and trying to correct the DNA repair defect in laboratory-grown cells from XP patients. Clinical studies on skin cancer prevention with oral medications and evaluation of XP patients with unusual features are being conducted at the National Institutes of Health.

Information about symptoms, treatment, and progress of patients with XP is being collected by the Xeroderma Pigmentosum Registry at the following address:

Department of Pathology
UMDNJ—New Jersey
Medical School
100 Bergen Street,
Newark, New Jersey 07013

Where can I get more information about XP?

Your dermatologist can supply answers to specific questions about this disease. Additional information may be obtained from these sources:

Task Force on Xeroderma Pigmentosum
American Academy of Dermatology
1567 Maple Avenue
Box 3116
Evanston, Illinois 60204

National Cancer Institute
Office of Cancer Communications
9000 Rockville Pike
Bethesda, Maryland 20892
(for cancer information)

Local Branches of the American Cancer Society (for cancer information)

Content contributed by Kenneth H. Kraemer, M.D. Research Scientist, National Cancer Institute, in cooperation with Alan D. Andrews, M.D., Department of Dermatology, Columbia University, School of Medicine; Arthur R Rhodes, M.D., Department of Dermatology, Harvard University, School of Medicine; and the Task Force on Xeroderma Pigmentosum of the American Academy of Dermatology.

Part Five

Infectious Organisms, Parasites, and Fungi

Chapter 35

Fever Blisters and Canker Sores

Fever blisters and canker sores are two of the most common disorders of the mouth, causing discomfort and annoyance to millions of Americans. Both cause small sores to develop in or around the mouth, and often are confused with each other. Canker sores, however, occur only inside the mouth—on the tongue and the inside linings of the cheeks, lips and throat. Fever blisters, also called cold sores, usually occur outside the mouth—on the lips, chin, cheeks or in the nostrils. When fever blisters do occur inside the mouth, it is usually on the gums or the roof of the mouth. Inside the mouth, fever blisters are smaller than canker sores, heal more quickly, and often begin as a blister.

Both canker sores and fever blisters have plagued mankind for thousands of years. Scientists at the National Institute of Dental Research, one of the federal government's National Institutes of Health, are seeking ways to better control and ultimately prevent these and other oral disorders.

Fever Blisters

In ancient Rome, an epidemic of fever blisters prompted Emperor Tiberius to ban kissing in public ceremonies. Today fever blisters still occur in epidemic proportions. About 100 million episodes of recurrent fever blisters occur yearly in the United States alone. An

NIH Publication No. 92-247.

estimated 45 to 80 percent of adults and children in this country have had at least one bout with the blisters.

What causes fever blisters?

Fever blisters are caused by a contagious virus called herpes simplex. There are two types of herpes simplex virus. Type 1 usually causes oral herpes, or fever blisters. Type 2 usually causes genital herpes. Although both type 1 and type 2 viruses can infect oral tissues, more than 95 percent of recurrent fever blister outbreaks are caused by the type 1 virus.

Herpes simplex virus is highly contagious when fever blisters are present, and the virus frequently is spread by kissing. Children often become infected by contact with parents, siblings or other close relatives who have fever blisters.

A child can spread the virus by rubbing his or her cold sore and then touching other children. About 10 percent of oral herpes infections in adults result from oral-genital sex with a person who has active genital herpes (type 2). These infections, however, usually do not result in repeat bouts of fever blisters.

Most people infected with the type 1 herpes simplex virus became infected before they were 10 years old. The virus usually invades the moist membrane cells of the lips, throat or mouth. In most people, the initial infection causes no symptoms. About 15 percent of patients, however, develop many fluid-filled blisters inside and outside the mouth three to five days after they are infected with the virus. These may be accompanied by fever, swollen neck glands and general aches. The blisters tend to merge and then collapse. Often a yellowish crust forms over the sores, which usually heal without scarring within two weeks.

The herpes virus, however, stays in the body. Once a person is infected with oral herpes, the virus remains in a nerve located near the cheek bone. It may stay permanently inactive in this site, or it may occasionally travel down the nerve to the skin surface, causing a recurrence of fever blisters. Recurring blisters usually erupt at the outside edge of the lip or the edge of the nostril, but can also occur on the chin, cheeks, or inside the mouth.

The symptoms of recurrent fever blister attacks usually are less severe than those experienced by some people after an initial infection. Recurrences appear to be less frequent after age 35. Many people who have recurring fever blisters feel itching, tingling or burning in the lip one to three days before the blister appears.

Fever Blisters and Canker Sores

What causes a recurrence of fever blisters?

Several factors weaken the body's defenses and trigger an outbreak of herpes. These include emotional stress, fever, illness, injury and exposure to sunlight. Many women have recurrences only during menstruation. One study indicates that susceptibility to herpes recurrences is inherited. Research is under way to discover exactly how the triggering factors interact with the immune system and the virus to prompt a recurrence of fever blisters.

What are the treatments for fever blisters?

Currently there is no cure for fever blisters. Some medications can relieve some of the pain and discomfort associated with the sores, however. These include ointments that numb the blisters, antibiotics that control secondary bacterial infections, and ointments that soften the crusts of the sores.

Is there a vaccine for fever blisters?

Currently there is no vaccine for herpes simplex virus available to the public. Many research laboratories, however, are working on this approach to preventing fever blisters. For example, scientists at the National Institute of Dental Research and the National Institute of Allergy and Infectious Diseases have developed a promising experimental herpes vaccine. In tests on laboratory mice, the vaccine has prevented the herpes simplex virus from infecting the animals and establishing itself in the nerves.

Although these findings are encouraging, the scientists must complete more animal studies on the safety and effectiveness of the vaccine before a decision can be made whether to test it in humans. The vaccine would be useful only for those not already infected with herpes simplex virus.

What can the patient do?

If fever blisters erupt, keep them clean and dry to prevent bacterial infections. Eat a soft, bland diet to avoid irritating the sores and surrounding sensitive areas. Be careful not to touch the sores and spread the virus to new sites, such as the eyes or genitals. To make sure you do not infect others, avoid kissing them or touching the sores and then touching another person.

There is good news for people whose fever blister outbreaks are triggered by sunlight. Scientists at the National Institute of Dental Research have confirmed that sunscreen on the lips can prevent sun-induced recurrences of herpes. They recommend applying the sunscreen before going outside and reapplying it frequently during sun exposure. The researchers used a sunblock with a protection factor of 15 in their studies. Little is known about how to prevent recurrences of fever blisters triggered by factors other than sunlight. People whose cold sores appear in response to stress should try to avoid stressful situations. Some investigators have suggested adding lysine to the diet or eliminating foods such as nuts, chocolate, seeds or gelatin. These measures have not, however, been proven effective in controlled studies.

What research is being done?

Researchers are working on several approaches to preventing or treating fever blisters. As mentioned earlier, they are trying to develop a vaccine against herpes simplex virus. Several laboratories are developing and testing antiviral drugs designed to hamper or prevent fever blister outbreaks. Researchers also are trying to develop ointments that make it easier for antiviral drugs to penetrate the skin.

Acyclovir is an antiviral drug that prevents the herpes simplex virus from multiplying. The U.S. Food and Drug Administration has approved the drug for use in treating genital herpes, and is considering its approval for use in treating oral herpes. Researchers have found that acyclovir taken in pill-form reduces the symptoms and frequency of fever blister recurrences in some patients. In one study, 50 percent of patients who took four acyclovir pills daily for four months had no fever blister outbreaks. Before taking the drug, they had an average of one recurrence every two months. In separate studies, pills taken at the onset of symptoms or acyclovir cream applied to the blisters or to areas of the lip that tingled or itched were found to be only minimally effective. The long-term effects of daily oral doses of acyclovir are not known, nor are the effects the drug might have on an unborn child.

Basic research on how the immune system interacts with herpes simplex viruses may lead to new therapies for fever blisters. The immune system uses a wide array of cells and chemicals to defend the body against infections. Scientists are trying to identify the immune components that prevent recurrent attacks of oral herpes.

Fever Blisters and Canker Sores

Scientists are also trying to determine the precise form and location of the inactive herpes virus in nerve cells. This information might allow them to design antiviral drugs that can attack the herpes virus while it lies dormant in nerves.

In addition, researchers are trying to understand how sunlight, skin injury and stress can trigger recurrences of fever blisters. They hope to develop methods for blocking reactivation of the virus.

Canker Sores

Recurrent canker sores afflict about 20 percent of the general population. The medical term for the sores is *aphthous stomatitis*.

Canker sores are usually found on the movable parts of the mouth such as the tongue or the inside linings of the lips and cheeks. They begin as small oval or round reddish swellings, which usually burst within a day. The ruptured sores are covered by a thin white or yellow membrane and edged by a red halo. Generally, they heal within two weeks. Canker sores range in size from an eighth of an inch wide in mild cases to more than an inch wide in severe cases. Severe canker sores may leave scars. Fever is rare, and the sores are rarely associated with other diseases. Usually a person will have only one or a few canker sores at a time.

Most people have their first bout with canker sores between the ages of 10 and 20. Children as young as 2, however, may develop the condition. The frequency of canker sore recurrences varies considerably. Some people have only one or two episodes a year, while others may have a continuous series of canker sores.

What causes canker sores?

The cause of canker sores is not well understood. More than one cause is likely, even for individual patients. Canker sores do not appear to be caused by viruses or bacteria, although an allergy to a type of bacterium commonly found in the mouth may trigger them in some people. The sores may be an allergic reaction to certain foods. In addition, there is research suggesting that canker sores may be caused by a faulty immune system that uses the body's defenses against disease to attack and destroy the normal cells of the mouth or tongue.

British studies show that, in about 20 percent of patients, canker sores are due partly to nutritional deficiencies, especially lack of vitamin B_{12}, folic acid and iron. Similar studies performed in the United

States, however, have not confirmed this finding. In a small percentage of patients, canker sores occur with gastrointestinal problems, such as an inability to digest certain cereals. In these patients, canker sores appear to be part of a generalized disorder of the digestive tract.

Female sex hormones apparently play a role in causing canker sores. Many women have bouts of the sores only during certain phases of their menstrual cycles. Most women experience improvement or remission of their canker sores during pregnancy. Researchers have used hormone therapy successfully in clinical studies to treat some women. Both emotional stress and injury to the mouth can trigger outbreaks of canker sores, but these factors probably do not cause the disorder.

Who is susceptible?

Women are more likely than men to have recurrent canker sores. Genetic studies show that susceptibility to recurrent outbreaks of the sores is inherited in some patients. This partially explains why the disorder is often shared by family members.

What are the treatments for canker sores?

Most doctors recommend that patients who have frequent bouts of canker sores undergo blood and allergy tests to determine if their sores are caused by a nutritional deficiency, an allergy or some other preventable cause. Vitamins and other nutritional supplements often prevent recurrences or reduce the severity of canker sores in patients with a nutritional deficiency. Patients with food allergies can reduce the frequency of canker sores by avoiding those foods.

There are several treatments for reducing the pain and duration of canker sores for patients whose outbreaks cannot be prevented. These include numbing ointments such as benzocaine, which are available in drug stores without a prescription. Anti-inflammatory steroid mouth rinses or gels can be prescribed for patients with severe sores.

Mouth rinses containing the antibiotic tetracycline may reduce the unpleasant symptoms of canker sores and speed healing by preventing bacterial infections in the sores. Clinical studies at the National Institute of Dental Research have shown that rinsing the mouth with tetracycline several times a day usually relieves pain in 24 hours and allows complete healing in five to seven days. The U.S. Food and Drug Administration warns, however, that tetracycline given to pregnant

Fever Blisters and Canker Sores

women and young children can permanently stain youngsters' teeth. Both steroid and tetracycline treatments require a prescription and care of a dentist or physician.

Patients with severe recurrent canker sores may need to take steroid or other immuno-suppressant drugs orally. These potent drugs can cause many undesirable side effects, and should be used only under the close supervision of a dentist or physician.

What can the patient do?

If you have canker sores, avoid abrasive foods such as potato chips that can stick in the cheek or gum and aggravate the sores. Take care when brushing your teeth not to stab the gums or cheek with a toothbrush bristle. Avoid acidic and spicy foods. Canker sores are not contagious, so patients do not have a worry about spreading them to other people.

What research is being done?

Researchers are trying to identify the malfunctions in patients' immune systems that make them susceptible to recurrent bouts of canker sores. By analyzing the blood of people with and without canker sores, scientists have found several differences in immune function between the two groups. Whether these differences cause canker sores is not yet known.

Researchers also are developing and testing new drugs designed to treat canker sores. Most of these drugs alter the patients' immune function. Although some of the drugs appear to be effective in treating canker sores in some patients, the data are still inconclusive. Until these drugs are proven to be absolutely safe and effective, they will not be available for general use.

Chapter 36

Scabies

Scabies is highly contagious and is usually transmitted by direct personal contact. It typically presents as an intensely pruritic eruption. Atypical presentations are common in Norwegian scabies and in childhood scabies. Infestation is documented by visualizing the mite, its eggs or scybala on low-power microscopy. The treatment of choice is 5-percent permethrin cream, used in a single application at bedtime and removed the next morning.

Scabies is a highly contagious, pruritic dermatosis caused by infestation with the *Sarcoptes scabiei* mite. Although this disorder is well characterized, scabies can present in many different forms and can baffle even the most astute clinician. A predisposition to widespread infestation (Norwegian scabies) occurs in institutionalized patients and in patients with immune system deficiency, including those with human immunodeficiency virus (HIV) infection.

History and Epidemiology

The scabies mite, *S. scabiei*, is an arachnid of the genus Acarus. Clinical descriptions of scabies infestation date back many centuries, but Bonomo, in 1687, was the first to identify the mite using light microscopy.[1]

Historically, scabies infestations were believed to occur in cycles, with epidemics occurring during World Wars I and II. More recently,

---

©1992 *American Family Physician* October 1992. Reprinted with permission.

scabies has made a resurgence, especially in the HIV-infected population.[2]

The scabies mite is predominantly transmitted by direct personal contact. Indirect contact with clothing or bedding is believed to lead to infestation infrequently. Scabies mites are often found in the inter-digital spaces of the hand, which suggests that infection can occur by simple hand-to-hand contact. The scabies mite can survive without a human host for several days.

The female scabies mite is fertilized on the skin surface and begins to burrow into the stratum corneum epidermis. The male mite, which has a shorter life span, remains on the skin surface or produces only shallow burrows. The female mite is uniquely equipped to burrow into human epidermis. Utilizing its jaws and the cutting claws of its forelegs, the mite completes its descent within 20 minutes. About 40 hours after fertilization, the female mite begins to deposit eggs behind her as she burrows. The eggs, laid in groups of two or four daily, can number up to 40 per mite. Also found in the scabietic burrows are fecal pellets, called scybala. The female completes its five-week life cycle and dies at the terminal end of a burrow.

The eggs produce larvae after four days of incubation. The larvae travel to the skin surface and pass through a nymph stage; the adult mite develops two weeks after the eggs hatch.[3]

Clinical Manifestations

Scabies infestation typically presents as an intensely pruritic eruption. Often the pruritus is worse at night. The classic lesion of scabies is the burrow, a thread-like, wavy, gray-white papule several millimeters in length. The end of the burrow may be marked by a small vesicle, which indicates the presence of the mite. Burrows are most likely found in inter-digital spaces of the hand, and on the flexor surfaces of the wrists and elbows, the belt line, the areola in women and the genitalia in men.

Atypical presentations are common in Norwegian scabies and in neonatal scabies. Norwegian scabies, seen in immunocompromised and institutionalized individuals, presents as crusted scaling lesions with varying degrees of pruritus. Additional sites where Norwegian scabies may appear include the head and neck and, in homosexual men, the buttocks and perianal regions. While the mite population in a typical scabies infestation averages about 12, in Norwegian scabies the crusted lesions are teeming with mites and the total mite population extends to the hundreds of thousands.[4]

Pediatric scabies, seen in infants as young as two months of age, presents with erythematous crusted lesions and burrows similar to those seen in Norwegian scabies. In addition, scabies in infants and children may involve the face, an extremely uncommon finding in adults. Other symptoms associated with scabies in infants include irritability and poor feeding.[5]

Diagnosis

Proof of scabies infestation is achieved by visualizing the mite, its eggs or scybala. If classic burrows are seen, simple skin scraping and visualization under low-power microscopy is the diagnostic method of choice. Use of a number 15 scalpel blade to uncover a burrow is the preferred method. Some authors advocate placing immersion oil on the blade before scraping to prevent scattering of epidermal fragments.[3] Alternatively, potassium hydroxide solutions may be used on the glass slide, particularly if tinea infections are included in the differential diagnosis.

The yield of skin scrapings is highest for new, nonexcoriated burrows. If clinical suspicion warrants, multiple scrapings may be obtained to increase the likelihood of making a positive identification. The yield of skin scrapings is highest in Norwegian scabies because of the great extent of infestation.

Differential Diagnosis

The differential diagnosis of scabies includes atopic dermatitis, dermatitis herpetiformis and other insect infestations. Atopic dermatitis is common and is often seen in persons who also have asthma and hay fever. Although burrows are not seen in atopic dermatitis, a linear arrangement of lesions may be confused with scabietic lesions. Dermatitis herpetiformis is an uncommon autoimmune disorder in which patients present with widespread, intensely pruritic papules, vesicles or excoriations.

The cutaneous findings of some other insect infestations require distinction from scabies. Fleas, bedbugs and the parasites of cats and dogs may produce an intensely pruritic eruption, usually referred to as papular urticaria. Dogs and other animals have their own species of scabies. Fortunately, scabies is species-specific (i.e., canine scabies are unable to burrow and breed in man). However, dog scabies can produce an unpleasant papulovesicular eruption in humans. It has been noted that a dog with sarcoptic mange is analogous to a human with Norwegian scabies, with thousands of organisms present. *Pediculosis corporis* and *pediculosis pubis* may also at times require distinction from human scabies.

Less common disorders to consider are numerous. Linear IgA bullous dermatosis, herpes gestationis and vesicular bullous pemphigoid are three autoimmune diseases that are somewhat similar to dermatitis herpetiformis and may mimic scabies infestations. Additionally, in pregnant women, the clinician must consider the pruritic eruptions of pregnancy, namely papular urticarial papules and plaques of pregnancy.

Differential Diagnosis of Scabies

Atopic dermatitis
Dermatitis herpetiformis
Other insect infestations
Linear IgA bullous dermatosis
Herpes gestationis
Bullous pemphigoid
Pruritic urticarial papules and plaques of pregnancy (PUPPP)
Lichen planus
Folliculitis
Syphilis
Seborrheic dermatitis
Nodular prurigo
Pityriasis Rosea

Other disorders in the differential diagnosis include lichen planus, folliculitis, syphilis, seborrheic dermatitis, nodular prurigo and pityriasis rosea. Rarely, occult malignancy may produce generalized pruritus. Finally, in patients with HIV infection, any chronic crusted dermatosis should be evaluated for scabies, whether or not pruritus is present.

Treatment

Dried chrysanthemum flowers have been used as an insecticide since 1840. They were first marketed commercially in Dalmatia (now Croatia) and exported to America by 1870 as Dalmatian "insect

Scabies

powder."[6] The common name for the active ingredient is pyrethrum, and pyrethrins are the active insecticidal ingredients.

In 1989, a synthetic pyrethrin-like chemical, permethrin, was approved as a treatment for scabies. Marketed as a 5-percent cream (Elimite), this agent is now considered the treatment of choice for scabies. A single application of 5-percent permethrin cream is used on all cutaneous surfaces (particularly the fingernails, waist and genitalia). Application at bedtime is preferred, and the cream is washed off the next morning. Close family members should also be treated. This treatment has been found to be very effective and is safe in children over the age of two months. However, overuse of the product is common. The physician should stress that only one application is necessary to kill mites and eggs.

Other permethrin products are available without a prescription. These low-strength formulations are designed to treat pediculosis and are not effective in the treatment of scabies. The primary care physician may be fooled when a pruritic rash is not responsive to the low-strength products used by the patient before the office visit. Nix cream rinse and Rid spray and shampoo are two commonly available 0.5-percent permethrin formulations.

Lindane (Kwell [gamma benzene hexachloride]) has long been a favored treatment for scabies; however, reports of neurotoxicity in children have occurred.[8] Ten-percent crotamiton cream (Eurax), a rarely used pediculicide, has been criticized for its low rate of effectiveness in children (less than 50 percent) and for its unknown toxicity.[7] Topical sulfur preparations have been reported to be effective but may be toxic in infants and children.

Pruritus may persist for several weeks after adequate therapy. Patients should be informed in advance to anticipate this continued discomfort and to avoid over-application of medication. Calamine lotion may be used for persistent pruritus. However, one must first attempt to verify the correct and vigorous application of topical medication and to examine the patient for persistent infestation by identification of viable mites.

It is essential that all members of a household be treated at the same time, including regular guests. If secondary impetigo occurs, which is common, oral antibiotics may also be used simultaneously. Fresh undergarments and sheets should be used after the last applications of scabicidal medication.

References

1. Parlette HL. "Scabietic infestations of man." *Cutis* 1975;16:47-52.
2. Sirera G, Rius F, Romeu J, et al. "Hospital outbreak of scabies stemming from two AIDS patients with Norwegian scabies" [Letter]. *Lancet* 1990;335:1227.
3. Lyell A. "Diagnosis and treatment of scabies." *Br Med J* 1967:2:223-5.
4. Burkhart CG. "Scabies: an epidemiologic reassessment." *Ann Intern Med* 1983:98:498-503.
5. Sterling GB, Janniger CK, Kihiczak G. Neonatal scabies. Cutis 1990:45:229-31.
6. Taplin D, Meinking TL. "Pyrethrins and pyrethroids in dermatology." *Arch Dermatol 1990*. 126:213-21.
7. Taplin D, Meinking TL, Chen JA, Sanchez R. "Comparison of crotamiton 10% cream (Eurax) and permethrin 5% cream (Elimite) for the treatment of scabies in children." *Ped Dermatol* 1990:7:67-73.
8. Schultz MW, Gomez M, Hansen RC, et al. "Comparative study of 5 percent permethrin cream and 1 percent lindane lotion for the treatment of scabies." *Arch Dermatol l990*;126:167-70.

— by Glenn B. Sterling, M.D.,
University of Pennsylvania
School of Medicine
Philadelphia, Pennsylvania;

Camila Krysicka Janniger, M.D.,
George Kihiczak M.D.,
and Robert A. Schwartz, M.D. M.P.H.,
UMDNJ-New Jersey Medical School,
Newark, New Jersey;

Michael D. Fox, M.D.,
San Mateo County Hospital,
San Mateo, California

The Authors

Glenn B. Sterling, M.D. is director of the Western Dermatology Center. Western-Fort Lauderdale, Fla. He received his medical degree from the State University of New York at Stony Brook School of Medicine and completed a residency in dermatology at the Hospital of the University of Pennsylvania, Philadelphia.

Camila Krysicka Janniger, M.D. is clinical assistant professor of dermatology at UMDNJ-New Jersey Medical School, Newark. She received her medical degree from the Medical Academy of Warsaw,

Poland, and completed a residency in dermatology at UMDNJ-New Jersey Medical School.

George Kihiczak, M.D. is clinical associate professor of dermatology at UMDNJ-New Jersey Medical School, Newark. He received his medical degree from UMDNJ-New Jersey Medical School and completed a residency in dermatology at New York Medical College, Valhalla.

Robert A. Schwartz. M. D., M.P.H. is professor and chief of dermatology service at UMDNJ-New Jersey Medical School, Newark. He received his medical degree from New York Medical College, Valhalla, and completed a residency in dermatology at the University of Cincinnati (Ohio) College of Medicine. He completed a fellowship in dermatologic oncology at Roswell Park Memorial Institute, Buffalo, N.Y. Dr. Schwartz is a member of AFP's editorial advisory board.

Michael D. Fox, M.D. is associate director of emergency room services at San Mateo County Hospital, San Mateo, Calif. He received his medical degree from New York Medical College, Valhalla, and completed a residency in family practice at the University of Connecticut School of Medicine, Farmington.

Chapter 37

Dermatophyte Infections: The Tinea Fungus (Ringworm)

Superficial infections caused by dermatophytes fungi that invade only dead tissues of the skin or its appendages (stratum corneum, nails, hair). Microsporum, Trichophyton, and *Epidermophyton* are the genera most commonly involved. Fomites are probably not responsible for transmission. Some dermatophytes produce only mild or no inflammation; in such cases, the organism may persist indefinitely, causing intermittent remissions and exacerbations of a gradually extending lesion with a scaling, slightly raised border. In other cases an acute infection may occur, typically causing a sudden vesicular and bullous disease of the feet or an inflamed boggy lesion of the scalp (**kerion**) that is due to a strong immunologic reaction to the fungus; the infection is usually followed by remission or cure.

Types of Dermatophyte Infections by Infection Site

Four communicable diseases caused by fungus growth on the body's surface are:

- **Tinea Pedis.** Ringworm of the feet,
- **Tinea Unguium**. Ringworm of the nails,
- **Tinea Corporis**. Ringworm of the body,
- **Tinea Capitis**. Ringworm of the scalp.

Excerpted from *The Merck Manual of Diagnosis and Therapy* ©1992, Sixteenth Edition. Reprinted with permission. NIH Publication No. 80-8239.

Ringworm of the Feet ("Athlete's Foot")

The most common of the fungus diseases that involve the skin is ringworm of the feet, more commonly known as "athlete's foot." This disease develops on a person's feet when certain fungi known as dermatophytes, contaminate the skin and begin to grow and multiply there. These fungi grow best on warm, moist, poorly ventilated areas of the feet such as the skin between the toes. Athlete's foot is usually most severe in hot weather in individuals who wear heavy shoes or boots, or in athlete's who do not properly wash and dry their feet after swimming or participation in active sports that cause excessive perspiration.

The signs and symptoms of infection are itching, cracking or scaling of the skin, and sometimes the development of small blisters that contain a watery fluid. If the disease is allowed to continue without treatment, the infection may spread over large areas of the feet and legs, and the individual may become incapacitated due to the irritation and soreness of the affected skin. Secondary bacterial infection may occur leading to further pain and incapacitation.

Ringworm of the Nails

Ringworm of the nails occurs when the dermatophyte fungi grow on or in the nails. It frequently begins in a nail that has been injured, but may spread to all the nails. It often is secondary to ringworm of the skin. The fungus growth may penetrate the entire nail, causing it to become thickened and misshapened, discolored, chalky, pitted, grooved and brittle. This is the most chronic and difficult form of ringworm infection to cure.

Ringworm of the Body

Ringworm of the body may result from spread of ringworm of the feet, or may be acquired by direct contacts with other infected persons, or indirectly by wearing contaminated clothing or articles, such as towels previously used by infected individuals.

Certain types of ringworm of the body may be acquired from cats, dogs, or other animals that have ringworm.

Indication of infection is usually the development of red, flat, frequently circular sores that may be dry and scaly or crusted and moist. As the sores enlarge, the center of the areas frequently clears, leaving

Dermatophyte Infections: The Tinea Fungus (Ringworm)

apparently normal skin surrounded by an infected edge. Such ring-shaped lesions have led to the name "ringworm" for this disease. Ringworm of the body can be transmitted from one person to another or from animals to persons as long as the disease is untreated.

Ringworm of the Scalp

Ringworm of the scalp is another skin disease that can be spread from person to person or from animals to people. Children are more likely to develop the infection than are adults, but the disease can occur at any age.

Clothing contaminated by an infected pet or person, barber's unsterilized tools, backs of theater seats, toilet articles including combs and brushes—all these are possible sources of the fungus.

Scalp ringworm generally begins in the form of a small pimple or sore, then spreads into a ringlike shape. Infected hairs become brittle and break easily, or fall out leaving bald patches that may be permanent.

Ringworm Prevention

Ringworm of the skin can be prevented by observing simple rules of hygiene.

Athlete's foot and ringworm of the toenails can be prevented by keeping the feet clean and dry; by wearing a clean pair of hose each day; by dusting the feet frequently with a fungicidal powder; and by using only gymnasium, swimming pool, and clubhouse locker rooms that are cleaned and disinfected daily. Wear shoes and stockings that are comfortably roomy, so that air can get to the feet.

Ringworm of the scalp and ringworm of the body, can be prevented by detection and treatment of infected persons or pets; by effective sterilization of barber's tools; by not wearing an infected person's hat, cap, or other clothing; and by not using their toilet articles.

Parents who have children of school age should notify the school authorities if ringworm develops in the family.

Ringworm Treatment

The types of ringworm described in this chapter can be cured in a short time if proper treatment is begun early and followed faithfully. Because improper self-treatment can make the infection worse, and because the several forms may require differing kinds of treatment, let your doctor tell you what to do to eliminate the infection. S/he can identify the fungus, recommend the proper medication, and help prevent a recurrence of the disease.

If family pets or livestock have ringworm, be sure to have them treated by a veterinarian.

Chapter 38

Shingles—or Chickenpox, Part Two

Illness often begins with a vague feeling of malaise—mild aches and pains, maybe a touch of nausea, chills, and fever. Those symptoms might signal the onset of food poisoning, the flu, or any of a dozen other complaints. But for 300,000 Americans each year they herald the reappearance of one of nature's most unwelcome guests—the varicella-zoster virus (VZV)—and with it a formidable disease with a humble name: shingles.

All of these unfortunate people have met VZV before, when it gave them chickenpox as children or (rarely) young adults. But the second time around, VZV produces not another case of chickenpox, but an acute infection of the central nervous system, known formally as Herpes zoster. (The medical name for chickenpox is Herpes varicella, hence the V-Z virus or VZV.) And, in its repeat onslaught, VZV is capable of causing nerve and organ damage and severe pain that can last months or years.

Fortunately, most cases of shingles are self-limiting; the illness spontaneously subsides after a few weeks and reappears in no more than 2 percent of otherwise healthy patients. But more than half, and perhaps as many as 75 percent, of shingles patients beyond age 60 develop a condition called post-herpetic neuralgia (PHN)—excruciating pain that persists long after the viral infection is over.

PHN is reported to be the principal cause of intractable, debilitating pain in the elderly and the leading cause of suicide in chronic pain sufferers over age 70. While shingles and PHN can strike at any age

FDA Consumer, July/August 1991.

(and equally among males and females), the risk increases with advancing years. About 50 percent of people who reach age 85 will have had shingles, and most of them will also suffer the protracted pain of post-herpetic neuralgia.

A Drama in Two Acts

Because shingles may start with nonspecific signs and symptoms, it can mimic conditions ranging from muscle strain to heart attack. The most common initial complaint is burning or shooting pain in the area served by the nerves infected by VZV, usually near the waist or on the head and face. Patients describe the pain as pulsating, stabbing, piercing, unbearable, and some experts have described it as second only to the pain produced by certain forms of cancer. (Some shingles victims have severe itching or aching rather than pain, and a blessed few, chiefly young patients, experience no discomfort at all.)

Within a couple of days, the pain or discomfort is accompanied by a rash: small, clear blisters (lesions) that form on inflamed skin in the painful area. New blisters continue to appear for about seven days. They gradually get larger, become cloudy, and form crusts that fall off with little or no scarring. The whole episode of pain, rash and healing is generally over in three to five weeks.

Once the rash appears, its cause is obvious to a trained eye. The pattern of lesions follows very closely the path in the skin taken by the VZV-infected nerves.

Since individual nerve ganglia serve either the left or right side of the body, but not both sides, the rash and pain of shingles are almost always confined to a rather narrow band on one side only. "Shingles" is in fact a misnomer. It comes from the Latin *cingulum*, which means a belt or girdle. (*Zoster* means the same thing in Greek.) But a case of shingles that actually encircles the body is rare.

One of the more frequent and painful targets of shingles is the area around one eye and the nose. Lesions on the eyelid pose no threat to the eye itself. On the other hand, the appearance of a shingles lesion on the tip of the nose means that the cornea will be affected, with the possibility of temporary loss of vision and permanent scarring in the involved eye. Glaucoma is a common late complication of ophthalmic shingles.

Strictly speaking, shingles is not a second bout with the varicella-zoster virus. It's more like Act II of a show with a long intermission.

Shingles—or Chickenpox, Part Two

After VZV has entered the body and caused chickenpox, it doesn't go away, even after the patient recovers. Instead, the virus takes up residence in nerve cells next to the spinal cord and cranial nerves. Years later, for reasons that scientists don't fully understand, VZV again becomes active. It infects nerve fibers to their very ends, causing them to send impulses that the brain interprets as severe pain, burning or itching. The skin in the area served by that nerve also becomes highly sensitive. The softest touch, even a gentle breeze, can cause agonizing pain. Act II of the VZV performance is under way.

There is good circumstantial evidence that the reactivation of dormant VZV is related to a weakening of the immune system. That would explain the increased occurrence of shingles among older people, whose immune systems are not as active as they once were. It might also explain why cancer patients, especially those with Hodgkin's disease or leukemia, diseases that impair the immune system, are especially susceptible to reactivation of VZV. About 10 percent of leukemia patients and one out of three persons with Hodgkin's disease develop shingles.

People with AIDS whose immune systems are severely compromised appear to be at increased risk of developing shingles, and they tend to have especially severe cases, involving internal organs as well as peripheral nerves and skin. Other people at increased risk include those who take powerful immunity-suppressing drugs used to prevent rejection following organ or bone marrow transplants. The use of cortisone and certain anti-cancer agents—drugs that interfere with the immune response—also appears to be linked with an increased risk of shingles. In immune-compromised patients, shingles and its aftermath can be devastating. The disease can spread throughout the skin and attack internal organs, such as the lungs and kidneys. If it goes unchecked, disseminated shingles can cause temporary or permanent injury, such as paralysis and loss of sight or hearing, depending on which part of the body is served by the infected nerves. Death can result from viral pneumonia or secondary bacterial infection.

Patients facing these extreme risks require extraordinary care. They may receive serum or other biological products obtained from the pooled blood of recent shingles victims to help their own immune systems resist the VZV. Large doses of anti-viral drugs may be administered intravenously to try to destroy or cripple the virus. The skin lesions associated with ophthalmic zoster are usually treated with cortisone applied to the skin to control local inflammation.

Acyclovir and Red Pepper

There is no specific treatment for shingles. Care is aimed at shortening the acute phase of pain and rash, making the patient as comfortable as possible, and preventing or minimizing complications. In otherwise healthy patients under 50, mild analgesics, such as aspirin (alone or with codeine); wet, cool compresses; and sedatives help relieve pain and itching. Antibacterial salves or lotions are used to control possible skin infection that can cause scarring.

If conservative measures aren't successful in managing pain, drugs that combat depression, such as amitriptyline (Elavil is one of several brand-name products), are sometimes used, especially among older patients. These drugs not only ease the emotional impact of unrelenting pain, they appear to act directly to lessen the pain itself.

In severe cases, especially in elderly patients, an oral corticosteroid such as prednisone (Deltasone and other brand names), if used in large amounts early in the course of the disease, may relieve pain during the acute phase of the illness and prevent or reduce post-herpetic pain.

In 1990, FDA broadened the approved use of the anti-herpesvirus drug acyclovir (Zovirax) to include treatment of acute shingles. The drug had previously been approved for use in genital herpes. Controlled clinical trials showed that acyclovir reduced the period during which new shingles lesions formed and shortened the times to scabbing, healing, and complete cessation of pain in patients with uncomplicated shingles. Patients receiving acyclovir were less likely to suffer pain and other discomfort during the acute phase of illness. Taken orally over a period of 7 to 10 days, acyclovir also lessened the time during which patients "shed" VZV and thus could infect people who had never had chickenpox. A person with active shingles can give chickenpox to someone who has not had the disease, but shingles itself is not contagious.

Although some drugs can reduce the pain, neither acyclovir nor any other treatment lowers the risk of post-herpetic neuralgia following an acute attack of shingles. But research over the last several years has focused attention on a drug that seems to offer pain relief for many patients afflicted by PHN. The drug is capsaicin, not a product of chemical conjuring, but a derivative of the plant family from which we get red pepper.

Capsaicin cream (Zostrix) has been reported by investigators at the pain clinic of Toronto General Hospital to reduce pain in a significant percentage of PHN victims. The researchers say that more than half (56 percent) of PHN patients who received capsaicin cream for four weeks had good or excellent pain relief, and that 78 percent noted at least some improvement in pain.

Although capsaicin is an over-the-counter drug sold for muscular aches and pains, patients should consult a physician before using it to treat PHN. The drug should not be applied until the lesions caused by shingles have completely healed.

The Canadian investigators pointed out that burning was a common adverse effect in most patients receiving capsaicin, about one-third of whom had to stop the treatment early because of an intolerable burning sensation. But other investigators have reported that the burning caused by capsaicin subsides if patients stay on the drug beyond 72 hours, by which time it has measurably lowered their sensitivity to both heat and pain.

Although the drug may seem to be merely a counterirritant, laboratory and clinical studies suggest that capsaicin directly reduces the amount of substance P, a chemical responsible for the transmission of pain impulses. It apparently depletes substance P from nerve fibers and prevents the nerves from taking up a fresh supply of the chemical.

Without substance P, nerves can't pass pain signals to the brain. Ease of administration—the cream is applied to the skin three or four times a day—and the fact that capsaicin does not interact with other drugs make it especially suitable for use in elderly patients.

Unanswered Questions

While drug treatment can shorten the duration of shingles and ease the pain of both shingles and post-herpetic neuralgia in otherwise healthy patients, VZV infection remains a serious, even life-threatening, problem for people with damaged immune systems and hence a substantial challenge for biomedical research.

The virus itself is far from well understood. A leading investigator remarked a few years ago that less is known about VZV than any other herpesvirus, despite the fact that this family of viruses is responsible not only for chickenpox and shingles but also for cold sores, fever blisters, mononucleosis, and genital herpes.

A vaccine against chickenpox might theoretically prevent shingles, because someone who has never had chickenpox can't come down with shingles. Studies are being conducted in this country and abroad on an experimental live virus vaccine against chickenpox. However, there are questions about the potential usefulness of a chickenpox vaccine in preventing shingles. If the vaccine introduced live viruses into the body to induce immunity to chickenpox, might not some of those viruses take refuge in the central nervous system and cause shingles years or decades later?

One reason there are still many unanswered questions about VZV is that no good, economical animal model exists in which the virus can be studied extensively. VZV grows poorly in laboratory cell cultures and does not infect animals other than humans. One type of monkey develops a condition similar to chickenpox when injected with a virus that closely resembles VZV. But that's less than an ideal situation for research on either VZV or the diseases it causes. Nonetheless, a good deal of research is under way at the National Institutes of Health and in other laboratories and clinics around the world to learn more about the biology of VZV itself, how the immune system keeps it under control, and better ways to ease the suffering caused by shingles and post-herpetic neuralgia.

—*by Ken Flieger*

Ken Flieger is a free-lance writer in Washington. D.C.

Chapter 39

New Treatment Helps Ease Pain of Shingles

Use of Antiviral Drugs at Onset Shortens Ailment's Duration, Complications

Almost half of the 600,000 people diagnosed with shingles every year suffer the complication of agonizing pain that can last from months to years. Until now doctors have had few treatments to control this pain described by some as akin to being jabbed repeatedly with an ice pick.

But there's growing evidence that immediate treatment with new antiviral drugs shortens the duration of shingles and its most painful complication known as post-herpetic neuralgia. Some of the newest research also suggests what doctors have only hoped for: that the drugs may reduce the risk of post-shingles pain.

University of Texas researcher Stephen Tyring and a team of scientists from the United States and Australia in a report published July 1995 in the *Archives of Internal Medicine* found that the drug famciclovir shortened the duration of post-herpetic neuralgia by approximately two months as compared with a group of shingles patients who received a placebo.

Another study published by University of California researcher Karl Beutner in the July 1995 issue of the journal *Antimicrobial Agents and Chemotherapy* showed that shingles sufferers who took the drug valacyclovir decreased the initial bout of shingles by as much

©1995 *Washington Post. Reprinted with permission.*

as two weeks. Use of the drug also cut by 6 percent the number of patients experiencing long-term pain after shingles. Valacyclovir a chemical cousin of the widely used acyclovir received Food and Drug Administration approval June 23, 1995.

The recent findings "represent an important advance" in treating the severe pain after shingles said Michael Oxman professor of medicine at the University of California at San Diego and a member of the scientific advisory board of the VZV Foundation, a nonprofit group that provides information to shingles patients and supports research on the disease.

Many doctors now routinely prescribe acyclovir a widely used antiviral that shortens the course of shingles but has mixed results in reducing complications. "There's been a feeling for more than a decade that acyclovir should make a difference [in post-herpetic neuralgia] but it's been hard to show," said Ronda Kost a researcher at the National Institute of Allergy and Infectious Diseases.

The latest findings suggest that famciclovir and valacyclovir could help bridge the gap. Both are newer types of antiviral medications known as pro-drugs. They are administered in an inactive form that is more easily absorbed by the body than acyclovir. Only as the drugs are metabolized do they change to the more potent chemical structure.

Another advantage of the new antivirals is that they can be taken less frequently—three times a day as opposed to the up-to-five daily doses needed for acyclovir. But doctors won't know for sure how the newer medications compare with acyclovir or with each other until head-to-head trials are completed. "You can't compare them because the studies have not been completed," Beutner said. "The key message to consumers is that there is therapy to shorten the duration of shingles and decrease the number of patients with pain."

Shingles—a common illness that strikes one in five Americans—is caused by a reactivation of a viral infection with varicella zoster virus the same virus that produces chicken pox. The name shingles comes from the Latin word cingulum meaning belt or girdle. Sufferers frequently experience tingling and pain before a sore blistery rash appears that runs like a line or belt around one half of their middle. Other common sites for shingles lesions include the face and scalp and the chest. The rash lasts for several weeks. It feels painful sometimes itchy, crusts, and then disappears in uncomplicated cases.

But for others shingles can lead to bizarre sensations that can linger for years. Johns Hopkins University neurologist Richard Johnson for example experienced a phantom feeling called dysesthesia, in

New Treatment Helps Ease Pain of Shingles

which he had the sensation of cold water running down the side of his face.

"During lectures I would be picking up my handkerchief and dabbing at my face even though I as a neurologist knew that it was dysesthesia" Johnson said. "But when you feel something cold running down the side of your face it can be very irritating."

For about half of people age 60 and older and those with compromised immune systems, shingles results in post-herpetic neuralgia. In this condition, the skin where the rash had appeared becomes extremely sensitive. Sufferers complain that a light breeze can feel like torture, a drop of water like a third-degree burn and even the softest clothing becomes unbearable where the rash appeared. "I wanted to float away and leave my burning left leg behind," wrote a 71-year-old man in a letter to the VZV Research Foundation.

The virus is crafty. After a bout of chicken pox, a small amount of virus takes refuge in nerve bundles near the spine, remaining dormant for years. As a person ages the odds of the virus reactivating into a full-blown case of shingles increases, probably because of a declining immune system. "By age 85, you have a 50-50 chance of getting shingles," Johnson said.

Scientists think that a decline in the activity of white blood cells in the immune system may allow the virus to re-emerge. As evidence, they point to the increased incidence of shingles not just among the elderly, but in children with leukemia, cancer patients undergoing chemotherapy, organ transplant recipient who take immunosuppressive drugs and people with HIV infection. "These patients have a 20- to 200-fold increase" in the rate of shingles for their age, Oxman said. "All of this makes a wonderful case to say shingles is due to a decline in cellular immunity."

If shingles is left untreated, the risk of complications greatly increases, particularly for older people and those with compromise immune systems. Three different studies have shown that without treatment, a quarter of people age 55 and older with shingles will develop post-herpetic neuralgia, as will half of those age 60 and older and nearly three-quarters of those age 70 and older.

The message, Oxman said, is that "you want to get antiviral drugs as fast as you can to stop the virus from replicating."

Findings from the most recent studies show why. The University of Texas' Tyring teamed with researchers at 36 medical centers in the United States and Australia to test the effectiveness of giving famciclovir to 419 adults with uncomplicated shingles. Within 72 hours of developing a rash, participants were randomly assigned to receive three doses daily for seven days of famciclovir or placebo for seven days. People in the drug group experienced complications for a shorter time.

The University of California study involved more than 1,100 patients treated at 107 study sites in 13 countries for up to 14 days, and it found that therapy beyond seven days "does not confer additional benefit."

Once post-shingles pain develops, doctors may prescribe small amounts of antidepressants and anti-convulsant medications such as tegretol to help ease the discomfort.

There may be more options in the future for controlling the pain after it starts. At the National Institutes of Health Pain Clinic, Mitchell Max and his colleagues are working with a new class of drugs known as NMDA blockers that inhibit the perception of pain by the brain.

A small preliminary pain clinic study involving eight patients and published earlier this year in the journal *Clinical Neuropharmacology* found that NMDA blockers "have promise for the treatment of neuropathic pain," Max reported. But he noted that more work needs to be done to figure out the most effective way to administer these medications.

Shingles at a Glance

Shingles is caused by a reactivation of a varicella zoster viral infection, the same virus that causes chicken pox. After the body recovers from chicken pox, the virus takes refuge in bundles of nerves, called ganglia, near the spine. There, it remains dormant for years. For reasons not completely understood but probably having to do with a decline in the immune system, the virus then reactivates itself. The result: a painful case of shingles.

- **Estimated Number of Annual Cases:** 600,000 in the U.S.

- **Symptoms:** Malaise and feeling under the weather as well as burning, tingling sensations on the skin before rash appears. Rash appears blistery, similar to chicken pox, but is much more limited, and tends to occur in a ring or line. Sores are very painful, extremely sensitive to heat and cold. Even a slight breeze can make them hurt. Symptoms last up to a month.

New Treatment Helps Ease Pain of Shingles

- **Treatment:** Antiviral medications, administered within the first 72 hours after the rash emerges, help reduce the risk of complications. Over-the-counter medications and prescription painkillers can help control discomfort.

- **Complications:** Debilitating pain called post-herpetic neuralgia. This pain on the site of the shingles lesions can last for years. Treatment includes low doses of antidepressants and sometimes anticonvulsives.

- **Prevention:** None except avoiding ever contracting chicken pox. Studies are underway to test whether a chicken pox vaccine can help prevent the development of shingles in older patients.

Resources

VZV Research Foundation, Inc., 40 E. 72nd Street, New York, N.Y., 800-472-VIRUS.

For information on pain studies underway at the National Institutes of Health Pain Research Clinic, run by the National Institute of Dental Research 301-496-5483. ext 434.

—by Sally Squires, Washington Post Staff Writer

Chapter 40

Group A Streptococcal Infections

Organism: Streptococcus Pyogenes

Group A beta-hemolytic streptococcus is responsible for most cases of streptococcal illness. Other serogroups (B, C, D, and G) may also cause infection. Group B streptococci cause the majority of streptococcal infections in newborns and maternal post-labor/delivery infections.

Syndromes

- streptococcal pharyngitis or "strep throat" (scarlet fever and rheumatic fever are uncommon complications, most often preceded by sore throat)

- rheumatic heart disease

- skin infections (erysipelas/cellulitis, impetigo)

- bacteremia/sepsis, toxic shock-like syndrome

- pneumonia

- myositis, necrotizing fasciitis (gangrene)

National Institute of Allergy and Infectious Diseases, April 1995, and *FDA Consumer*, April 1991.

Strep Throat

Signs & Symptoms: Red, sore throat with white patches on tonsils; swollen lymph glands in neck; fever, headache. Nausea, vomiting, and abdominal pain more common in children.

Transmission: Direct, close contact with patient or carrier via respiratory droplets. Casual contact rarely results in transmission. Contaminated food, especially milk and milk products can result in outbreaks. Untreated patients are most infectious for 2-3 weeks after onset of infection.

Incubation: 2-4 days. Patient is no longer infectious within 24-48 hrs, after treatment begins.

Diagnosis: Throat is swabbed for a rapid strep test (10-20 minutes) to detect antibodies, and a follow-up culture (24-48 hrs.) to confirm infection. A negative culture suggests a viral or minor bacterial infection, and antibiotic treatment should be withheld or discontinued.

Treatment: Antibiotic treatment may reduce symptoms, minimizes spread (transmission), and reduces likelihood of complications. Treatment consists of penicillin (oral=10 days; or single intramuscular injection of penicillin G). Erythromycin for penicillin-allergic patient. Second line antibiotics include amoxicillin, dicloxacillin, clindamycin, oral cephalosporins. Although symptoms subside within four days even without treatment, it is very important to complete the full course of antibiotics to prevent complications and the development of antibiotic-resistant strains of streptococcus.

Complications of Strep Throat

Scarlet Fever (scarlatina): An uncommon strep infection that may follow untreated strep throat. Scarlet fever may develop within two days of sore throat, producing fever and a fine red, rough-textured rash over the upper body and in skin folds. It may also follow impetigo or minor skin infection or trauma. Rash blanches upon pressure. Scarlet fever also produces a bright red tongue with "strawberry" appearance. With antibiotics, recovery is complete within two weeks. Skin often "desquamates" or peels after recovery, usually on tips of fingers and toes. A severe form of scarlet fever can cause serious illness, including high fever, convulsions and death.

Group A Streptococcal Infections

Rheumatic Fever: While outbreaks are rare, isolated cases occur in susceptible persons due to particular strains of Group A strep. It is most common among children between 5-15 years of age. A family history predisposes to rheumatic fever. An acute attack lasts approximately three months. Symptoms often occur 18 days after untreated strep throat, including high fever and joint pain.

Rheumatic Heart Disease (carditis): The most serious complication is carditis, or heart inflammation (rheumatic heart disease), as this may lead to chronic heart disease, and disability or death years after an attack. Other symptoms include nosebleeds, bumps or nodules under the skin (usually over spine or other bony areas), and a red expanding rash on trunk and extremities that recurs over weeks to months. Because of the different ways rheumatic fever presents itself, the disease may be difficult to diagnose.

Chorea: Chorea, a neurological disorder, can occur months after an initial attack, causing jerky, involuntary movements, muscle weakness, slurred speech, and personality changes. Rheumatic fever is treated with antibiotics, anti-inflammatories, and sedatives, depending on the severity of symptoms.

Prevention: Both scarlet fever and rheumatic fever can be prevented by prompt recognition and treatment of strep throat. However, some cases follow a mild or inapparent sore throat.

Superficial Skin Infections

IMPETIGO: A superficial skin infection most common among young children, age 2-6 years. Skin infections are usually caused by different strains than those that cause strep throat.

Signs & Symptoms: One or more pimple-like lesions, surrounded by reddened skin. Lesions fill with pus, then break down over 4-6 days and form a thick crust. Exposed areas are more susceptible, e.g., face, legs, arms. Itching is common. Scratching may spread the lesions.

Transmission: Direct contact with lesions or with nasal carriers. Incubation: 1-3 days. Dried streptococci in the air are not infectious to intact skin.

Diagnosis: Because both staphylococci and streptococci can cause impetigo, lesions are cultured to distinguish between the two organisms.

Treatment: Same as for strep throat—penicillin. Untreated impetigo may progress to glomerulonephritis (kidney inflammation), after several weeks.

CELLULITIS/ERYSIPELAS: Inflammation of skin and underlying tissues.

Signs & Symptoms: Skin is painful, red, and tender. Patients experience fever, chills. Lymph glands may be swollen. Skin may blister and then scab over. Perianal cellulitis may also occur with itching and painful bowel movements. The erysipelas rash may occur on face, arms, or legs and has raised borders. Infection may recur, causing chronic swelling of extremities (lymphadenitis).

Transmission: Cellulitis begins with minor trauma, usually to an extremity.

Diagnosis: The organism is difficult to culture from skin lesions, but may be recovered from blood. Immunofluorescence detects antibodies in blood serum.

Treatment: Infection may resolve spontaneously. Cold compresses and aspirin provide relief. With oral penicillin, infection usually resolves in two weeks. At onset of antibiotic treatment, symptoms may worsen briefly due to abrupt death of many organisms.

Severe Streptococcal Infections

Some strains of Group A streptococci (GAS) cause severe infection only in susceptible hosts. All severe GAS infections may lead to shock, multi-system organ failure, and death. Early recognition and treatment are critical. Diagnostic tests include blood and urinalysis, cultures of blood or fluid from wound site. Antibiotics of choice include penicillin, erythromycin, and clindamycin.

BACTEREMIA: An invasion of bacteria into the bloodstream. An uncommon complication of strep throat or streptococcal skin infection. Infection can spread, via the bloodstream, to other parts of body, producing abscesses, peritonitis (inflammation of abdominal cavity), endocarditis (inflammation of membrane covering the heart), or meningitis. Bacteremia may lead to sepsis, or shock, causing a systemic illness with high fever, blood coagulation (thickening) and eventually organ failure. Those at greatest risk include children with chickenpox;

Group A Streptococcal Infections

persons with suppressed immune systems; burn victims; elderly persons with cellulitis, diabetes, blood vessel disease, cancer; persons taking steroid treatments or chemotherapy. Intravenous drug users are at highest risk. Bacteremia may also occur in healthy young adults with no known risk factors.

TOXIC SHOCK-LIKE SYNDROME: A syndrome that begins with flu-like symptoms (fever, chills, muscle aches). Pain is common, usually in an extremity; sometimes in abdomen or chest. Condition progresses to confusion, coma. Blood pressure drops, kidneys malfunction, soft tissues may be infected and develop gangrene (necrotizing fasciitis or myositis). The source of streptococcus, when identified, is most often the site of a minor wound or bruise. The syndrome occurs most often in healthy adults between the ages of 20-50.

PNEUMONIA: Pneumonia resulting from GAS is uncommon, but may follow influenza (flu), measles, pertussis, or chickenpox. Begins with chills, fever, cough, progressing to labored breathing, chest pain and bloody sputum. Lungs rapidly accumulate fluid causing adult respiratory distress syndrome (ARDS). Bacteremia may occur. Infection may extend to the heart. Treatment consists of intravenous or intramuscular injections of penicillin G every 6-12 hours and fluid drainage from lung.

NECROTIZING FASCIITIS AND MYOSITIS: A serious, but rare, invasive strep infection of the skin and subcutaneous tissues. Myositis involves muscle tissue. Both conditions may exist at the same time. Most cases of necrotizing fasciitis are caused by organisms other than Group A streptococci.

The infection rarely starts with a sore throat. It more often begins at site of minor, or no apparent, trauma, or with pulmonary symptoms. Affected skin is very painful, red, hot and swollen. Skin may progress to violet discoloration and blister formation, with necrosis (death) of subcutaneous tissues. Fever and systemic toxicity, e.g., bacteremia, tachycardia (rapid heart rate). Impeded blood flow may lead to GAS gangrene. Most severe cases progress within hours and mortality is high. It is diagnosed by either blood cultures or aspiration of pus from tissue. Surgical exploration may be necessary. Early medical treatment is critical. Penicillin is the treatment of choice, along with aggressive surgical debridement (removal of infected tissue). Limb amputation may be necessary. Clindamycin combined with a beta-lactam drug may also be effective.

Erythromycin

For eyes:

- erythromycin (Ilotycin)

For skin:

- erythromycin (EryDerm, Erygel, Erymax, T-STAT)
- erythromycin and benzoyl peroxide (Benzamycin)

Oral:

- erythromycin base (E-Base, ERYC, Ery-Tab, PCE)
- erythromycin estolate (Ilosone)
- erythromycin ethylsuccinate (E.E.S., EryPed)
- erythromycin stearate (Erythrocin, Wyamycin S)
- erythromycin and sulfisoxazole (Pediazole)

Intravenous:

- erythromycin gluceptate (Ilotycin)
- erythromycin lactobionate (Erythrocin)

How you take a drug can affect how well it works and how safe it will be for you. Sometimes it can be almost as important as what you take. Timing, what you eat and when you eat, proper dose, and many other factors can mean the difference between feeling better, staying the same, or even feeling worse. This drug information page is intended to help you make your treatment work as effectively as possible. It is important to note, however, that this is only a guideline. You should talk to your doctor about how and when to take any prescribed drugs.

Erythromycin is an antibiotic used alone or in combination with other chemicals or drugs to treat various infections. Erythromycins also are used as part of a preoperative bowel preparation that suppresses the normal bacterial flora, thus reducing the chances of infection following bowel surgery.

Group A Streptococcal Infections

Conditions These Drugs Treat

Erythromycin was first isolated in 1952. Like other antibiotics, it is produced by a microorganism—in this case, Streptomyces erythraeus—and has the capacity to inhibit the growth of or to kill other microorganisms. It is effective against a number of common bacteria, including *Chlamydia trachomatis, Corynebacterium diphtheriae, Neisseria gonorrhoeae, Listeria monocytogenes, Streptococcus pneumoniae, Bordetella pertussis, Legionella pneumophilia,* and *Mycoplasma pneumoniae.*

It is used to treat conditions caused by those organisms, such as diphtheria, gonorrhea, Legionnaires' disease, pneumonia, sinusitis caused by *S. pneumoniae,* pertussis (whooping cough), rheumatic fever, and chlamydial infections of the eyes and genitourinary tract and, in infants, lungs. It also is used for penicillin-allergic patients who have syphilis.

The skin preparations are prescribed for acne.

Erythromycin will not cure or combat colds, flu, or other viral infections.

How to Take

Erythromycin may be applied to the eyes (eye ointment) or to the skin (topical gels, ointments, swabs or liquids), swallowed (liquid, tablet or capsule), or administered intravenously (fluid).

The doctor determines the dosage, including the dose and treatment period, depending on the type and severity of the infection.

The medication should be taken for the full time prescribed, even if symptoms are no longer present, to ensure that the infection does not recur. The exception might be if side effects occur, in which case the doctor should be consulted. For patients with "strep" infection, it is important that the medicine be taken for at least 10 days, or as prescribed by the doctor. Serious heart problems, such as rheumatic fever, could develop later if the infection isn't cleared up completely.

In general, the eye ointment is applied at least twice daily, the skin preparations twice daily (in the morning and at night), and erythromycin taken by mouth is taken daily at 6- or 12-hour intervals. Intravenous erythromycin is given continuously.

Most oral forms of erythromycin are absorbed best on an empty stomach and therefore should be taken at least one-half hour before or two hours after a meal. They may be taken with food, however, if they upset the stomach.

Of special note:

- Chewable tablets, such as Ilosone and EryPed chewable tablets, must be chewed or crushed before they are swallowed.

- Delayed-release capsules or tablets such as Ery-Tab and E-Base delayed-release tablets, should be swallowed whole; they should not be broken or crushed.

- Specially marked spoons or other measuring devices that come with liquid oral forms should be used to ensure accurate doses. Household teaspoons should not be used because they may not hold the right amount of liquid.

Missed Doses

Erythromycin taken by mouth works best if it circulates in the blood at a constant level. Therefore, it is important that doses not be missed and that they be taken at regular intervals.

If a dose is missed and just a short time has passed, it should be taken as soon as possible. However, if it is time for the next dose, a physician should be consulted before making up the dose.

Relief of Symptoms

Erythromycin usually clears infections within days. However, because it does not relieve symptoms immediately, the doctor may prescribe other medicines, such as aspirin or acetaminophen, to ease pain and fever until the erythromycin takes effect.

Side Effects and Risks

Erythromycin taken by mouth may cause mild stomach cramps, diarrhea, nausea and vomiting, and sore mouth or tongue. These problems are usually minor and may go away as the body adjusts to the medicine. If they persist, however, the doctor should be consulted.

Although relatively rare, other side effects that may occur are:

Group A Streptococcal Infections

- **with eye ointment:** eye irritation not present before therapy.

- **with skin preparations:** dry or scaly skin; itching, stinging, peeling, or redness of the skin.

- **with medications taken by mouth:** skin rash, hives, or itching; dark or amber urine; pale stools; severe stomach pain; unusual tiredness or weakness; or yellow eyes or skin (jaundice).

- **with intravenous administration:** pain, swelling or redness at the injection site.

The doctor should be consulted if any of these side effects occurs.

Precautions and Warnings

Because various adverse drug interactions between erythromycin and other medications can occur, patients should inform their doctors of all prescription and nonprescription drugs they are taking before starting this medicine.

Patients also should tell their doctors:

- if they have ever had an unusual reaction to erythromycin.

- if they are pregnant or could possibly become pregnant. Although erythromycin has not been shown to cause birth defects or other problems in humans, it does cross the placenta.

- if they are breast-feeding. Because erythromycin passes into breast milk, a nursing mother should consult her doctor before taking the drug.

- if they are on a low-sodium, low-sugar, or other special diet, or if they are allergic to any foods, sulfites, or other preservatives or dyes that also may be present in an erythromycin-based drug.

- if they have ever had liver disease or hearing loss. Although very rare, patients with kidney problems who take erythromycin may suffer hearing loss, which is reversible after the drug is stopped.

— by Paula Kurtzweil

Chapter 41

Warts

People once thought that handling toads caused warts and getting rid of them required any one of a number of solemn magical rites. Folklore aside, warts are now known to be common, generally harmless skin growths caused by a group of viruses known as human papillomaviruses. Warts can be spread by direct contact from one person to another. Warts can develop, disappear rapidly and may then appear again.

Warts occur most frequently in individuals as they reach puberty, with the incidence falling off sharply in the late teens. Common warts occur frequently in children below the age of six or in adults above the age of fifty.

Types of Warts

These small growths may develop either singly or, if the virus spreads, in groups. They can be classified by their appearance and location into four general categories:

Common warts. Common warts are round or irregular, rough and gray in color. They are found most often on the fingers, elbows, knees, face and scalp, but they may spread elsewhere from those sites.

Plantar warts. Plantar warts are warts that have been flattened by pressure and are surrounded by hardened skin. This type of wart

---

NIH Publication *Backgrounder*. June 1992.

is commonly found on the soles of the feet, which may be quite tender. **Mosaic warts** are patches of closely set plantar warts.

Flat warts. Flat warts are smooth, flat and yellow-brown in color. They usually occur on the faces of children or young adults.

Anogenital warts. Anogenital warts (*condylomata acuminata* or venereal warts) develop initially in the anal and genital regions, but may spread into the vagina or rectum. They often occur in groups and may accumulate into large patches that resemble a cauliflower. Anogenital warts are transmitted by sexual contact with an infected partner. (The National Institute of Allergy and Infectious Diseases Sexually Transmitted Diseases Fact Sheets contain more information on anogenital warts.)

Other warts. Other warts may grow in unusual shapes such as thread-like or stemmed. These types are found more frequently on the head and neck. **Filiform warts** are thread-like warts on the eyelids, face, neck or lips.

Treatment

There are many forms of treatment, most directed at destroying the wart, but none are entirely effective. In fact, since most warts are not malignant and even regress or disappear in time, treatment for one or two warts is usually considered unnecessary. Even when warts are removed, the virus may remain in the skin ready to form new warts at a later time. When therapy is indicated, doctors often prefer to treat all family members who have warts (other than genital warts) at the same time, since warts can be transmitted from one person to another. Anyone with a wart in the beard or scalp areas should consult a physician for treatment, as shaving and combing the hair may spread the wart or cause infection.

Unlike other warts, genital warts caused by certain types of human papillomaviruses are of concern because they are associated with an increased risk of cancer, especially cervical cancer in women. Anyone with genital warts should consult a doctor to determine if treatment is needed.

Cryotherapy. Cryotherapy is one of the most common treatments for warts. It involves "freezing" the wart by briefly applying dry ice or liquid nitrogen. After about a week, the wart can usually be lifted out.

Surgery. Surgery, such as electrocautery (burning), is sometimes performed under local anesthesia if warts are not numerous. Warts can also be removed by total excision, which usually involves cutting superficially along the sides of the wart and then scraping to dislodge the wart. Most surgical techniques are not recommended for plantar or genital warts. Laser surgery, however, is sometimes used for plantar or genital warts. But because it is expensive, doctors often hesitate to use this technique for initial treatment.

Chemotherapy. Chemotherapy can also be used. The wart is painted with a salicylic acid or cantharidin preparation. Occasionally, some people may develop a hypersensitivity to these chemicals. Podophyllum resin or podophyllotoxin is used for treating plantar as well as anogenital warts. 5-Fluorouracil cream is also used for anogenital warts. Podophyllum, podophyllotoxin and 5-fluorouracil should not be used, however, in pregnant women. Trichloracetic acid (TCA) may also be used.

Repeated applications of these chemicals over several weeks is often necessary. If warts continue to recur after using other treatments, interferon injected directly into the warts may be successful.

X-ray therapy. Treatment with x-rays is **not recommended** for warts of any type.

Over-the-counter treatments. Although there are many over-the-counter remedies available for removing warts, most of them contain some kind of acid and can be harmful if directions are not followed carefully. It is best to consult a physician for effective removal of warts because there are many different methods of treatment, and, with any method, several treatments may be required. The method the doctor chooses will depend on the type, number and location of the warts.

Chapter 42

Herpes Simplex Virus and Genital Herpes

Genital herpes is a contagious viral infection that affects an estimated 30 million Americans. Each year, as many as 500,000 new cases are believed to occur. The infection is caused by the herpes simplex virus (HSV). There are two types of HSV, and both can cause the symptoms of genital herpes. HSV type 1 most commonly causes sores on the lips (known as fever blisters or cold sores), but it can cause genital infections as well. HSV type 2 most often causes genital sores, but it can also infect the mouth.

HSV 1 and 2 can both produce sores in and around the vaginal area, on the penis, around the anal opening, and on the buttocks or thighs. Occasionally, sores also appear on other parts of the body where broken skin has come into contact with HSV. The virus remains in certain nerve cells of the body for life, causing periodic symptoms in some people. Most people who are infected with HSV never develop any symptoms.

Genital herpes infection is usually acquired by sexual contact with someone who has an outbreak of herpes sores in the genital area. People with oral herpes can transmit the infection to the genital area of a partner during oral-genital sex. Herpes infections can be transmitted by a person who is infected with HSV but has no noticeable symptoms. The virus is rarely spread by contact with objects such as a toilet seat or hot tub.

National Institute of Allergy and Infectious Diseases, August 1992, and *NIAID Update*, February 1995.

Symptoms

The symptoms of genital herpes vary widely from person to person. When symptoms of a first episode of genital herpes occur, they usually appear within 2 to 10 days of exposure to the virus and last an average of 2 to 3 weeks. The early symptoms can include an itching or burning sensation; pain in the legs, buttocks, or genital area; vaginal discharge; or a feeling of pressure in the abdominal region.

Within a few days, sores (also called lesions) appear at the site of infection. Lesions can also occur on the cervix in women or in the urinary passage in men. These small red bumps may develop into blisters or painful open sores. Over a period of days, the sores become crusted and then heal without scarring. Other symptoms that may accompany a primary episode of genital herpes can include fever, headache, muscle aches, painful or difficult urination, vaginal discharge, and swollen glands in the groin area.

Recurrences

In genital herpes, after invading the skin or mucous membranes, the virus travels to the sensory nerves at the end of the spinal cord. Even after the skin lesions have disappeared, the virus remains inside the nerve cells in an inactive state. In most people, the virus reactivates from time to time. When this happens, the virus begins to travel along the nerves to the skin, where it multiplies on the surface at or near the site of the original herpes sores, causing new sores to erupt. It can also reactivate without causing any visible sores. At these times, small amounts of the virus may be shed at, or near, sites of the original infection, in genital or oral secretions, or from inapparent lesions. This shedding is infrequent, however, and usually lasts only a day, but it is sufficient to infect a sex partner.

The symptoms of recurrent episodes are usually milder than those of the first episode and typically last about a week. A recurrent outbreak may be signaled by a tingling sensation or itching in the genital area or pain in the buttocks or down the leg. These are called prodromal symptoms, and, for some people, they can be the most painful and annoying part of a recurrent episode. Sometimes only the prodrome is present, and no visible sores develop. At other times, blisters appear that may be very small and barely noticeable or may break into open sores that crust over and then disappear.

Herpes Simplex Virus and Genital Herpes

The frequency and severity of the recurrent episodes vary greatly. While some people recognize only one or two recurrences in a lifetime, others may experience several outbreaks a year. The number and pattern of recurrences often change over time for an individual. Scientists do not know what causes the virus to reactivate. Although some people with herpes report that their recurrences are brought on by other illness, stress, or menstruation, recurrences often are not predictable. In some cases, exposure to sunlight is associated with recurrences.

Diagnosis

The sores of genital herpes in its active stage are usually visible to the naked eye. Several laboratory tests may be needed, however, to distinguish herpes sores from other infections. The most accurate method of diagnosis is by viral culture, in which a new sore is swabbed or scraped and the sample is added to a laboratory culture containing healthy cells. After one or two days, when examined under a microscope, the cells will begin to show changes that indicate growth of the herpes virus.

A newer, more rapid, but somewhat less accurate way of diagnosing herpes involves detection of viral protein components in lesion swabs.

These tests should be done when the sores first appear to ensure reliable results. Other laboratory tests are also available to physicians to confirm the presence of HSV in the blood and to determine whether HSV 1 or 2 is present.

A blood test cannot determine whether a person has an active genital herpes infection. A blood test can, however, detect antibodies to the virus, which indicate that the person has, at some time, been infected with HSV and produced antibodies to it. (Antibodies are proteins made by a person's immune system to light infections.) Unlike antibodies to some other viruses, however, antibodies to HSV do not totally protect an individual against another infection with a different strain or a different type of herpes virus, nor do they prevent a reactivation of the latent virus. Antibody tests are the best way to determine if a person is an HSV carrier. New blood tests have been developed that can distinguish whether a person has had prior type 1 or type 2 infection, or both. However, these tests are available mainly in research hospitals and are not used routinely in the doctor's office.

Treatment

During an active herpes episode, whether primary or recurrent, it is important to follow a few simple steps to speed healing and to avoid spreading the infection to other sites of the body or to other people:

- Keep the infected area clean and dry to prevent the development of secondary infections.

- Try to avoid touching the sores; wash hands after contact with the sores.

- Avoid sexual contact from the time symptoms are first recognized until the sores are completely healed, i.e., scab has fallen off and new skin has formed over the site of the lesion.

In 1982, the first antiviral drug for genital herpes, acyclovir, was approved by the Food and Drug Administration for use as a topical ointment in persons suffering from an initial episode of infection. Over the next few years, investigators at the National Institute of Allergy and Infectious Diseases (NIAID) and elsewhere subsequently proved that an oral form of acyclovir is a superior treatment capable of benefitting persons with first or recurrent episodes of genital herpes. The oral form of the drug markedly shortens the course of a first episode and limits the severity of recurrences if taken within 24 hours of onset of symptoms. People who have very frequent recurrent episodes of the disease can also take oral acyclovir daily for up to one year to suppress the virus' activity and prevent most recurrences. Acyclovir is not a cure for herpes—the virus remains in the body, but while taken regularly, the drug interferes with the virus' ability to reproduce itself.

Complications

Genital herpes infections do not cause permanent disability or long-term damage in healthy adults. However, in people who have suppressed immune systems, HSV episodes can be long-lasting and unusually severe. A pregnant woman who develops a first episode of genital herpes can pass the virus to her fetus and may be at higher risk for premature delivery. Newborns rarely become infected with herpes; however, half of those who do either die or suffer neurologic

Herpes Simplex Virus and Genital Herpes

damage. With early detection and therapy, many serious complications can be lessened.

The newborn's chances of infection depend on whether the mother is having a recurrent or a first outbreak. If the mother is having her first outbreak at the time of a vaginal birth, the baby's risk of infection is approximately one in three. If the outbreak is a recurrence, the baby's risk is very low. Because of the danger of infection to the baby, however, the physician will perform a cesarean section if herpes lesions are detected in or near the birth canal during labor. Some physicians also perform a viral culture at the time of delivery to detect shedding in women known to have had genital herpes outbreaks in the past. A baby born with herpes can develop encephalitis (inflammation of the brain), severe rashes, and eye problems. Acyclovir can greatly improve the outcome for babies with neonatal herpes, particularly if they receive immediate treatment.

HSV and AIDS

Genital herpes, like other genital ulcer diseases, increases the risk of acquiring HIV, the virus that causes AIDS, by providing an accessible point of entry for HIV. Persons with HIV can have severe herpes outbreaks, and this may help facilitate transmission of both herpes and HIV infections to other persons.

Prevention

People with early signs of a herpes outbreak or with visible sores should not have sexual intercourse until the sores have completely healed. Between outbreaks, use of condoms (rubbers) during sexual intercourse is the best way to prevent infecting a partner.

Counseling and help for those who have genital herpes is often available from local or state health departments. The American Social Health Association (ASHA) maintains the Herpes Resource Center (HRC). ASHA's Herpes hotline is (919) 361-8488, Monday through Friday, 9:00 a.m. to 7:00 p.m. Eastern time. For further information on HRC programs and their literature regarding herpes, send a self-addressed stamped envelope to: HRC, P.O. Box 13827, Research Triangle Park, North Carolina 27709.

Research

Scientists supported by NIAID are concentrating their efforts in several areas of investigation. One important goal is the development of a safe and effective vaccine for genital herpes. Results from early, small-scale testing of a promising new vaccine showed it to be safe and capable of stimulating an immune response in both infected and uninfected study participants. Current studies being conducted by researchers at NIAID and elsewhere are determining whether it will greatly reduce or eliminate genital herpes outbreaks in infected persons.

Other scientists have developed an experimental test that can be used to screen blood samples for evidence of herpes infection and can accurately distinguish type 1 from type 2 infections. Rapid diagnostic tests have been developed that can detect active virus in a pregnant woman at the time of delivery. These tests may be able to identify exposed infants who should be observed carefully or receive immediate care. Researchers are still studying the potential of acyclovir for treating HSV while continuing to search for other antiviral drugs that may be effective against the herpes simplex virus. Several new drugs are being tested now to determine whether they would be more effective than acyclovir.

For most people, genital herpes rarely progresses to serious consequences, except in newborns or in people with suppressed immune systems such as AIDS patients. Recurrences can, however, be distressing, inconvenient, and sometimes painful. Concern about transmitting the disease to others and disruption of sexual relations during active outbreaks of the sores can affect personal relationships. Although the fact that genital herpes can be a chronic condition may at first sound frightening, it is reassuring to know that with proper counseling, treatment, and preventive measures, the disease can be coped with and managed effectively.

Herpes Vaccine Tests

NIAID is currently conducting clinical trials of the first genetically engineered herpes vaccine to be tested in people. The research is being carried out under the leadership of Stephen E. Straus, M.D., chief of NIAID's Laboratory of Clinical Investigation.

This vaccine shows promise not only in preventing people from getting genital herpes, but also as a treatment that will greatly reduce or even eliminate herpes outbreaks in people who already have the disease.

The first phase of testing in people showed that the vaccine was safe and capable of stimulating a strong immune response in both infected and uninfected study participants. The 18-month treatment trial (described below), for people with frequent outbreaks, is now under way, and all of the volunteers have received the vaccine.

Enrollment for the prevention trial is also completed. This study is designed to determine the vaccine's ability to prevent infection in people who are at high risk.

The Need for a Vaccine

For the estimated 20 percent of the world's population already infected with the genital herpes virus, a therapeutic vaccine that reduces the number of outbreaks could have a very significant impact on their lives. Such a vaccine would not eliminate the virus from the body, but it might help the immune system keep the virus in check.

In the case of newborns, a vaccine could be a lifesaver. Each year, 1,600 U.S. babies are born infected with herpes. The infant contracts the infection at delivery as it passes through the infected mother's birth canal. At present, up to 50 percent of these infected babies either die or suffer neurologic damage. In the future, it is possible that a vaccine could either protect women at risk for infection or, if used as a treatment, prevent an outbreak at delivery time.

Acyclovir Treatment

In a study published in 1984, Dr. Straus and his colleagues showed that the number of outbreaks could be reduced by the antiviral drug acyclovir. It was a much-hailed breakthrough, but to prevent reactivations, the drug must be taken daily, perhaps for years. Acyclovir has proved to be very safe, but it is costly and does not resolve the problem of infection in newborns. As with many viral diseases, prevention with a vaccine is the ultimate solution.

Using the Virus's Genes to Make a Vaccine

With genetic engineering, researchers can now identify and separate out molecules in a virus that are essential to the formulation of a vaccine. This technology made it possible to obtain the HSV-2 genetic proteins that signal the immune system to make antibodies.

When the body is faced with a real viral invasion, these antibodies are already primed to go into action to protect us from the virus.

Cloning the Genes

At Chiron Corporation, a biotechnology company in Emeryville, California, scientists identified which proteins on the outer coat of the virus trigger the strongest signal to the immune system. HSV-2 glycoprotein D (gD2) and glycoprotein B (gB2) emerged as the best candidates. The researchers then used what they refer to as "recombinant" technology to molecularly clone the genes for these two proteins. To mass produce the proteins for a vaccine, the scientists used Chinese hamster ovarian cells as a growth medium.

Vaccine Studies in Animals

When tested in healthy guinea pigs, the gD2 and/or gB2 vaccines did induce an immune response strong enough to protect the animals from HSV-2 infection. Next, variations of the gD2 and gB2 formulas were developed and tested in guinea pigs that had already been infected with HSV-2. The refined formulations reduced the number of herpes outbreaks in the animals by as much as 43 percent.

Initial Trial

Testing the vaccine for safety and immune response in humans was the next step. In a collaborative effort between government and industry, Dr. Straus worked with Chiron to design a protocol for the vaccine's first clinical trial. It began in August of 1989 and was conducted at the NIH Clinical Center. Twenty-four volunteers were immunized with a vaccine formulation containing gD2 alone. Alum was used as the adjuvant (a component commonly used to augment the effects of vaccines). The study took two years and involved participants who were and were not infected with HSV-2. Each volunteer was given three injections, the first two administered one month apart, with a booster injection at month 12. The study also compared the effects of two different dosages.

The initial trial ended with very encouraging results. The formulation proved to be extremely well tolerated—even at the higher, more immunogenic dose. But more significantly, antibody levels in the volunteers approached those seen after natural infection.

Initial Studies of a Second-generation Preventive Vaccine

In the fall of 1992, 80 volunteers not infected with HSV-2 were given a more advanced vaccine formulation. It combines both the gD2 and the gB2 proteins with a new, even more potent adjuvant known as MF59. This new formulation, gD2/gB2/MF59, proved to be safe and even more immunogenic than the gD2/alum vaccine.

Therapeutic Trial

The first trial designed to test the effectiveness of herpes vaccine as a therapeutic agent began in 1991. The study involved 98 HSV-2-infected volunteers, who each received two injections. Half the group received the first-generation vaccine containing gD2 alone and the other half an alum placebo. The results showed that those who received the gD2 vaccine had about 30 percent fewer herpes outbreaks per month than had the placebo group.

Extended Therapeutic Trial

In early 1994, NIAID completed screening of 200 volunteers with recurrent genital herpes for a study of the gD2/gB2/MF59 vaccine as a treatment. The hope is that it will be more effective than the earlier gD2 vaccine. At the two study sites, NIH and the University of Washington, half of the patients received injections of the vaccine at entry and again two months later. The other half received placebo injections. Follow-up of the volunteers after the injections should provide the researchers with a relatively simple gauge of success: the number of outbreaks in the vaccinated group compared to outbreaks in the placebo group. One year after the initial vaccination, all of the volunteers—including the placebo group—will be offered a booster injection and followed for an additional six months.

Prevention Trial

NIAID and Researchers at other sites around the country are also participating in a Chiron-sponsored trial of gD2/gB2/MF59 as a preventive vaccine. The study population consists of 400 people who are not infected with HSV-2 but are at high risk for acquiring it, i.e., they are in a monogamous, long-term relationship with a sex partner who has genital herpes. At the same time, Chiron is conducting a similar study for people who have multiple partners and have had at least one sexually transmitted disease other than herpes.

Screening of the volunteers and their partners included a blood test (Western blot) to confirm their HSV-2 status. Half of the volunteers received the vaccine and half the placebo (MF59 alone). The protocol entails three injections to be given over six months, after which all volunteers will be carefully followed for one year. The participants will undergo routine blood tests to monitor for HSV-2 infection and will report any outbreaks.

The Future

The studies continue to show that the vaccine is well tolerated. If the current trials proceed as expected, the vaccine's effectiveness as a treatment and as a preventive will need to be verified in trials involving even larger numbers of people. Testing at this level could take three to four more years. If the vaccine trials continue to demonstrate effectiveness, the manufacturer could apply to the Food and Drug Administration for approval of the vaccine.

Applying for Participation in Future Studies

Now that the current trials are under way, NIAID is no longer seeking volunteers who have genital herpes or are partners of people with herpes. We do not maintain a waiting list for future trials because screening criteria for study populations change.

Once these studies are completed, and if analysis of the results shows that further trials are warranted, protocols will be designed for larger follow-up studies. It is impossible to predict how quickly any new trials might begin. To recruit volunteers, NIAID will notify the Herpes Hotline (919-361-8488) and place advertisements in the health sections of local newspapers. Call 301-496-1836 for taped updates on recruitment. People with herpes are encouraged to join herpes support groups, which are also likely to be sources of information about ongoing research.

Chapter 43

Human Papillomavirus and Genital Warts

It may not grab as many headlines as AIDS and herpes, but genital warts, another sexually transmitted disease, is also a current concern. Half a million new cases of genital warts are diagnosed in the United States each year. Visits to physicians for treatment of genital warts have increased tenfold since 1986, perhaps because of increased awareness of sexual health issues.

Technically known as *condyloma acuminata*, genital warts are small growths, resembling cauliflower, that occur on or near the genitals. Like other warts, the genital variety is caused by a virus, called human papilloma virus (HPV). This virus comes in 60 forms, two of which account for nearly all cases of genital warts.

The wart itself is actually "the tip of an iceberg," says Katherine Stone, M.D., medical epidemiologist with the division of sexually transmitted diseases at the national Centers for Disease Control and Prevention in Atlanta. This is because the virus lurks in cells of the normal-appearing skin around the visible wart, and also possibly in other urogenital areas. The viral nature of the condition also has important implications for transmission and treatment.

Sexual Transmission

Because active virus is on the genitals, sexual contact can spread the infection. Studies show that 60 to 90 percent of people whose partners have visible warts also have warts within three months.

FDA Consumer, May 1995.

However, many people may harbor this virus and not know it. The virus may infect cells but not cause warts for many years, erupting into visible lesions when the immune system is suppressed. Several studies of women receiving routine Pap smears, which can reveal HPV infection, show that many women without a recent history of exposure harbor the virus, suggesting that it may have been acquired earlier.

The viral nature of genital warts suggests that anti-viral therapies may be effective. Standard treatments burn, scrape, freeze, or use a laser to remove affected tissue. A newer treatment, alpha interferon, attacks the virus, the underlying source. In 1988, the Food and Drug Administration licensed alpha interferon to treat genital warts in patients who have not been helped by other therapies.

"Interferon is an anti-viral agent, and warts are caused by viruses. It also has other effects—it is an anti-proliferative, blocking cell division, and has immunomodulatory effects. It is an effective therapy," says David Finbloom, M.D., chief of the Laboratory of Cytokine Research at FDA. In development are several biologic agents that attack the virus' genetic material. Although these new approaches make scientific sense, whether or not they offer better relief than traditional treatments remains an important question.

A genital wart may appear externally on the genitalia, in the anal area, internally in the upper vagina or cervix, and in the male urethra. The lesion is typically raised and pinkish. This condition may produce no symptoms at all, or cause itching, burning, tenderness, pain during intercourse, or frequent urination.

But because of a wart's location and sexual mode of transmission, it may cause emotional and social problems. "Genital warts can inflict extreme psychological turmoil, and patients often feel embarrassed, angry, and even guilty," says Robert Brodell, M.D., head of the dermatology section, Northeastern Ohio Universities College of Medicine in Warren, Ohio. He has a large private practice and uses many techniques to treat genital warts. Although the warts themselves may not hurt, treatment does, and the high frequency of recurrence, even with treatment, can be very frustrating, he adds.

Concern about genital warts has increased because of an association between HPV and genital cancers. But cancer risk is not elevated for people with visible genital warts, says CDC's Stone. Of the 60 known types of HPV, five are seen in nearly all surface cancers of the cervix, vagina, vulva, anus, penis, and perianal area—but these are not the forms of the virus that cause visible warts. Cancer is linked to types 16, 18, and 31; genital warts to types 6 and 11.

Risk Factors

Anyone who has ever had sex is at risk for harboring HPV. The virus seems to cause visible lesions when a person's immune system is suppressed, but may flare up even without an obvious trigger. This may occur because of illness (particularly other sexually transmitted diseases), or from taking certain drugs, such as cancer chemotherapy or drugs to prevent rejection of an organ transplant. Deficiencies of folic acid and vitamin A also may trigger genital warts. Smoking raises risk twofold, partly because nicotine byproducts attack immune system cells in the cervix, says Stone.

Preventing spread of HPV is difficult, because many people have the virus without visible signs of it. "Condoms will not completely prevent transmission of genital warts. This is a virus that may exist outside the area protected by a condom—even if the warts are not visible," says Marcia Bowling, M.D., clinical assistant professor in the division of gynecologic oncology at the University of Cincinnati.

Diagnosis

Finding a cauliflower-like growth on the genitals is reason to see a dermatologist, urologist or gynecologist, who can tell if it is genital warts or a different kind of growth, such as a cancer or ulcer. A gynecologist may use a type of microscope called a colposcope to examine a woman's cervix to see if there are internal outbreaks.

When acetic acid (vinegar) is swabbed on the cervix, HPV lesions appear whitish. Colposcopy can be valuable in detecting flat lesions that are not visible to the unaided eye, but only two-thirds of white areas seen in a colposcope are due to HPV infection. Sampling cells with a biopsy and testing for HPV genetic material may be necessary to confirm a diagnosis.

Treatment

People with genital warts have a variety of treatments to choose from, but none is a perfect cure, and all have side effects. The treatments also vary widely in cost. In the March 1995 issue of *Clinical Infectious Diseases*, Stone writes that several treatment studies have demonstrated that warts treated with placebo preparations completely regressed within three months in 10 to 30 percent of patients, and that no studies have followed persons with warts longer than five months to assess spontaneous regression. The problem, of course, is that there is no way to know who the lucky patients will be.

Genital wart treatments fall into three categories—prescription topical preparations that destroy wart tissue; surgical methods that remove wart tissue; and biological-based approaches that target the virus causing the underlying condition. (Each treatment must be applied to individual warts—none is taken systemically.)

FDA has approved Condylox (podofilox) as a topical treatment for genital warts. Some doctors also prescribe Podocon-25 and Podofin (podophyllin), which are approved for other uses.

Podocon-25 and Podofin are made from resin of the mandrake plant, or May apple. A physician applies the drug to warts, where it causes the skin to ulcerate. Typically the drug is left in place for only 30 to 40 minutes the first time to see how the patient reacts. In subsequent treatments, podophyllin is left on for up to four hours but no longer, or surrounding skin may ulcerate. Side effects include pain, redness, itching, burning, and swelling of the treated area.

Warts that are extensive, scaly in appearance, or have been present for a long time are not likely to respond well to podophyllin. Patients who are pregnant, have diabetes, or are taking steroid drugs or have poor circulation are not good candidates for this treatment.

Condylox also is a plant extract, derived from mandrake or juniper plants. The patient can use it at home, after a doctor demonstrates how to apply it with a cotton-tipped stick. The patient applies the drug every 12 hours for three consecutive days, does not use it for four days, then repeats the three-day regimen, for a total of not more than four cycles. If it hasn't worked by then, another treatment should be tried.

Most Condylox users experience a burning sensation, pain, inflammation, itching, or erosion of the affected area. Although Condylox has not been shown to harm fetuses, it is not advised for pregnant women because similar drugs are harmful.

Physicians sometimes use other topical treatments, such as trichloroacetic acid. This is a very caustic chemical that has not been tested very extensively on genital warts. Some physicians also use bichloroacetic acid or 5-fluorouracil, but FDA has not approved any of these for treating genital warts.

Human Papillomavirus and Genital Warts

Removal and Recurrence

Visible genital warts can be physically removed using cold, heat, or excision by a scalpel or a laser. All of these techniques are uncomfortable, and the warts tend to recur because HPV is still present in surrounding cells.

Carbon dioxide laser vaporization and conventional surgical excision are best reserved for extensive warts, especially for patients who haven't responded to other treatments, according to CDC's 1993 *Sexually Transmitted Disease Treatment Guidelines*. These guidelines are not requirements, according to CDC medical epidemiologist Stuart Berman, M.D.

Stephen K. Tyring, M.D., Ph.D, associate professor at the University of Texas Medical Branch, and colleagues, including Brodell, writing in the June 1993 issue of *The Female Patient*, say that laser vaporization may require general anesthesia, is painful, and may require months to heal, sometimes leaving a whitish, scarred area. Surgical excision requires local anesthesia, and may produce scarring and lead to infection.

Cryotherapy is performed on less extensive lesions. This method uses liquid nitrogen or a device called a cryoprobe to freeze wart tissue, which then crumbles away. It is inexpensive, does not require an anesthetic, and is less likely to leave a scar than excision using a scalpel. However, most patients experience pain during and after the procedure. Cryotherapy with liquid nitrogen is especially well suited for warts in hard-to-reach places, such as in the vagina, anus, or the area where the urethra contacts the outside of the body.

With electrocautery, a metal loop heated by an electric current is used to burn off the lesion. Like the other surgical techniques, electrocautery requires a very skilled physician to avoid damaging surrounding or underlying tissue. CDC advises against using electrocautery to treat warts on the external genitalia or anal area.

Interferon

Interferon is a natural immune system biochemical. In treating genital warts, unlike other approaches, interferon attacks the responsible virus. One brand of alpha interferon used to treat genital warts, Alferon N, is obtained from white blood cells. The interferon is acid-treated and carefully screened for contaminants and viruses, says FDA's Finbloom. Another brand of alpha interferon licensed to treat genital warts, Intron A, is manufactured through genetic engineering.

Interferon was discovered in 1957, and its varied effects on immunity led scientists to hail it as a potential miracle cure for many conditions. However, it was difficult to obtain in sufficient amounts to test. With the advent of recombinant DNA technology in the 1970s, abundant, pure supplies of interferon became available to researchers. Not quite the magic elixir some expected, alpha interferon nevertheless is used today in the United States to treat hepatitis B and C, hairy cell leukemia, AIDS-associated Kaposi's sarcoma, and genital warts. Another form of interferon, Betaseron (or beta interferon), is approved to treat multiple sclerosis.

Treatment with interferon involves the doctor injecting the substance with a very small needle directly into each wart. Alferon N is injected twice a week, and Intron A three times a week. Treatment usually lasts eight weeks, with the lesions beginning to shrink by the fourth week. In one study, interferon was given along with podophyllin. The combination increased efficacy, but also raised recurrence rate.

About 30 percent of patients develop mild flu-like symptoms about two to four hours following treatment. For this reason, many doctors using interferon treat patients in the late afternoon, so that the patients feel well enough to go to work by the next morning. This side effect mimics the natural role of interferon in the body. The fever, aches and pains of a viral infection are actually caused by interferon and other immune system biochemicals readying the immune system to attack infecting virus, not by the bug itself.

Interferon therapy is expensive, usually costing from $1,100 to $1,200 for the entire treatment, counting office visits. CDC's 1993 treatment guidelines state, "Interferon therapy is not recommended because of its cost and its association with a high frequency of adverse side effects, and efficacy is no greater than that of other available therapies." Stone explains that the guidelines were based on analysis of published reports up until August 1992 of interferon's efficacy. "The bottom line was that the clearance rate [efficacy] and recurrence are not better than what you see with less invasive, less expensive therapies," she says.

Stone and others at CDC were particularly concerned about a woman who called them saying she had gone to a clinic in Atlanta and been asked to pay $2,000 up front for interferon treatment of a single wart. This was the first treatment the woman was offered.

Human Papillomavirus and Genital Warts

Yet Brodell reports that he has "patients whom I can't make better using traditional approaches, and I see 70 percent of them get better using interferon."

"My patients typically have had two laser treatments, cryotherapy twice, and at home treatment with Condylox. I freeze the warts, use bichloroacetic acid, say magic words and bury a potato in the backyard, but it doesn't help," he says. Brodell finds the recurrence rate of genital warts using interferon to be about 25 percent.

Treatments Under Investigation

Elsewhere, other biological approaches are attempting to treat the underlying cause of genital warts. ISIS Pharmaceuticals in Carlsbad, Calif., is conducting clinical trials of a biologic called afovirsen that blocks HPV from using one of its key genes, disarming it from infecting human cells. Like interferon, afovirsen is injected into individual warts.

Researchers at Gilead Sciences in Foster City, Calif., are testing a topical drug called GS504 that blocks the virus from duplicating its genetic material. They are trying to see if this experimental drug, by entering nearby cells that are not yet infected, can prevent the virus from taking hold, according to company spokeswoman Lana Lauher. GS504 is currently being tested in people who are HIV positive or who have AIDS. Genital warts are especially severe in such people because their immune systems are suppressed. Therefore, if a treatment helps them, chances are good that it will also work on less severe cases.

Although genital warts are not life-threatening, they can cause great mental anguish. "Fortunately, a patient has many treatment options," says FDA's Finbloom.

—by Ricki Lewis, Ph.D.

Ricki Lewis is a geneticist and textbook author.

Part Six

Skin Traumas and Treatments

Chapter 44

Anatomy of a Scar

You hurt yourself and then you heal, leaving a scar as a reminder of your injury and your recovery. The most familiar kind of scar forms on the skin, and is made of connective tissue known as collagen. There also can be scar formation beneath the skin's surface. And when internal organs are traumatized, as in surgery, scar tissue forms there as well.

Formation of an External Scar

Injury leads to production of a blood clot, which holds the edges of the wound together. A dry crust, called a scab, forms over the top of the wounded area. As healing begins, reddish "granulation tissue" moves into the wound, replacing the clot and also producing collagen which then replaces the granulation tissue. Reddish color begins to fade. When the edges of the wound are held together during healing, the resulting scar may be barely visible; wider scars develop where edges of skin are further apart during healing.

Complications

- **Proud flesh:** Granulation tissue can push up through the surface of the wound.

©July 9, 1991 Gerri Kobren, *The Baltimore Sun*. Reprinted courtesy of *The Baltimore Sun* and ©May 22, 1991 *New York Times*. Reprinted with permission.

- **Keloids:** Excess collagen protrudes above the surface of the wound.

- **Contracture:** Scar tissue can shorten over time, causing disfigurement or limiting movement.

- **Stricture:** Internal scar tissue can tighten around body passages, impeding or preventing normal function.

- **Adhesions:** Internal scar tissue can form abnormal bonds between different structures, impeding or preventing normal functions.

Research by Gerri Kobren of The Baltimore Sun

When Healing Backfires

When the skin has been injured, cells adjacent to the injury produce collagen, a fibrous connective tissue. Sometimes far more new tissue grows than is needed to heal a wound. Tumor-like growths of excess tissue are called keloids. A more common condition, raised tissue within the confines of the original wound, is called a hypertrophic scar. The more collagen fibers that form, the larger and stiffer the scar. When the scar forms under a scab, the scar can be indented.

New Methods to Counter Serious Scarring.

Even under the best of circumstances injuries and operations are not readily forgotten. When they leave behind a scar that is disfiguring or that limits mobility the legacy can be emotionally scarring as well. In recent years, plastic surgeons and dermatologists have devised promising preventives and treatments for these ugly and uncomfortable scars. In some cases, the remedy can be successfully applied even to scars that are years old, but most work best when a scar is just forming, so patients should tell their doctors about past scarring problems.

Anatomy of a Scar

The Scarring Problem

Living tissues of all kinds form scars, which represent new cells laid down to close a gap in the skin, whether from a kitchen knife or surgeon's scalpel, a burn or blister, a scrape or a chemical. Whether the wound is superficial or deep, the process is basically the same.

After an injury whether accidental or deliberate, the body musters an inflammatory response bringing white blood cells and antibodies to the area to help destroy or expel intruders like infectious organisms and dead cells.

As the inflammation subsides, scar tissue begins to form. It includes tiny new blood vessels called capillaries to restore circulation. Then cells in the adjacent skin called fibroblasts start producing a fibrous connective tissue, collagen, similar to the tissue inside the end of the nose. Linkages form between the fibers increasing the strength of the scar: the more fibers, the firmer and less flexible the scar.

For unknown reasons, in some people scar tissue grows far beyond the amount needed to heal a wound, forming a benign tumor-like growth called a keloid that is uncomfortable and unsightly. For a person who forms keloids, ear piercing can cause a scar the size of a golf ball. The tendency to form keloids is especially common among Blacks and Asians, strongly suggesting a genetic factor. People who form keloids are usually advised to avoid cosmetic surgery.

In another more common type of abnormal scarring called hypertrophic scars the scar tissue overgrows but stays within the confines of the original wound. The raised portion may subside with time but many of these scars remain an ugly problem, causing pain, itchiness or irritation and sometimes interfering with body movements.

Far more troublesome are the big, angry-looking hypertrophic scars that can develop when extensive burns heal. These scars can impede movement, especially around a joint. According to Dr. William W. Monafo, a professor of surgery at Washington University School of Medicine in St. Louis, hypertrophic scars are neither predictable nor preventable. They most often form in children, adults under 40, and dark-skinned people after deep wounds or incisions as well as burns.

Even people who do not scar abnormally often develop cosmetically undesirable scars after a deeply scraped knee or elbow. If the scrape bleeds, a scab will soon form to cover the wound. But when the scab falls off, the scar beneath it typically forms a depression and may remain indented indefinitely.

Getting Help

Let's start with the easy ones first. The trick to avoiding indented scars is to prevent scabbing. This can be done by covering the cleaned wound with a non-stick or other semi-permeable bandage that keeps the wound warm and moist but allows air to penetrate.

Ordinary surgical scars can some times be removed by a popular technique called dermabrasion often used to minimize acne scars. Dr. Bruce E. Katz and colleagues in the department of dermatology at Columbia University College of Physicians and Surgeons in New York recently reported good results from scarabrasion, as they call it. In a study of 48 patients, half the scars treated at eight weeks after injury disappeared.

Scar abrasion, which can be an outpatient procedure, involves numbing the area with an anesthetic spray, abrading the scar, applying an antibiotic ointment and keeping it covered with gauze for about one week.

Hypertrophic scars are more challenging. Surgical remedies often leave a worse scar, although there has been some success with skin grafts, which have more stretch than the scar tissue.

More recently Dr. Thomas A. Mustoe, a plastic surgeon at Washington University School of Medicine, in studies with Dr. Monafo and their colleagues, tested a treatment for hypertrophic scars that is moderately to greatly effective in two-thirds of patients. The treatment works best with scars that are a few months old, but even when the scars are a year to four years old, the St. Louis team has reported beneficial results in many patients. The treatment involves placing a sheet of silicone gel over the scarred area for 12 or more hours a day for several months. The area can be hidden by clothing; the gel is best left in place all day, except for brief daily cleaning.

In patients who are helped, the raised scars become flatter, lighter in color and more flexible. Studies thus far indicate that the improvements last at least six months. A few patients successfully treated several years ago have thus far retained the improvements, Dr. Mustoe said. He added that "you can tell within a month if the treatment is working," thus sparing patients who would not be helped the months of treatment.

Since the initial reports from the St. Louis team, there have been four other reports of success with the therapy from surgeons in other countries, and many physicians in burn centers in the United States have adopted the approach, Dr. Mustoe said. A self-adhering gel for large areas is now under development.

The most difficult scars to treat are keloids. While there has been a host of efforts, including the use of lasers to remove keloids, recurrences are extremely common.

Patients who know they form keloid scars and are anticipating surgery should tell the surgeon in advance. Treatment with antibiotics and corticosteroids either applied to the surface or injected into the scar as it forms can often inhibit keloid formation, reduce pain and even cause the keloid to shrink, said Dr. Ted Rosen, a dermatologist at Baylor College of Medicine in Houston. Some patients are helped by repeated freezing of the scar with liquid nitrogen, followed by corticosteroid injections.

When all else fails and a keloid is disfiguring or debilitating, surgical removal may be attempted, followed by periodic corticosteroid injections as the wound heals.

Chapter 45

Help for Cuts, Scrapes, and Burns

A half-inch scar on my left knee is a graphic reminder of a painful scrape at age 7. Also painful was the burn of Merthiolate antiseptic, applied as first aid to ward off infection.

Today's approved over-the-counter (OTC) topical (used on the skin) first-aid antimicrobials are less irritating and more effective than Merthiolate, which contains the mercury drug thimerosal. The Food and Drug Administration has approved seven topical OTC antibiotics (see "OTC Antibiotics below") and is evaluating OTC topical antiseptics under a proposed rule. The proposal would ban numerous antiseptics, including mercurials, as ineffective and some, including thimerosal, as also unsafe.

Antibiotics are also available by prescription as injectable and oral medicines and medicines for the eye and ear. They are used to treat infections. While some can kill a limited number of bacteria, other varieties affect many bacteria.

Antiseptics weaken microbes, but don't usually kill them. Health-care antiseptics in soaps and other products help prevent the spread of infection in medical facilities.

OTC first-aid antibiotics and antiseptics are applied to the skin to help prevent infection in minor cuts, scrapes and burns.

"Used topically, OTC antimicrobials inhibit the growth of bacteria, but don't necessarily kill them all," says Audrey Love, a microbiologist with the division of OTC drug evaluation in FDA's Center for Drug Evaluation and Research. "If an injury is extensive," Love says,

FDA Consumer, May 1996.

"it should be taken care of by a doctor. But consumers have to consider for themselves, based on reading the labeling, whether a product is something they should use."

FDA has published rules (monographs) establishing adequate labeling for OTC antimicrobials, and conditions under which products would be generally recognized as safe and effective for use without medical supervision. The final antibiotics rule (1987) and proposed antiseptics rule (1991) specify active ingredients and concentrations, as well as labeling information such as product identification, indications for use, warnings, and directions for use. All drugs must meet the agency's good manufacturing practice requirements for product identity, strength, quality, and purity.

Some Restrictions

OTC first-aid antimicrobials are for use only up to one week. If an injury persists or worsens after this time, the label warns consumers to stop use and consult a doctor.

The products are not for existing infections, animal bites, sunburn, punctures, or eye injuries. Nor should they be used for cuts, scrapes or burns needing medical care, such as:

- cuts that are deep, continue bleeding, or may require stitches
- scrapes with imbedded particles that can't be flushed away
- large wounds
- burns more serious than a small reddened area.

Use of an antibiotic or antiseptic does not in itself constitute first-aid treatment of a minor wound.

A panel of experts convened by FDA defined first aid as "a process that includes initial adequate cleansing which may or may not be followed by application of a safe, nonirritating product which does not interfere with normal wound healing and which may reduce the bacterial numbers and help prevent infection." (From 1972 to 1981, at FDA's request, 16 outside panels evaluated marketed OTC drugs. Their charge completed, the panels no longer meet.)

FDA requires that labels for antibiotics advise users to first "clean the affected area." Antiseptics also would be labeled with the advice.

Because topical antimicrobials are not totally effective in killing bacteria, FDA does not allow firms to place the claim "Helps kill bacteria" in the same area as the required information. FDA believes the

Help for Cuts, Scrapes, and Burns

term "kill" implies the product will eliminate all bacteria and could be misleading if appearing with the required term "infection" (or alternate term "bacterial contamination") in the label's indications section. The claim may be used, though, as additional information elsewhere in the label.

More about Antibiotics

In its final rule, FDA listed these antibiotic active ingredients as safe and effective: bacitracin, bacitracin zinc, chlortetracycline hydrochloride, tetracycline hydrochloride, neomycin sulfate, oxytetracycline hydrochloride, and polymyxin B sulfate—the latter two only for combination products because of their limited effectiveness against certain microorganisms when used alone.

The rule does not allow the previously marketed antibiotic gramicidin, because it has the potential to break down red blood cells when absorbed through fresh wounds. The agency called for a well-designed, double-blind study (where neither patient nor doctor knows who gets the drug) to show gramicidin's effects.

The data on which FDA based its approval of the other antibiotics included a well-controlled study of minor skin injuries or insect bites in 59 children. Streptococcal infection developed in 15 of the 32 receiving a topical placebo and in three of the 27 receiving a topical antibiotic. Twelve of the 15 receiving placebos eventually needed oral antibiotics, and one of the three using antibiotics did as well.

The agency agreed with comments that many such injuries are self-healing, but that some do not heal without treatment and it is impossible to make this distinction at the time of injury.

Also, says FDA's Love, there's always a chance someone can be allergic to a drug—prescription or OTC. "People who tend to be allergic," she says, "should talk to their doctor or pharmacist before trying any OTC medicine for the first time."

About 1 in 20 people is allergic to neomycin, according to an article in the August 1995 *Harvard Health Letter*. If a reaction such as redness, itching or burning occurs, the article advises, "Stop using the preparation immediately, and consult a physician if symptoms worsen or persist for more than 48 hours."

Hypersensitivity reactions may also occur with bacitracin, according to the *Handbook of Nonprescription Drugs* (10th edition), published by the American Pharmaceutical Association and The National Professional Society of Pharmacists, Washington, D.C. The handbook also states that tetracycline products may trigger reactions in allergic patients, "some of whom may have severe reactions even if exposure is by topical application only."

With repeated use on large areas, neomycin also fosters development of neomycin-resistant strains of Staphylococci bacteria. Neomycin products that include polymyxin B and bacitracin guard against this.

To prevent neomycin overuse, FDA limits the drug to ointments and creams, the most likely dosage forms for small wounds. Also, all OTC antimicrobials must be labeled for short-term use. The agency believes short-term use of neomycin ointments or creams on small wounds would not risk overuse. To reduce the risk even further, FDA requires labels for ointments and creams to identify a dose as "an amount equal to the surface area of the tip of a finger."

Another issue is the combination of a product with a local "caine" anesthetic, such as benzocaine, as is allowed for bacitracin ointment or a combination ointment of bacitracin, neomycin, or polymyxin B. The review panel was concerned an anesthetic might mask symptoms of infection, delaying treatment by a doctor. But FDA believes the required warnings on the label adequately inform consumers when to consult a doctor. (See "Labeling Final Rule below.")

OTC Antibiotics

The following antibiotic products have been approved by FDA for use without a prescription. They are ointments unless otherwise noted:

Single-ingredient Products

- bacitracin—Baciguent
- bacitracin zinc—Bacitracin Zinc
- chlortetracycline hydrochloride—Aureomycin
- neomycin sulfate—Neomycin, Myciguent Cream
- tetracycline hydrochloride—Achromycin

Combination Products

- Bacitracin-neomycin—none currently marketed

- bacitracin-polymyxin B aerosol—none currently marketed

Help for Cuts, Scrapes, and Burns

- bacitracin-neomycin-polymyxin B—Lanabiotic, Medi-Quik Triple Antibiotic, Clomycin Cream (with lidocaine anesthetic), Mycitracin Plus Pain Reliever (with lidocaine)

- bacitracin zinc-neomycin—none currently marketed

- bacitracin zinc-polymyxin B ointment, aerosol or powder—Polysporin, Polysporin Powder

- bacitracin zinc-neomycin-polymyxin B—Neomixin, Neosporin Original

- neomycin-polymyxin B ointment or cream—Neosporin Plus Maximum Strength Cream (with lidocaine)

- oxytetracycline-polymyxin B ointment or powder—none currently marketed.

More about Antiseptics

In its proposed rule, FDA listed these active antiseptic ingredients as tentatively safe and effective: ethyl alcohol (48 to 95 percent), isopropyl alcohol, benzalkonium chloride, benzethonium chloride, camphorated metacresol, camphorated phenol, phenol, hexylresorcinol, hydrogen peroxide solution, iodine tincture, iodine topical solution, povidone-iodine, and methylbenzethonium. Five ingredients listed as tentatively effective only in combination products are ethyl alcohol (26.9 percent), eucalyptol, menthol, methyl salicylate, and thymol.

The proposal would ban numerous mercury ingredients and cloflucarban, fluorosalan and tribromsalan antiseptics as not generally recognized as safe and effective for OTC use.

FDA had requested study data on whether use of topical povidone-iodine affected thyroid function. In submitted data, iodine blood levels did increase after two weeks' use, but returned to normal when use was stopped. There was no effect on thyroid function.

Antiseptics would be labeled similarly to antibiotics, but with some differences.

Labels on camphorated metacresol, camphorated phenol, and phenol, for example, would warn, "Do not bandage."

"The drugs can be hard on the skin," says Debbie Lumpkins, a microbiologist in FDA's division of OTC drug evaluation. She explains that "when bandaged, the skin gets damp, increasing absorption. Therefore, more drug enters the skin and may cause more damage than if you just left the wound uncovered."

Labels for ethyl alcohol (48 to 95 percent) and isopropyl alcohol (50 to 91.3 percent) would warn: "Flammable, keep away from fire or flame."

For liquid antiseptics, labels would direct users to let the product dry before bandaging.

Comments on the proposal were minimal, Lumpkins says, emphasizing that FDA's evaluation of the ingredients is still very much an evolving process.

"Frequently," she says, "we find that one study or one article says one thing, and there's another study or article on the other side. We have to determine the facts. Literature searches that we can now do so easily help, but we won't find everything. We rely on people to bring things to our attention."

Recent publications advise against two currently marketed antiseptics. The National Safety Council's *1996 First Aid Pocket Guide* states: "DO NOT use hydrogen peroxide. It does not kill bacteria, and it adversely affects capillary blood flow and wound healing." And the *Handbook on Nonprescription Drugs* states ethyl alcohol "is not a desirable wound antiseptic because it irritates already damaged tissue. The coagulum [crust] formed may, in fact, protect the bacteria."

The final rule will reflect FDA's evaluation of all the data, Lumpkins says. Thus, antiseptic ingredients proposed as safe and effective could be found unsafe or ineffective, or new ingredients could be added, depending on new information.

Whether using an OTC antibiotic or antiseptic, consumers should realize "there are limits to what the products can do," Lumpkins says. "People should read the label, and use the product appropriately. If they notice a change in their condition, or if there's redness or swelling, they shouldn't continue to try to treat it. They should see a doctor."

Labelling Final Rule

Under the final rule, labels for topical antibiotics must:

- state the established name of the drug

- identify the drug as a "first-aid antibiotic"

Help for Cuts, Scrapes, and Burns

- state the drug's approved use—for example: "First aid to help protect against infection in minor cuts, scrapes, and burns." (Allowed alternative wording includes "help prevent skin infection" or "help reduce the risk of bacterial contamination." Other descriptive statements may be added, provided they are truthful and not misleading)

- warn:

  —*"For external use only. Do not use in the eyes or apply over large areas of the body. In case of deep or puncture wounds, animal bites, or serious burns, consult a doctor."*

  —*"Stop use and consult a doctor if the condition persists or gets worse. Do not use longer than one week unless directed by a doctor."*

- advise to clean the area, to use a small amount one to three times daily, and to cover with a sterile bandage if desired

- specify on ointments and creams to use *"an amount equal to the surface area of the tip of a finger."* Combination products must give the established name of each active ingredient. Labels must identify any added anesthetic as such, include the directions and warnings in its monograph, and state: *"First aid for the temporary relief of pain* [or other approved alternative] *in minor cuts, scrapes, and burns."*

—by Dixie Farley

Dixie Farley is a staff writer for FDA Consumer.

Chapter 46

Keloids and Hypertropic Scars: When Skin Repairs Run Amok

When a freshman at Fisk University in Nashville decided to have her ears pierced, she expected her father would be angry. What she did not expect were the unsightly lumps of continuously growing scar tissue that developed at the wound. In response to the piercing, her skin-repairing mechanism had gone into overdrive. She, like one in every thirty African Americans, carried a gene that derails skin healing, producing benign tumors known as keloids.

When skin is broken, a battalion of specialized cells springs into action, laying down collagen and elastin fibers that form new scar tissue to close the wound. In normal scars, rapid tissue formation stops once the wound is closed, and the slower process of strengthening and consolidating the new tissue takes over. But in carriers of the keloid gene, primarily blacks and Asians, the initial wound-closing does not stop. Scar tissue continues to form well after the original need has passed, piling up to produce thick, hard, unsightly keloids that often become infected and are almost impossible to get rid of.

Perhaps because keloid tumors are not cancerous, they have attracted relatively little attention from the scientific community. But at the NCRR-supported research center at Meharry Medical College in Nashville, Tennessee, investigators are trying to understand why keloids form and how they might be prevented. Their studies may also help shed light on the details of wound healing. "The initiation of wound healing has been fairly well studied, but the process by which

---

NCRR Reporter November/December 1994, and the Office of Scientific and Health Communications 7/94.

wound healing terminates has not been that well defined," Dr. Shirley Russell says.

Several matrix proteins—proteins that cells secrete into surrounding tissue—play an important structural role in wound healing. The various forms of collagen, which are the most abundant structural proteins, provide strength to new tissue. Elastin keeps it supple, and a host of other substances provide cushioning and regulate matrix protein production. Both elastin and collagen are made by a type of cell called a fibroblast. "Fibroblasts are recruited into the wound area by a variety of factors produced by immune cells," says Dr. Shirley Russell. "It is not quite clear where they come from." She explains that the new matrix may play a role in limiting its own formation by interacting with the fibroblasts. Keloid cells, which are abnormal fibroblasts, do not appear to be similarly regulated. "One of the questions we are asking is: Do keloid cells respond abnormally to matrix?"

To study how fibroblast proliferation is regulated, Dr. Shirley Russell and her colleagues Drs. James Russell and Joel S. Trupin grow fibroblasts in culture and monitor how various hormones and cell growth factors affect collagen and elastin production. The scientists recently found that the hormone hydrocortisone, which helps regulate skin repair, inhibits the synthesis of elastin in normal fibroblasts but has no effect on keloid cells. The researchers had earlier seen the same effect in studies on the synthesis of collagens.

"The finding that elastin does not respond to hydrocortisone is exciting because we now know that the deranged regulatory program at work in keloids affects at least four different matrix protein molecules: three collagens and elastin," says Dr. Trupin.

Recently, with support from NCRR's Research Centers in Minority Institutions (RCMI) Program, population geneticist Dr. Scott Williams joined the Meharry team to attack the problem from a different angle: tracking down the gene or genes responsible for keloids using linkage analysis. Also, in collaboration with Meharry epidemiologist Dr. Robert Levine, he is collecting information regarding familial incidences of keloids and other fibro-proliferative diseases—including uterine fibromas—from questionnaires used in a large hypertension study. Although no documented studies show that patients with keloids are prone to get other fibro-proliferative diseases, the high frequency of all of these diseases in populations of African descent makes the possibility worth examining. "It is speculation," says Dr. Shirley Russell, "but we began to wonder about similarities to keloid formation."

Keloids and Hypertropic Scars: When Skin Repairs Run Amok

"Keloids in general are tremendously understudied, and virtually nothing is known about the genetics of keloids," says Dr. Trupin. "Continued NCRR support via the RCMI Program has been a boon for this research."

A clue to the genetic and regulatory abnormalities in keloids came, rather unexpectedly, when Canadian scientists produced transgenic mice that overexpressed an oncogene—or cancer-causing gene—known as *v-jun*. Proteins encoded by *jun* and another gene called *fos* regulate the expression of many other genes. When these mice were marked for identification by notching their tails and ears, they developed growths that looked like keloids. This finding may implicate *Fos-Jun* proteins in abnormal collagen output.

Results of a California research team also suggest that *Fos-Jun* proteins could underlie abnormal collagen formation. Surprisingly, researchers found that glucocorticoids (a group of hormones that include hydrocortisone) could either increase or dampen collagen gene expression—depending on the ratio between *Fos* and *Jun* proteins in the experimental setup. These results might explain the Meharry finding that hydrocortisone inhibits collagen and elastin synthesis in normal fibroblasts and has no effect in keloid cells. In fact, Dr. Shirley Russell and her colleagues have found evidence of abnormal expression of *Fos-Jun* proteins in keloids, "but we don't know yet which member of the *Fos-Jun* family plays a role," she says.

Dr. Williams is now searching for a "keloid" regulatory genetic defect. At the same time, Meharry cell biologists are tracking down the activity and amounts of the *Fos-Jun* proteins in keloid cells. They hope that this double-barreled attack may reveal what happens when the healing process runs amok.

Dr. Shirley Russell says that African Americans should be made more aware of the risk of keloids from ear piercing, cosmetic surgery, and other seemingly harmless choices. "This is a potential problem for a large number of individuals."

— by Elisabeth J. Sherman, Ph.D.

This research was supported by the Research Centers in Minority Institutions Program of the National Center for Research Resources; the National Institute of General Medical Sciences, the National Cancer Institute; the National Heart Lung, and Blood Institute; the National Institute on Aging, the National Science Foundation; and the Department of Veterans Affairs.

Additional Reading

Russell, S. B., Trupin, J. S., Kennedy, R. Z., et al., "Glucocorticoid regulation of elastin synthesis in human fibroblasts: Down-regulation in fibroblasts from normal dermis but not from keloids." *Journal of Investigative Dermatology*, in press.

Russell, S. B., Trupin, K.M., Rodriguez-Eaton, S., et al., "Reduced growth-factor requirement of keloid-derived fibroblasts may account for tumor growth." *Proceedings of the National Academy of Sciences USA* 85:587-591 1994.

Diamond, M. I., Miner, J. N., Yoshinaga, S. K., and Yamamoto, K. R., "Transcription factor interactions: Selectors of positive or negative regulation from a single DNA element." *Science* 249:1266-1272, 1990.

Russell, S. B., Trupin, J. S., Myers, J. C., et al., "Differential glucocorticoid regulation of collagen mRNA in human dermal fibroblasts." *Journal of Biological Chemistry* 264:13730-13735, 1989.

Keloids and Hypertrophic Scars Fact Sheet

What is a keloid and how does it differ from a hypertrophic scar?

A keloid is raised scar tissue. It is due to deposits of connective tissue (primarily collagen). Keloids may occur on any part of the body, but the areas most often affected are the face, earlobes, neck, breastbone, and upper back. They can be unattractive and uncomfortable.

A hypertrophic scar resembles a keloid. It involves the overgrowth of scar tissue during the first six to eight weeks of healing of a wound or puncture of the skin, which may then take many months to flatten. Caucasians (people with white skin) rarely have keloids; they are more likely to develop hypertrophic scars. The scars can cause pain, itchiness, and, if at a joint, interfere with movement.

What causes keloids?

Keloids may form when tissue injury affects the blood vessels and capillaries. This may occur following accidents, surgery, burns, exposure to toxic agents (e.g., acids) or other forms of wounding. Minor scratches, vaccinations, or even insect bites may produce keloids in some people. Ear piercing, particularly where cartilage (soft bone) is

Keloids and Hypertropic Scars: When Skin Repairs Run Amok

pierced, may result in keloids. Dark skinned people are more likely to produce keloids than light skinned people, and the tendency to form keloids may be inherited.

What treatments are available for these scars?

A broad range of treatment for keloids and hypertrophic scars has been investigated. However, more research is needed regarding the appropriate selection of each treatment and the circumstances under which each treatment is most effective.

Intralesional injections. The injection of medicines directly into the scar has been found to sometimes flatten the scar or improve its appearance. A corticosteroid is the usual substance injected because it reduces the making of collagen and inflammation (redness) in the tissues. Steroids may also be injected into the area of a scar that has been removed by surgery to prevent new scar formation.

Silastic gel sheeting (SGS). SGS looks like a large, clear, silicone bandage. When applied for 12 to 24 hours a day for two months, particularly early in the wound-healing process, scars are reduced in thickness, redness, and elevation. Scars of longer duration also improve with this treatment. The way in which SGS works is not clearly understand and is still being studied. The positive results may be due to maintaining moisture to the scar.

Surgery. Laser surgery is one means of removing a keloid scar. Because the scars tend to come back after surgery, steroid injections are sometimes combined with surgery to suppress reappearance of a scar. Surgery plus radiation therapy is another combination that has shown a range of effectiveness from 50 percent to 98 percent depending on dosage and kind of radiation.

Cryotherapy. Many patients with well-established, rather than new keloids, may be helped by repeated freezing of the scar with liquid nitrogen followed by corticosteroid injections.

Pressure therapy. Pressure was first proposed for treatment of burn scars in the 1800s. The pressure softens and flattens the scar. More recently, pressure applied for four to six months following surgery in those likely to develop keloids has been shown to suppress keloid formation. Pressure can be applied to the face by a specially designed mask or to other parts of the body by a bandage or custom-fitted garment.

Radiation therapy. Small doses of x-ray or other forms of radiation alone has been tried as treatment with varying results. Radiation is sometimes considered in keloids that are resistant to corticosteroids, surgery alone or pressure.

Skin grafts. Grafts (adding skin) are sometimes tried with hypertrophic scars because they provide more stretch than the scar tissue. This may relieve discomfort and bending and tightening of limbs.

Splints. Because tightening of the limbs tends to occur if keloids are located at a joint, splints have been used, especially at night, to prevent tightening and bending of the limbs.

Other treatments under investigation. A number of treatments that are being studied include injection of **interferon-gamma** (reduces production of collagen by fibroblasts), **chemotherapy** (chemicals usually used to treat cancer), and **retinoic acid** applied to the skin.

Chapter 47

Dog, Cat, and Human Bites

Abstract

It is estimated that half of all Americans will be bitten by an animal or another human being during their lifetimes. The vast majority of the estimated two million annual mammalian bite wounds are minor, and the victims never seek medical attention. Nonetheless, bite wounds account for approximately 1 percent of all emergency department visits and more than $30 million in annual health care costs. Infection is the most common bite-associated complication; the relative risk is determined by the species of the inflicting animal, bite location, host factors, and local wound care. Most infections caused by mammalian bites are polymicrobial, with mixed aerobic and anaerobic species. The clinical presentation and appropriate treatment of infected bite wounds vary according to the causative organisms. Human bite wounds have long had a bad reputation for severe infection and frequent complication. However, recent data demonstrate that human bites occurring anywhere other than the hand present no more of a risk for infection than any other type of mammalian bite. The increased incidence of serious infections and complications associated with human bites to the hand warrants their consideration and management in three different categories: occlusional/simple, clenched fist

©1995 American Academy of Dermatology. Reproduced from the *Journal of the American Academy of Dermatology*, Robert D. Greigo, MD, Ted Rosen, MD, Ida F. Orengo, MD and John Wolf, MD, "Dog, Cat and Human Bites: Review." 1995, vol.33 no.6, pp.1019-1029. With permission from Mosby Year-Book.

injuries, and occlusional bites to the hand. This chapter reviews dog, cat, and human bite wounds, risk factors for complications, evaluation components, bacteriology, antimicrobial susceptibility patterns, and recommended treatments. Epidemiology, clinical presentation, and treatment of infections caused by *Pasteurella multocida, Capnocytophaga canimorsus, Eikenella corrodens,* and *rhabdovirus* (rabies only) receive particular emphasis. (J AM ACAD DERMATOL 1995; 33:1019-29.)

It is estimated that half of all Americans will be bitten by either an animal or another human being during their lifetimes. The vast majority of the estimated two million annual mammalian bite wounds are minor, and the victims never seek medical attention. However, bite wounds still account for approximately 1 percent of all emergency department visits and for more than $30 million in annual health care costs. The dermatologist may be the first medical professional called on to treat bite wounds; therefore an understanding of the different wound types, risk factors, evaluation components, bacteriology, antimicrobial susceptibility patterns, and recommended treatments are essential to avoid serious complications. It must be acknowledged that almost all studies of bite wounds, and therefore this review, are likely to be biased because they are based on data from patients who seek medical attention. This self-selected group is more likely to have serious wounds and the resultant complications.

Table 47.1. Risk factors for bite infection

Location on hand, foot, over major joint
Location on scalp or face of infant
Puncture wounds
Crush injuries
Treatment delay greater than 12 hours
Patient age greater than 50 years
Patient immunosuppression: Immune disorders, corticosteroids, asplenism
Chronic alcoholism
Diabetes mellitus
Vascular disease
Preexisting edema of the affected extremity

Dog, Cat, and Human Bites

Dog Bites

The most common animal bite injuries in the United States are inflicted by dogs, accounting for 80 percent to 90 percent of all bites. The high incidence of dog bites reflects a canine population that has grown four times faster than the human population; over half of all households own at least one dog. Approximately 1 in 20 dogs will bite a human being during the dog's lifetime; the pet is known to the victim in approximately 90 percent of such cases. The risk of being bitten varies with age, with bites occurring much more frequently in persons 2 through 19 years of age. Provocation of dogs by teasing or by the unintentionally threatening behavior of children has been suggested as the precipitating factor in many attacks.

Dog bites most often affect the extremities (54 percent to 85 percent), with upper extremity bites occurring slightly more frequently than lower extremity bites. Specifically, bites to the hand occur in 18 percent to 68 percent and are at increased risk for tenosynovitis, septic arthritis, and abscess formation. Bites to the head and neck occur second most commonly (15 percent to 27 percent) followed by bites to the trunk (0 percent to 10 percent). However, the smaller the victim, the more likely a facial or scalp injury will occur; nearly two-thirds of bites in children younger than four years old involve the head and neck. Bite injuries may consist of punctures, avulsions, tears, and abrasions. The overall infection rate for dog bites is among the lowest of all mammalian bites, estimated at 2 percent to 20 percent. The risk for infection of any type of bite wound is determined by local wound care, host factors, and bite location (Table 47.1). It is the interrelation between the crush injury, resultant edema, ecchymosis, devitalized tissue, other host factors, and bacterial inoculation that results in serious bites. Serious and fatal dog bites have increased in incidence as owners acquire larger, more aggressive breeds for home protection, with a recently reported annual mortality rate from dog bites of 6.7 per 100 million population. Fatal bites typically occur with small children, secondary to involvement of the head and neck resulting in exsanguination from a major blood vessel. Doberman pinschers, German shepherds, and pit bull terriers are all more prone to attack without provocation, with pit bulls perpetrating the majority of deaths. Bites from these large dogs routinely inflict serious wounds because their jaws are capable of exerting forces in excess of 450 pounds per square inch, which is sufficient to penetrate light sheet metal.

Cat Bites

Cat bites are the second most common type of mammalian bites in the United States, accounting for an estimated 5 percent to 15 percent, with an estimated annual incidence of 400,000. Again, most cat bites result in minor injuries and the victims do not seek medical attention. Of those patients with problematic bites who seek medical attention, puncture wounds, frequently affecting the hand or extremities, occur. Studies have shown that 60 percent to 67 percent of cat bite injuries occur on the upper extremity, whereas 15 percent to 20 percent occur on the head and neck 10 percent to 13 percent on the lower extremities, and fewer than 5 percent on the trunk. These factors help to account for an associated infection rate of 30 percent to more than 50 percent, more than double the rate for dog bites. The sharp, slender teeth of cats may penetrate bones, resulting in septic arthritis and osteomyelitis. Cat scratches typically inoculate the same organisms as bites and should be treated similarly.

Human Bites

Human bites are the third most frequent type of mammalian bite, accounting for 3.6 percent to 23 percent of bite wounds examined by urban physicians. Most human bites result from overtly aggressive behavior; however, accidental bites associated with sports, school-related activities, and sexual activity also occur. Male victims are most frequently bitten on the hand, arm, and shoulder; female victims are most frequently bitten on the breast, genitalia, leg, and arm.

Human bite wounds have a bad reputation for severe infection and frequent complication. In the preantibiotic era, 33 percent of bite victims seen more than one hour after injury required amputation of the affected part because of severe infection; a majority of patients suffered from permanent residual disability. Recently, the validity of this dogma has been questioned. As with other bites, reports on human bites reflect a selection bias for those that have not healed from self-treatment by patients or that occur in victims of crimes or unprovoked attacks. Thus more severe wounds, with frequent involvement of the hand and specifically the metacarpophalangeal (MCP) joint, and patients seen with infection already present, are typically treated by medical personnel. Such factors increase the risk for severe wound infection, regardless of the cause.

Dog, Cat, and Human Bites

Recent data demonstrate an overall human bite infection rate ranging from 10 percent to 50 percent. However, because of the variable risk for infection depending on wound type, it is useful to consider human bites as three different categories: occlusional/simple, clenched fist injuries, and occlusional bites to the hand. Occlusional/simple bites occur when the teeth are sunk into the skin. This type of bite, when occurring anywhere other than the hand, is considered by some to be no more dangerous than any other laceration or bite. A study of the natural course of 434 human bites and 803 lacerations in an institution for the developmentally disabled revealed an infection incidence of 17.7 percent for bite wounds compared with 13.4 percent for lacerations. The same study also demonstrated that hand wounds of any cause had greater than a twofold increased risk for infection compared with wounds elsewhere. As human bites occur most frequently on the upper extremities (60 percent to 75 percent), particularly the hands and fingers, more frequent infection is to be expected. Thus it is valuable to consider occlusional bites to the hand, which do not involve a clenched fist, to be of higher risk for infection and complication than simple occlusional bites to other areas.

The clenched fist injury or "fight bite" is the most serious of all human bite wounds. This injury results from one person punching another in the mouth with a clenched fist, usually causing a 3 to 8 mm puncture or laceration of the skin overlying the third MCP joint or the back of the hand. This wound is often inflicted with considerable force, frequently resulting in MCP joint capsule perforation, and rarely tendon or nerve laceration, or phalangeal or metacarpal fracture. The benign appearance of this wound often results in delays in seeking treatment until infection is already present as evidenced by swelling, discharge, and severe pain. These injuries may result in simple cellulitis. However, because of frequent penetration of the MCP joint capsule with resultant bacterial inoculation, more serious infection such as septic arthritis and osteomyelitis may result. The complex anatomy of the hand increases the likelihood for spread of infection into the various compartments of the hand and for abscess formation. Clenched fist injuries, particularly those overlying joints, should be evaluated by a hand surgeon with possible surgical exploration/assessment for joint injury and tendon involvement.

Paronychia occurring among children who suck their fingers should also be regarded as bite wounds with respect to their microbiology because of the normal oral flora involved. However, bite wounds inflicted by children have a reduced rate of infection compared with those of adults, possibly a reflection of fewer diseased teeth or less gingivitis.

Microbiology

Dog and Cat Bites (See Table 47.2)

Most infections that develop from dog and cat bites are polymicrobial, with a mean of 2.8 to 3.6 bacterial species isolated per wound culture, including an average of one anaerobic species per wound. *Staphylococcus* sp., *Streptococcus* sp., and *Corynebacterium* sp. are the most commonly isolated aerobic organisms from infected dog bites. Anaerobic bacteria are present in 38 percent to 76 percent of dog and cat bites. The most frequently isolated anaerobes include *Bacteroides fragilis, Prevotella, Porphyromonas, Peptostreptococcus,* and *Fusobacterium* sp., as well as *Veillonella parvula*. These anaerobes only rarely produce, ß-lactamase.

Pasteurella multocida, the major pathogen isolated from cat bites, is also associated with bites from dogs and many other animals. *P. multocida* is a small aerobic, facultatively anaerobic, gram-negative coccobacillus, which can be difficult to culture. It is a component of the normal oral flora in 70 percent to 90 percent of cats and 50 percent to 66 percent of dogs. *P. multocida* has been found in 50 percent to 80 percent of cat bite wound infections and in 25 percent of dog bite wounds. A recent article by Holst et al. noted that *P. multocida* has several different subspecies with differences in host animals, propensities for infection, and severity of associated infections. This will become important in the future because these organisms may become separate species. Clinical infection with *P. multocida* is characterized by the rapid development of an intense inflammatory response with prominent pain and swelling developing within 24 hours of the initial injury in 70 percent of cases and by 48 hours in 90 percent. This organism has been associated with abscess formation, septic arthritis, osteomyelitis, meningitis, sepsis, endocarditis and pneumonia. The preferred antibiotics for oral treatment are penicillin V, amoxicillin, amoxicillin-clavulanate, cefuroxime, tetracycline, and ciprofloxacin. Although some isolates are exceptions, *P. multocida* is generally resistant to levels of erythromycin attainable by oral therapy. Penicillin G, ß-lactam—ß-lactamase inhibitor combinations or second- or third-generation cephalosporins are recommended for intravenous therapy.

AEROBES

Acinetobacter sp.	EF-4, EF-7	Pasteurella multocida
Actinobacillus actinomycetemcomitans	Eikenella corrodens	Other Pasteurella sp.
Actinobacillus lignieresii	Enterobacter sp.	Proteus mirabilis
Aeromonas hydrophila	Escherichia coli	Pseudomonas aeruginosa
Bacillus subtilis	Flavobacterium sp.	Other Pseudomonas sp.
Other Bacillus sp.	Haemophilus aphrophilus	Serratia marcescens
Bordetella sp.	Haemophilus felis	Staphylococcus aureus
Branhamella catarrhalis	Haemophilus influenzae	Staphylococcus epidermidis
Brucella canis	Haemophilus parainfluenzae	Staphylococcus intermedius
Capnocytophaga canimorsus (formerly CDC group DF-2)	II-R	Staphylococcus saprophyticus
	Klebsiella pneumoniae	Streptococci
Capnocytophaga cyanodegmi	Micrococcus sp.	α-Hemolytic
Chromobacterium sp.	Moraxella sp.	β-Hemolytic
Clostridium perfringens	Neisseria weaveri (formerly M-5)	γ-Hemolytic
Corynebacterium sp.	Neisseria sp.	Weeksella zoohelicum (formerly (II-j)

ANAEROBES

Actinomyces sp.	Leptotrichia sp.	Propionibacterium acnes
Arachnia propionica	Peptococcus sp.	Other Propionibacterium sp.
Bacteroides fragilis (isolated from dog bites)	Peptostreptococcus sp.	Veillonella sp.
Eubacterium sp.	Porphyromonas sp.	
Fusobacterium sp.	Prevotella sp.	

RARE PATHOGENS

Afipia felis (formerly the cat-scratch bacillus)	Leptospira sp.	Sporotrichia sp.
Blastomyces dermatitidis	Rabies	Streptobacillus sp.
Clostridium tetani	Rio Bravo virus	Yersinia pestis
Francisella tularensis	Spirilum minus	Other Yersinia sp.

Table 47.2. Microorganisms isolated from animal bite wounds

A rare, but potentially fatal, bacterial infection strongly associated with dog bites, and rarely from cat bites or scratches, is that of *Capnocytophaga canimorsus* (formerly Centers for Disease Control group DF-2). Since the first case in 1976, more than 50 cases have been reported. *C. canimorsus* is a fastidious, thin, gram-negative rod, isolated as part of the normal oral flora of 16 percent of dogs and 18 percent of cats. Approximately 80 percent of reported cases have had a predisposing condition, most commonly splenectomy; other cases have been associated with trauma, Hodgkin's disease, idiopathic thrombocytopenic purpura, steroid therapy, alcohol abuse, and chronic lung disease.

Clinical infection with *C. canimorsus* most often presents with overwhelming sepsis characterized by fever, positive blood cultures, leukocytosis, petechiae, macular/papular rash, disseminated intravascular coagulation, cellulitis, hypotension, renal failure, meningitis, or pneumonia. This infection carries a fatality rate of approximately 25 percent; there have been several fatal cases in immunocompetent hosts. Penicillin G is considered the antibiotic of choice; in vitro susceptibility to ampicillin, carbenicillin, cephalothin, cefoxitin, cefotaxime, clindamycin, chloramphenicol, ciprofloxacin, erythromycin, and tetracycline has also been reported.

Cat bites are rarely associated with the transmission of tularemia, plague, sporotrichosis, blastomycosis, and rabies.

Human Bites (See Table 47.3)

More than 42 different species of bacteria have been isolated from the normal human mouth, and up to 190 species in the presence of gingivitis or periodontitis. Human saliva has been found to contain anaerobes in concentrations of 1×10^8 organisms/ml, *Streptococcus* species measure 2×10^7 organisms/ml, and *Staphylococcus* species measure 5×10^3 organisms/ml.

The bacteriology of human bite wounds is complex. Early bacteriologic studies of human bites did not employ suitable methods for the recovery of anaerobic bacteria. Therefore the isolation of α-hemolytic streptococci and *Staphylococcus aureus* most commonly from wound infections may not accurately reflect the true microbiology of such infections. Recent studies that include cultures for both aerobic and anaerobic bacteria have revealed that the majority of human bite wounds demonstrate an average of five different microorganisms isolated per wound, three of these being anaerobes. The

AEROBES

Acinetobacter sp.	Haemophilus parainfluenzae
Branhamella catarrhalis	Klebsiella pneumoniae
Corynebacterium sp.	Micrococcus sp.
Eikenella corrodens	Moraxella sp.
Enterobacter cloacae	Neisseria gonorrhoeae
Other Enterobacter sp.	Other Neisseria sp.
Escherichia coli	Nocardia sp.
Haemophilus aphrophilus	Proteus mirabilis
Haemophilus influenzae	Pseudomonas aeruginosa
	Other Pseudomonas sp.
	Serratia marcescens
	Staphylococcus aureus
	Staphylococcus epidermidis
	Staphylococcus intermedius
	Staphylococcus saprophyticus
	Streptococci
	α-Hemolytic
	β-Hemolytic
	γ-Hemolytic

ANAEROBES

Acidaminococcus sp.	Eubacterium sp.
Actinomyces sp.	Fusobacterium nucleatum
Arachnia propionica	Peptostreptococcus anaerobius
Bacteroides fragilis	Peptostreptococcus prevotii
Clostridium sp.	Other Peptostreptococcus sp.
	Prevotella sp.
	Propionibacterium acnes
	Other Propionibacterium sp.

Table 47.3. Microorganisms isolated from human bite wounds

most frequently isolated anaerobic bacteria are similar to those recovered from dog and cat bites, and include *Bacteroides fragilis, Prevotella, Porphyromonas, Peptostreptococcus, Fusobacterium, Veillonella,* and *Clostridium* species. However, unlike the anaerobes recovered from animal bites, the organisms found in human bites, particularly *B. fragilis*, frequently produce ß-lactamase, comprising up to 41 percent to 45 percent of isolates in some studies. The predominant aerobic organisms recovered from human bite wounds are α- and ß-hemolytic streptococci, *S. aureus, Staphylococcus epidermidis, Corynebacterium* sp., and *Eikenella corrodens. S. aureus* has historically been associated with more severe bite wound infections; it frequently produces ß-lactamase and is generally resistant to penicillin.

Another organism found in 10 percent to 29 percent of human bite wounds is the fastidious, slow-growing, gram-negative, facultatively anaerobic rod *E. corrodens. E. corrodens* is present in approximately 25 percent of clenched fist injuries and frequently results in serious, chronic, indolent infections. This organism may coexist with α-hemolytic streptococci, demonstrating a synergistic relation. Its growth may actually depend on concomitant streptococcal infection. *E. corrodens* is typically susceptible to penicillin, amoxicillin/clavulanic acid, cefoxitin, trimethoprim-sulfamethoxazole, ceftriaxone, tetracycline, and ciprofloxacin. Resistance has characteristically been found to penicillinase-resistant penicillins, such as dicloxacillin and nafcillin, as well as first-generation cephalosporins, clindamycin, aminoglycosides, and erythromycin.

Table 47.4. Rare organisms transmitted by human bites

Actinomyces sp.
Clostridium tetani
Hepatitis B and C
Herpes simplex virus
Mycobacterium tuberculosis
Treponema pallidum

Transmission of herpesvirus types 1 and 2 and hepatitis B and C, as well as several other serious infectious diseases, has also been documented through human bites (Table 47.4). Although the presence of low levels of HIV has been detected in the saliva of up to 44 percent

Dog, Cat, and Human Bites

of infected persons, unequivocal evidence for transmission of HIV through human bites has not been documented. Two retrospective cases of possible HIV transmission through human bites have been published; however, one of these cases had other risk factors, making implication of the bite wound unscientific. On the basis of the prospective analysis and follow-up of patients bitten by HIV-infected persons, such transmission appears unlikely. However, the presence of HIV in saliva makes disease transmission biologically possible, and bites from infected or high-risk persons should be regarded as conveying a very low but genuine risk for viral transmission. Although use of prophylactic oral antiviral agents is controversial, thorough and vigorous wound irrigation with virucidal agents such as 1-percent povidone-iodine is appropriate, and a baseline HIV serologic test with a six-month follow-up test may be prudent to obtain.

Table 47.5. Bite management: Diagnosis

A. History

1. Type of offending animal
2. Animal's behavior, provocation, location, ownership
3. Time elapsed since injury
4. Specific complaints
5. Victim's medical condition (immunosuppression by medication or disease, splenectomy, diabetes, arterial or venous disease)
6. Allergies (anesthetics, analgesics, antibiotics)
7. Tetanus immune status

B. Examination

1. Evaluate skin site for depth and crush injury
2. Evaluate nerve, tendon function
3. Evaluate vascular supply
4. Evaluate underlying joints for penetration
5. Photograph or diagram wounds

C. Laboratory

1. Culture, aerobic and anaerobic (if infected)
2. X-ray: crush injuries, suspected fracture, foreign body

Table 47.6. Bite management: Therapy

A. Immediate treatment

1. Copious irrigation (normal saline or 1 percent povidone-iodine solution, with a 20 ml or larger syringe and 19-gauge needle)
2. Cautious debridement if indicated
3. Prophylactic antibiotics (human bites)
4. Therapeutic antibiotics (signs of infection)
5. Immobilization (position of function)
6. Elevation
7. Tetanus toxoid if indicated (with or without tetanus immune globulin as necessary)
8. Rabies prophylaxis (if indicated)
9. Primary closure (controversial)

B. Long-term issues

1. Report to health department (if indicated)
2. Exercise rehabilitation program
3. Follow-up appointments

Bite Wound Management

The management of mammalian bite wounds should include the elements of history, physical examination, documentation, laboratory investigation, therapeutic intervention, and prophylactic measures. These elements are listed in Tables 47.5 and 47.6. The prompt implementation of such appropriate medical and surgical therapy for bite wounds may serve to prevent associated complications. A focused history with attention to the specific features will serve to identify persons at highest risk for complications who may require hospital admission for intravenous antibiotics or careful outpatient follow-up, while also serving to identify animal behavior suggestive of rabies infection.

Because most animal bites do not become infected, bacterial cultures of bites without signs of clinical infection are not usually warranted. Wounds, including punctures, examined more than 24 hours after the bite and without signs of infection need not be cultured. When infection is present, both aerobic and anaerobic cultures should be obtained from deep within the wound, after removal of superficial crusts, but before debridement. Prompt, copious irrigation (greater than 150 ml) of all bite wounds, including punctures, through an 18- or 19-gauge needle or plastic catheter is indicated. Such irrigation provides a high-pressure jet, which serves to reduce the bacterial inoculum and debride the wound. However, irrigation should be in the direction of the puncture wound, and care must be taken not to inject into the tissue or inflict additional trauma. Although normal saline is the most commonly recommended solution for irrigation, a povidone-iodine-containing solution may be indicated in bites at high risk for rabies because animal data support a decreased transmission rate associated with its use. Although cautious debridement of devitalized or crushed tissue and foreign material is often necessary, debridement of puncture wounds is not advised because this can lead to a defect that cannot be closed.

Primary closure of bite wounds is controversial. There are data to support primary closure of dog bites in low-risk locations, after proper local wound care. However, because of the lack of reliable prospective scientific data, no consensus exists regarding which bites should be sutured. Callaham recommends suturing all bite wounds unless they are high risk and delaying primary closure of clinically uninfected high-risk wounds 72 hours after initial treatment. However, it is generally accepted that deep puncture wounds, wounds examined more than 24 hours after the bite, clinically infected wounds, and bites to the hand should not be sutured. All types of mammalian bites to the face and head are frequently closed, primarily by plastic surgeons, to minimize scarring. Good results are probably due to excellent blood supply, rarity of edema, meticulous irrigation, avoidance of multiple layered closures with buried sutures, and antibiotic prophylaxis.

When to administer antimicrobial therapy for bite wounds and the specific agents to use remain unsettled issues. The lack of a consensus results from the deficiency of large, prospective, blinded, randomized studies; heterogeneity of patients, wounds, and treatments among published studies; and the notoriously poor correlation between in vitro and in vivo antimicrobial sensitivities. Because of the wide range of potential pathogens and frequent coinfection by several bacteria with differing antimicrobial sensitivities, treatment can be challenging. A recent prospective, randomized study of 45 patients with uncomplicated human bites to the hand who were seen within 24 hours without evidence of infection and with no tendon injury or joint capsule perforation showed subsequent development of infection in 46.7 percent of those treated by mechanical wound care alone versus 0 percent in those treated with oral or parenteral antibiotics. Oral and intravenous antibiotics were found to be of equal efficacy for prophylaxis; therefore mechanical wound care and a broad-spectrum oral antibiotic were recommended as adequate care for uncomplicated human hand bites. Prophylactic antibiotics are also generally indicated in the situations listed in Table 47.7. A recommended course of the appropriate prophylactic antibiotic is 3 to 5 days. Because most studies have either noncomparable wounds, small numbers, or design flaws, there are no good data to support either side of the issue, and the decision is left to the clinical judgment of the treating physician. This determination should weigh the circumstances under which the patient has come for medical attention; it should also consider relative cost analysis of an appropriate 3-day course of therapy versus the potential expenses of medical treatment, lost time from work, and residual disability if infection develops. However, it is agreed that "minor" bite wounds do not require prophylaxis.

Table 47.7. Bite management: Indications for prophylactic antibiotics

Presentation more than eight hours after bite?
Moderate or severe wounds?
Cat bites (most)
Diabetes mellitus
Asplenic patient
Immunocompromised (disease or drugs)
Facial involvement
Hand involvement
Deep puncture wounds

Empiric treatment of overt infection should be directed at the aerobic and anaerobic oral flora of the offending animal, as well as at pathogens from the skin flora of the victim. Whenever possible, treatment should be directed according to the specific antibiotic sensitivities of pathogens isolated from infected wounds. Antibiotic regimens for empiric treatment of specific bites are listed in Table 47.8. The majority of patients with clinically infected bites can be managed as outpatients. Although no clear-cut criteria for hospitalization exist, situations requiring complicated wound management, surgical intervention, intravenous antibiotics, or close follow-up may warrant admission (see Table 47.9). Many of the specific therapies recommended

Dog, Cat, and Human Bites

for bite wounds are controversial with opinions on either side of most issues. Local standards of care should be followed, and appropriate consultation with an orthopedic surgeon, or infectious disease specialist should be considered.

Table 47.8. Bite management: antibiotics

Broad-spectrum antibiotics: Effective in most bites

- Amoxicillin/clavulanic acid (500 mg q 8 hr): Effective against *S. aureus, E. corrodens*, anaerobes, *P. multocida, C. canimorsus*
- Cefuroxime (500 mg b.i.d.), second-generation cephalosporin: Effective against *S. aureus*, most *E. corrodens*, anaerobes, *P. multocida*
- Ceftriaxone (one gm IM q.d.): Effective against *S. aureus, E. corrodens*, most anaerobes, *P. multocida, P. aeruginosa*

Antibiotics for specific bites

Dog bites (relatively low incidence of *P. multocida*)
- Penicillin V (500 mg q.i.d.) or amoxicillin (250 to 500 mg t.i.d.)
- If allergic to *penicillin* Doxycycline (100 mg b.i.d.) (cannot use in children or pregnant women)

Cat bites (high incidence of *P. multocida*)
- Amoxicillin/clavulanate (500 mg t.i.d.)
- Penicillin and/or dicloxacillin (500 mg q.i.d.) for both (penicillin is the drug of choice for *P. multocida* but has poor coverage for *S. aureus*; dicloxacillin is excellent for most *S. aureus*, but has poor coverage for *P. multocida*)
- If allergic to *penicillin*: Doxycycline (100 mg b.i.d.) (cannot use in children or pregnant women)

Human bites (pathogens include *S. aureus, E. corrodens*)
- Amoxicillin/clavulanate (500 mg t.i.d.) or
- Penicillin and/or dicloxacillin (500 mg q.i.d.) for both (penicillin is the drug of choice for *E. corrodens* but has poor coverage for *S. aureus*; dicloxacillin is excellent for most *S. aureus*, but has poor coverage for *E. corrodens*)
- If allergic to *penicillin*: Doxycycline (100 mg b.i.d.) (cannot use in children or pregnant women)

Table 47.9. Bite management: indications for hospital admission

Systemic manifestations of infection (fever, chills)
Severe cellulitis
Penetration of a joint, nerve, bone, tendon, or central nervous system
Likelihood for noncompliance
Presence of peripheral vascular disease
Immunocompromised by disease or drugs
Diabetes mellitus
Significant bites to the hand
Injuries requiring reconstructive surgery
Head injuries
Infection refractory to oral or outpatient therapy

Even when appropriate antibiotics have been administered, clinical failures have occurred, often because of edema of the affected leg or hand. Elevation of the involved area is an essential component of therapy; it should be stressed to the patient that it must be continued for several days, or until edema has resolved.

Rabies

Perhaps the most serious animal bite complication is infection with rabies. Although it is estimated that an untreated person has less than a 20 percent chance of contracting rabies from the bite of a rabid animal, the essentially uniform mortality associated with rabies once contracted makes this a grave illness. Rabies presently results in more than 20,000 deaths per year worldwide. However, because of the effective efforts of animal control and vaccination and easy access to medical care and rabies prophylaxis in this country, human rabies in the United States is rare, averaging only one case per year. Discussion of rabies outside the United States is beyond the scope of this review. Rabies is an acute encephalomyelitis caused by a neurotropic bullet-shaped RNA virus from the rhabdovirus family. It is most frequently transmitted to human beings by the inoculation of saliva into bite wounds or scratches; however, transmission through inhalation by laboratory workers and spelunkers as well as through infected corneal grafts has been documented.

The dog is the major animal reservoir for rabies worldwide. In the United States, however, the main vectors are wild animals with highly variable regional predominance. In 1988, skunks accounted for 38 percent of reported cases, raccoons 31 percent, bats 14 percent, foxes 4 percent, and other wild animals 2 percent. Raccoon rabies is currently an epizootic disease in the mid-Atlantic and south Atlantic states. From November 1989 to May 1994, 2,724 cases of rabies in terrestrial animals were confirmed by examination of animal heads in the state of New Jersey alone. [New Jersey Department of Public Health. Epizootic Hotline (recorded message; telephone. 609-292-5769). June 1, 1994.] Of these cases, 81 percent were raccoons, 12 percent were skunks, and 3 percent were domestic cats. Of domestic animal rabies in the United States, cats are the most frequently infected species (35 percent), followed by cattle (31 percent) and dogs (23 percent).

When a patient with possible rabies exposure is examined, consideration of the type of exposure, animal species, predominant local vectors, and circumstances of the incident are all important. The local health department should be contacted for information on the local prevalence of rabies in the specific offending animal species. Bite penetration of the skin and salivary contact with open wounds, scratches, abrasions, or mucous membranes should all be regarded as high-risk bite exposures. An unprovoked attack by an animal exhibiting bizarre or furious behavior should arouse suspicion. As with all bite wounds, local wound care is of paramount importance in cases at high risk for rabies. Irrigation, debridement, and evaluation as already outlined are all appropriate features of management. Prompt, thorough wound irrigation with soap or iodine solution reduces the development of rabies by up to 90 percent.

In addition to proper wound care, assessment of the likelihood that an exposure to rabies has occurred and the necessity for prophylaxis must be made. Algorithms to aid in this assessment have been published elsewhere. In the consideration of the need for rabies vaccination, it must be recognized that immunotherapy is purely prophylactic; once clinical signs of rabies have developed, the course is almost uniformly fatal. Therapy is based on the administration of passive immunization with human rabies immune globulin (HRIG) and active immunization with the human diploid cell vaccine (HDCV) or the rabies vaccine adsorbed (RVA). HRIG should be administered on day 0 as a single 20 IU/kg dose, half infiltrated around the site of exposure and the other half given intramuscularly. HDCV or RVA should be administered intramuscularly in a series of five 1-ml injections given on days 0, 3, 7, 14, and 28. The deltoid muscle of adults and the anterolateral thigh of small children are the recommended injection sites for HDCV and RVA; administration into the gluteal region has been associated with treatment failure and is not advised. To date, no cases of rabies development have been reported in the United States after appropriate immunization with the combination of HRIG and HDCV or RVA.

—by Robert D. Griego, MD,
Ted Rosen, MD, Ida F. Orengo, MD,
and John E. Wolf, MD Houston, Texas

Chapter 48

Preventing Pressure Ulcers

What Are Pressure Ulcers

A pressure ulcer is an injury usually caused by unrelieved pressure that damages the skin and underlying tissue. Pressure ulcers are also called bed sores and range in severity from mild (minor skin reddening) to severe (deep craters down to muscle and bone).

Unrelieved pressure on the skin squeezes tiny blood vessels, which supply the skin with nutrients and oxygen. When skin is starved of nutrients and oxygen for too long, the tissue dies and a pressure ulcer forms. Skin reddening that disappears after pressure is removed is normal and not a pressure ulcer.

Other factors cause pressure ulcers too. If a person slides down in the bed or chair, blood vessels can stretch or bend and cause pressure ulcers. Even slight rubbing or friction on the skin may cause minor pressure ulcers.

Pressure ulcers are serious problems that can lead to pain, a longer stay in the hospital or nursing home, and slower recovery from health problems. Anyone who must stay in a bed, chair, or wheelchair because of illness or injury can get pressure ulcers.

Fortunately, most pressure ulcers can be prevented, and when pressure ulcers do form, they do not have to get worse. This chapter describes where pressure ulcers form and how to tell if you are at risk of getting a pressure ulcer. It also lists steps to take to prevent them or

---

U.S. Department of Health and Human Services, AHCPR Publication Number 92-0048.

keep them from getting worse, and suggests how to work effectively with your health care team.

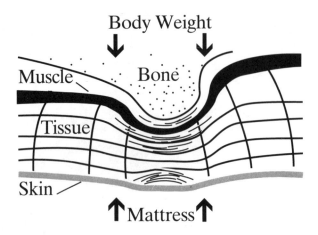

Figure 48.1. Tissue under pressure

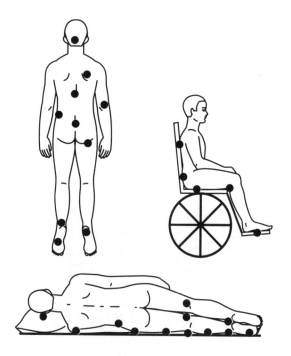

Figure 48.2. The Body's Pressure Points

Preventing Pressure Ulcers

Pressure ulcers form where bone causes the greatest force on the skin and tissue and squeezes them against an outside surface. This may be where bony parts of the body press against other body parts, a mattress, or a chair. In persons who must stay in bed, most pressure ulcers form on the lower back below the waist (sacrum), the hip bone (trochanter), and on the heels. In people in chairs or wheelchairs, the exact spot where pressure ulcers form depends on the sitting position. Pressure ulcers can also form on the knees, ankles, shoulder blades, back of the head, and spine.

Nerves normally "tell" the body when to move to relieve pressure on the skin. Persons in bed who are unable to move may get pressure ulcers after as little as one to two hours. Persons who sit in chairs and who cannot move can get pressure ulcers in even less time because the force on the skin is greater.

Risk Factors

Confinement to bed or a chair, being unable to move, loss of bowel or bladder control, poor nutrition, and lowered mental awareness are "risk factors" that increase your chance of getting pressure ulcers. Your risk results from the number and seriousness of the risk factors that apply to you.

Bed or chair confinement. If you must stay in bed, a chair, or a wheelchair, the risk of getting a pressure ulcer can be high.

Inability to move. If you cannot change positions without help, you are at great risk. Persons who are in a coma or who are paralyzed or who have a hip fracture are at special risk. Risks of getting pressure ulcers are lower when persons can move by themselves.

Loss of bowel or bladder control. If you cannot keep your skin free of urine, stool, or perspiration, you have a higher risk. These sources of moisture may irritate the skin.

Poor nutrition. If you cannot eat a balanced diet, your skin may not be properly nourished. Pressure ulcers are more likely to form when skin is not healthy.

Lowered mental awareness. When mental awareness is lowered, a person cannot act to prevent pressure ulcers. Mental awareness can be affected by health problems, medications, or anesthesia.

Fortunately, you can lower your risk. Following the steps in this chapter can help you and your health care provider to reduce your risk of pressure ulcers.

Prevention

The following steps for prevention are based on research, professional judgment, and practice. These steps can also keep pressure ulcers from getting worse. Some steps apply to all prevention efforts; others apply only in specific conditions. It may help to talk to a nurse or doctor about which steps are right for you.

Take Care of Your Skin

Your skin should be inspected at least once a day. Pay special attention to any reddened areas that remain after you have changed positions and the pressure has been relieved. This inspection can be done by yourself or your caregiver. A mirror can help when looking at hard-to-see areas. Pay special attention to pressure points shown in Figure 48.2. The goal is to find and correct problems before pressure ulcers form.

Your skin should be cleaned as soon as it is soiled. A soft cloth or sponge should be used to reduce injury to skin. Take a bath when needed for comfort or cleanliness. If a daily bath or shower is preferred or necessary, additional measures should be taken to minimize irritation and prevent dry skin. When bathing or showering, warm (not hot) water and a mild soap should be used.

To prevent dry skin:

- Use creams or oils on your skin.
- Avoid cold or dry air.

Minimize moisture from urine or stool, perspiration, or wound drainage. Often urine leaks can be treated. To obtain a copy of *Managing Urinary Incontinence: A Patient's Guide*, write to the AHCPR Publications Clearinghouse, P.O. Box 8547, Silver Spring, MD 20907.

When moisture cannot be controlled:

- Pads or briefs that absorb urine and have a quick drying surface that keeps moisture away from the skin should be used.

Preventing Pressure Ulcers

- A cream or ointment to protect skin from urine, stool, or wound drainage may be helpful.

Protect Your Skin from Injury

Avoid massage of your skin over bony parts of the body. Massage may squeeze and damage the tissue under the skin and make you more likely to get pressure ulcers.

Limit pressure over bony parts by changing positions or having your caregiver change your position.

- If you are in bed, your position should be changed at least every two hours.

- If you are in a chair, your position should be changed at least every hour. (If you are able to shift your own weight, you should do so every 15 minutes while sitting.)

Reduce friction (rubbing) by making sure you are lifted, rather than dragged, during repositioning. Friction can rub off the top layer of skin and damage blood vessels under the skin. You may be able to help by holding on to a trapeze hanging from an overhead frame. If nurses or others are helping to lift you, bed sheets or lifters can be used. A thin film of corn starch can be used on the skin to help reduce damage from friction.

Avoid use of donut-shape (ring) cushions. Donut-shape cushions can increase your risk of getting a pressure ulcer by reducing blood flow and causing tissue to swell.

If you are confined to bed:

- A special mattress that contains foam, air, gel, or water helps to prevent pressure ulcers. The cost and effectiveness of these products vary greatly. Talk to your health care provider about the best mattress for you.

- The head of the bed should be raised as little and for as short a time as possible if consistent with medical conditions and other restrictions. When the head of the bed is raised more than 30 degrees, your skin may slide over the bed surface, damaging skin and tiny blood vessels.

Skin Disorders Sourcebook

- Pillows or wedges should be used to keep knees or ankles from touching each other.

- Avoid lying directly on your hip bone (trochanter) when lying on your side. Also, a position that spreads weight and pressure more evenly should be chosen—pillows may also help.

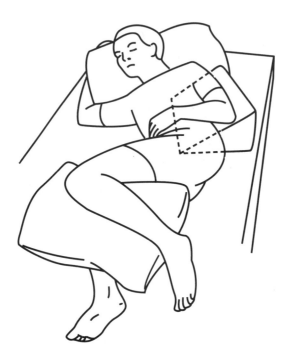

Figure 48.3. Adapted from J. Maklebust. Pressure ulcer update. RN, December 1991, pages 56-63. Original illustration by Jack Tandy. Used with permission.

- If you are completely immobile, pillows should be put under your legs from mid-calf to ankle to keep heels off the bed. **Never** place pillows behind the knee.

If you are in a chair or wheelchair:

- Foam, gel, or air cushions should be used to relieve pressure. Ask your health care provider which is best for you. Avoid do-nut-shape cushions because they reduce blood flow and cause

Preventing Pressure Ulcers

tissue to swell, which can increase your risk of getting a pressure ulcer.

- Avoid sitting without moving or being moved.

- Good posture and comfort are important.

Eat Well

Eat a balanced diet. Protein and calories are very important. Healthy skin is less likely to be damaged. If you are unable to eat a normal diet, talk to your health care provider about nutritional supplements that may be desirable.

Improve Your Ability to Move

A rehabilitation program can help some persons regain movement and independence.

Care of Pressure Ulcers by Risk Factor

Bed or Chair Confinement:

- Inspect skin at least once a day
- Bathe when needed for comfort or cleanliness
- Prevent dry skin.
- Reduce friction by:
  1. Lifting rather than dragging when repositioning.
  2. Using corn starch on skin.
- Avoid use of donut-shape cushions.
- Participate in a rehabilitation program

Bed Confinement:

- Change position at least every two hours.
- Use a special mattress that contains foam, air, gel, or water.
- Raise the head of bed as little and for as short a time as possible.

Chair Confinement:

- Change position every hour.

- Use foam, gel, or air cushion to relieve pressure.

Inability to Move

- Persons confined to chairs should be repositioned every hour if unable to do so themselves.
- For a person in a chair who is able to shift his or her own weight, change position at least every 15 minutes.
- Use pillows or wedges to keep knees or ankles from touching each other
- When in bed, place a pillow under the legs from mid-calf to ankle to keep the heels off the bed

Loss of Bowel or Bladder Control

- Clean skin as soon as soiled.
- Assess and treat urine leaks.
- If moisture cannot be controlled:
  1. Use absorbent pads and/or briefs with a quick-drying surface.
  2. Protect skin with a cream or ointment.

Poor Nutrition

- Eat a balanced diet.
- If a normal diet is not possible, talk to health care provider about nutritional supplements

Lowered Mental Awareness

- Choose preventive actions that apply to the person with lowered mental awareness. For example, if the person is chair-bound, refer to the specific preventive actions outlined in the Chair Confinement section above.

Communication with Your Doctor

This chapter tells how to reduce your risk of getting pressure ulcers. Not all steps apply to every person at risk. The best program for preventing pressure ulcers will consider what you want and be based on your condition.

Preventing Pressure Ulcers

Be sure you:

- Ask questions.

- Explain your needs, wants, and concerns.

- Understand what and why things are being done.

- Know what is best for you. Talk about what you can do to help prevent pressure ulcers, at home, in the hospital, or in the nursing home.

You can help to prevent most pressure ulcers. The extra effort can mean better health.

For More Information

National and international organizations provide a variety of resources for people concerned with pressure ulcers.

International Association of Enterostomal Therapy
(Will refer patients to local Enterostomal Therapy Nurses)
27241 La Paz Road, Suite 121
Laguna Niguel, CA 92656
714-476-0268

National Pressure Ulcer Advisory Panel
(Offers information for caregivers, families providing care at home, and others)
SUNY at Buffalo, Beck Hall
3435 Main Street
Buffalo, NY 14214
716-881-3558

The information in this chapter was taken from the *Clinical Practice Guideline on Pressure Ulcers in Adults: Prediction and Prevention*. The guideline was developed by an expert panel of doctors, nurses, other health care providers, and a consumer representative, and it was sponsored by the Agency for Health Care Policy and Research. Other guidelines on common health problems are being developed and will be released in the near future. For more information about the guidelines write to:

Agency for Health Care Policy and Research Publications Clearinghouse
P.O. Box 8547
Silver Spring, MD 20907

Chapter 49

Treating Pressure Sores

What Is a Pressure Sore

A pressure sore (or bed sore) is an injury to the skin and tissue under it. Pressure sores are usually caused by unrelieved pressure. If you sit or lie in the same position for a long time, the pressure on a small area of the body can squeeze shut tiny blood vessels that normally supply tissue with oxygen and nutrients. If tissue is starved of these "fuels" for too long, it begins to die, and a pressure sore starts to form.

Pressure sores are called pressure ulcers and decubitus ulcers as well as bed sores. How serious they are depends on the amount of damage to skin and tissue. Damage can range from a change in the color of unbroken skin (Stage I) to severe, deep wounds down to muscle or bone (Stage IV). In light-skinned people, a Stage I sore may change skin color to a dark purple or red area that does not become pale under fingertip pressure. In dark-skinned people, this area may become darker than normal. The affected area may feel warmer than surrounding tissue.

Treating Pressure Sores

A pressure sore is serious. It must not be ignored. With proper treatment, most pressure sores will heal. Healing depends on many

U.S. Dept. of Health and Human Services, AHCPR Publication Number 95-0654.

things: your general health, diet, relieving pressure on the sore, and careful cleaning and dressing of the sore.

This chapter gives the steps essential to helping a pressure sore heal. Although not all steps apply to everyone, it is important that you:

- Learn how to prevent and treat pressure sores.
- Ask questions if you do not understand.
- Explain your needs and concerns.
- Know what is best for you.
- Be active in your care.

Healing a pressure sore is a team effort. A team of health care professionals will work with you to prepare a treatment plan. Your team may include doctors, nurses, dietitians, social workers, pharmacists, and occupational and physical therapists. However, you and your caregiver are the most important team members. Feel free to ask questions or share concerns with other team members.

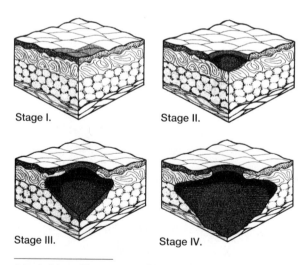

Adapted from *Statement on Pressure Ulcer Prevention.* Copyright, 1993. Used with permission of National Pressure Ulcer Advisory Panel.

Figure 49.1. Pressure sore stages

Treating Pressure Sores

Your Role

You and your caregiver need to:

- Know your roles in the treatment program.
- Learn how to perform the care.
- Know what to report to the doctor or nurse.
- Know how to tell if the treatment works.
- Help change the treatment plan when needed.
- Know what questions you want to ask.
- Get answers you understand.

Treatment Plan

To develop a treatment plan that meets your needs, the doctor or nurse must know about:

- Your general health.
- Illnesses that might slow healing (such as diabetes or hardening of the arteries).
- Prescription or over-the-counter medicines you take.
- The emotional support and physical assistance available from family friends, and others.

Your doctor or nurse will perform a physical exam and check the condition of your pressure sore to decide how to care for it. If you have had a pressure sore before, tell the doctor or nurse what helped it heal and what didn't help.

Your emotional health is also important. Be sure to share information about stresses in your life as well as health beliefs and practices. This will help your care team design a treatment plan that meets your personal needs. The treatment plan will be based on the results of your physical exam, health history, personal circumstances, and the condition of the sore (how it looks). This plan will include specific instructions for:

- Taking pressure off the sore.

- Caring for the pressure sore by cleaning the wound, removing dead tissue and debris, and dressing or bandaging the area to protect it while it heals.

- Aiding healing by making sure you get enough calories, protein, vitamins, and minerals.

Note to Caregivers

Although patients should be as active in their care as possible, you may need to provide much or all of their care. As a result, you may find you have questions or problems. If so, ask for help. Call doctors, nurses, and other professionals for answers and other support.

Remember that patients who must be in a bed or chair for long periods don't have to get pressure sores. Pressure sores can be prevented. And sores that have formed can be healed.

Three Keys to Helping Pressure Sores to Heal

Healing pressure sores depends on three principles: pressure relief, care of the sore, and good nutrition.

Pressure Relief

Pressure sores form when there is constant pressure on certain parts of the body. Long periods of unrelieved pressure cause or worsen pressure sores and slow healing once a sore has formed. Taking pressure off the sore is the first step toward healing.

Pressure sores usually form on parts of the body over bony prominences (such as hips and heels) that bear weight when you sit or lie down for a long time. Figure 48.2 in the previous chapter shows "pressure points" where sores often form. You can relieve or reduce pressure by:

- Using special surfaces to support your body.
- Putting your body in certain positions.
- Changing positions often.

Support Surfaces

Support surfaces are special beds, mattresses, mattress overlays, or seat cushions that support your body in bed or in a chair. These surfaces reduce or relieve pressure. By relieving pressure, you can help pressure sores heal and prevent new ones from forming.

Treating Pressure Sores

You can get different kinds of support surfaces. The best kind depends on your general health, if you are able to change positions, your body build, and the condition of your sore. You and your doctor or nurse can choose the surface best for you.

One way to see if a support surface reduces pressure enough is for the caregiver to do a "hand check" under the person (Figure 49.2). The caregiver places his or her hand under the support surface, beneath the pressure point, with the palm up and fingers flat. If there is less than 1 inch of support surface between the pressure point of the body and the caregiver's hand, the surface does not give enough support.

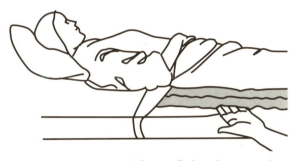

Slide hand (palm up and fingers flat) under support surface, just under pressure point. Do not flex fingers.

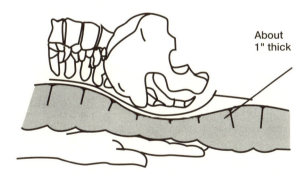

With good support, about 1 inch or more of uncompressed support surface is between caregiver's hand and patient.

Copyright, 1989. Used with permission of Gaymar Industries, Inc.

Figure 49.2. Hand Check to Assess Pressure Relief

If you need more support, your doctor or nurse will recommend a different support surface.

Caregivers should know that pressure sores are often painful, and a hand check may increase pain. Caregivers should ask if it will be okay to do a hand check, which should be done as gently as possible.

Good Body Positions

Your position is important to relieving pressure on the sore and preventing new ones. You need to switch positions whether you are in a bed or a chair.

In bed, follow these guidelines:

- Do not lie on the pressure sore. Use foam pads or pillows to relieve pressure on the sore, as shown in Figure 49.3.

- Change position at least every two hours.

- Do not rest directly on your hip bone when lying on your side. A 30-degree side-lying position is best (see Figure 49.3).

- When lying on your back, keep your heels up off the bed by placing a thin foam pad or pillow under your legs from mid-calf to ankle. The pad or pillow should raise the heels just enough so a piece of paper can be passed between them and the bed. Do not place the pad or pillow directly under the knee when on your back, because this could reduce blood flow to your lower leg.

- Do not use donut-shaped (ring) cushions; they reduce blood flow to tissue.

- Use pillows or small foam pads to keep knees and ankles from touching each other.

- Raise the head of the bed as little as possible. Raise it no more than 30 degrees from horizontal. If you have other health problems (such as respiratory ailments) that are improved by sitting up, ask your doctor or nurse which positions are best.

Treating Pressure Sores

- Use the upright position during meals to prevent choking. The head of the bed can be moved back to a lying or semi-reclining position one hour after eating.

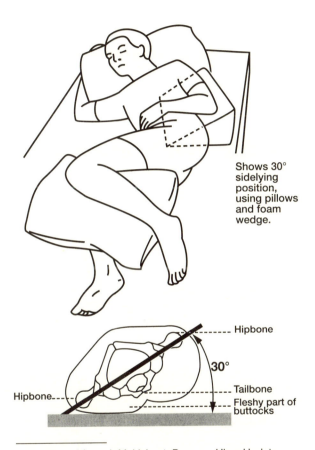

Top: Adapted from J. Maklebust. Pressure Ulcer Update. *RN,* Dec. 1991, pp. 56-63. Illustration by J. Tandy. Copyright, 1991. Used with permission of Medical Economics Publishing/J. Tandy.

Bottom: Adapted from J. Maklebust, M. Sieggreen. *Pressure Ulcers: Guidelines for Prevention and Nursing Management.* 1991. Copyright, 1991. Used with permission of Springhouse Corp. All rights reserved.

Figure 49.3. Best Position While on Side

463

In a chair or wheelchair, follow these guidelines:

When sitting, you should have good posture and be able to keep upright in the chair or wheelchair (Figure 49.4). A good position will allow you to move more easily and help prevent new sores.

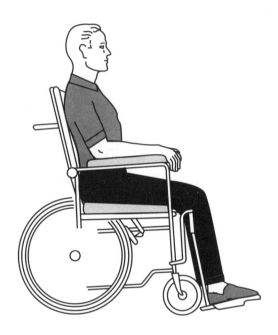

Figure 49.4. *Best Position While Sitting. Ankles should not be flexed or extended. Note the position of the thighs, hands and forearms. Use a specially designed 2 to 3 inch cushion.*

For your specific needs, use cushions designed to relieve pressure on sitting surfaces. Even if pressure can be relieved with cushions, your position should be changed every hour. Remember to:

- Avoid sitting directly on the pressure sore.

- Keep the top of your thighs horizontal and your ankles in a comfortable, "neutral" position on the floor or footrest (Figure 49.4). Rest your elbows, forearms, and wrists on arm supports.

Treating Pressure Sores

- If you cannot move yourself, have someone help you change your position at least every hour. If you can move yourself, shifting your weight every 15 minutes is even better.

- If your position in a chair cannot be changed, have someone help you back to bed so you can change position.

- Do not use donut-shaped or ring cushions, because they reduce blood flow to tissue.

Changing Positions

Change your body position often, at least every hour while seated in a chair and at least every two hours while lying in bed. A written turning schedule or a turn clock (with positions written next to times) may help you and your caregiver remember turning times and positions. You may want to set a kitchen timer. Be sure your plan works for you. It should consider your skin's condition, personal needs and preferences, and your comfort level.

Pressure Sore Care

The second principle of healing is proper care of the sore. The three aspects of care are: cleaning, removing dead tissue and debris (debridement), and dressing (bandaging) the pressure sore.

You should know about sore care even if only your caregiver is caring for the sore. Knowing about your care will help you make informed decisions about it.

Cleaning

Pressure sores heal best when they are clean. They should be free of dead tissue (which may look like a scab), excess fluid draining from the sore, and other debris. If not, healing can be slowed, and infection can result. A health care professional will show you and your caregiver how to clean and/or rinse the pressure sore. Clean the sore each time dressings are changed.

Cleaning usually involves rinsing or "irrigating" the sore. Loose material may also be gently wiped away with a gauze pad. It is important to use the right equipment and methods for cleaning the sore. Tissue that is healing can be hurt if too much force is used when rinsing. Cleaning may be ineffective if too little force is used.

Use only cleaning solutions recommended by a health care professional. Usually saline is best for rinsing the pressure sore. Saline can be bought at a drug store or made at home.

Caution: Sometimes water supplies become contaminated. If the health department warns against drinking the water, use saline from the drug store or use bottled water to make saline for cleaning sores.

Do not use antiseptics such as hydrogen peroxide or iodine. They can damage sensitive tissue and prevent healing.

Cleansing methods are usually effective in keeping sores clean. However, in some cases, other methods will be needed to remove dead tissue.

- Recipe for Making Saline (Salt Water)

    1. Use 1 gallon of distilled water or boil 1 gallon of tap water for five minutes. Do not use well water or sea water.

    2. Add eight teaspoons of table salt to the distilled or boiled water.

    3. Mix the solution well until the salt is completely dissolved. Be sure storage container and mixing utensil are clean (boiled). *Note: Cool to room temperature before using. This solution can be stored at room temperature in a tightly covered glass or plastic bottle for up to one week.*

Removing Dead Tissue and Debris

Dead tissue in the pressure sore can delay healing and lead to infection. Removing dead tissue is often painful. You may want to take pain-relieving medicine 30 to 60 minutes before these procedures. Under supervision of health care professionals, dead tissue and debris can be removed in several ways:

- Rinsing (to wash away loose debris).

- Wet-to-dry dressings. In this special method, wet dressings are put on and allowed to dry. Dead tissue and debris are pulled off when the dry dressing is taken off. This method is only used to remove dead tissue; it is never used on a clean wound.

- Enzyme medications to dissolve dead tissue only.

Treating Pressure Sores

- Special dressings left in place for several days help the body's natural enzymes dissolve dead tissue slowly. This method should not be used if the sore is infected. With infected sores, a faster method for removing dead tissue and debris should be used.

Qualified health care professionals may use surgical instruments to cut away dead tissue. Based on the person's general health and the condition of the sore, the doctor or nurse will recommend the best method for removing dead tissue.

Choosing and Using Dressings

Choosing the right dressings is important to pressure sore care. The doctor or nurse will consider the location and condition of the pressure sore when recommending dressings.

The most common dressings are gauze (moistened with saline), film (see-through), and hydrocolloid (moisture and oxygen-retaining) dressings. Gauze dressings must be moistened often with saline and changed at least daily. If they are not kept moist, new tissue will be pulled off when the dressing is removed.

Unless the sore is infected, film or hydrocolloid dressings can be left on for several days to keep in the sore's natural moisture.

The choice of dressing is based on:

- The type of material that will best aid healing,
- How often dressings will need to be changed, and
- Whether the sore is infected.

In general, the dressing should keep the sore moist and the surrounding skin dry. As the sore heals, a different type of dressing may be needed.

Storing and Caring for Dressings

Clean (rather than sterile) dressings usually can be used, if they are kept clean and dry. There is no evidence that using sterile dressings is better than using clean dressings. However, contamination between patients can occur in hospitals and nursing homes. When clean dressings are used in institutions, procedures that prevent cross-contamination should be followed carefully.

At home, clean dressings may also be used. Carefully follow the methods given below on how to store, care for, and change dressings.

To keep dressings clean and dry:

- Store dressings in their original packages (or in other protective, closed plastic packages) in a clean, dry place.
- Wash hands with soap and water before touching clean dressings.
- Take dressings from the box only when they will be used.
- Do not touch the packaged dressing once the sore has been touched.
- Discard the entire package if any dressings become wet or dirty.

Changing Dressings

Ask your doctor or nurse to show how to remove dressings and put on new ones. If possible, he or she should watch you change the dressings at least once.

Ask for written instructions if you need them. Discuss any problems or questions about changing dressings with the doctor or nurse.

Wash your hands with soap and water before and after each dressing change. Use each dressing **only once**. You should check to be sure the dressing stays in place when changing positions. After the used dressing is removed, it must be disposed of safely to prevent spread of germs that may be on dressings.

Basic Steps of Pressure Sore Care

Prepare

1. Wash hands with soap and water.

2. Get supplies: saline; irrigation equipment (syringe or other device, basin, large plastic bag); dressings and tape; disposable plastic gloves and small plastic [sandwich] bag; towel; glasses, goggles, and plastic apron (optional).

3. Move patient into comfortable position.

4. Place large plastic bag on bed to protect bed linen.

Treating Pressure Sores

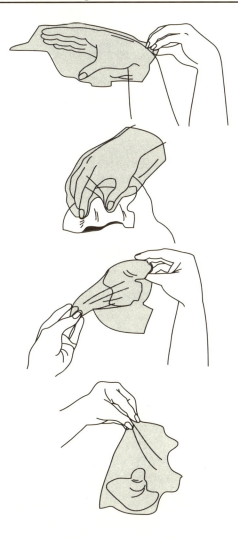

Figure 49.5. *Plastic Bag Method of Removing Bandages. A small plastic bag (such as a sandwich bag) can be used to lift the dressing off the pressure sore. Seal the bag before throwing it away. If you use gloves; throw them away after each use.*

    Place small, clean bag over hand like a mitten. Carefully lift dressing off sore and turn bag inside out to enclose dressing. Seal before throwing it away.

    Adapted from J. Maklebust, M.A. Magnan. Approaches to Patient and Family Education for Pressure Ulcer Management. Decubitus, *July 1992, pp. 18-26. Copyright, 1992. Used with permission of Springhouse Corp.*

Remove Dressing

1. Place hand into small plastic bag (see Figure 49.5).

2. Grasp old dressing with bag-covered hand and pull off dressing.

3. Turn bag inside-out over the old dressing.

4. Close the bag tightly before throwing it away.

Irrigate Sore

1. Put on disposable plastic gloves. (Wear glasses or goggles and plastic apron if drainage might splash.)

2. Fill syringe or other device with saline.

3. Place basin under pressure sore to catch drainage.

4. Hold irrigation device one to six inches from sore and spray it with saline.

5. Use enough force to remove dead tissue and old drainage, but not damage new tissue.

6. Carefully remove basin so fluid doesn't spill.

7. Dry the skin surrounding the sore by patting skin with soft, clean towel.

8. After assessing and dressing the sore, remove gloves by pulling them inside out. Throw away gloves properly.

Assess Sore

1. Assess healing. As sore heals, it will slowly become smaller and drain less. New tissue at the bottom of the sore is light red or pink and looks lumpy and glossy. Do not disturb this tissue.

2. Tell health care provider if the sore is larger, drainage increases, the sore is infected, or there are no signs of healing in two to four weeks.

Treating Pressure Sores

Dressing the Sore

Place a new dressing over the sore as instructed by the doctor or nurse. Remember to:

- Use dressings only once.
- Keep dressings in the original package or other closed plastic package.
- Store dressings in a clean, dry place.
- Throw out the entire package if any dressings get wet, contaminated, or dirty.
- Wash your hands before touching clean dressings.
- Do not touch packaged dressings once you touch the sore.

Good Nutrition

Good nutrition is the third principle of healing. Eating a balanced diet will help your pressure sore heal and prevent new sores from forming. You and your doctor, dietitian, or nurse should review any other medical conditions you have (such as diabetes or kidney problems) before designing a special diet.

Weigh yourself weekly. If you find you cannot eat enough food to maintain your weight or if you notice a sudden increase or decrease, you may need a special diet and vitamin supplements. You may need extra calories as part of a well-balanced diet.

Tell your doctor or nurse about any weight change. An unplanned weight gain or loss of 10 pounds or more in six months should be looked into.

Managing Pain and Infection

Even if you care for your pressure sore properly, problems may come up. Pain and infection are two such problems. Pain can make it hard to move or to participate in care. Infection can slow healing.

Managing Pain

You may feel pain in or near the pressure sore. Tell your doctor or nurse if you do. Covering the sore with a dressing or changing your body position may lessen the pain.

If you feel pain during cleaning of the pressure sore or during dressing changes, medicine may help. It may be over-the-counter or prescription medicine. Take medicine to relieve pain 30 to 60 minutes before these procedures to give it time to work. Tell your doctor or nurse if your pain medicine does not work.

Treating Infection

Healing may slow if the sore becomes infected. Infection from the sore can spread to surrounding tissue (cellulitis), to underlying bone (osteomyelitis), or throughout the body (sepsis). These serious complications demand immediate medical attention. **If you note any of the signs of infection described below, call your doctor right away.**

Signs of Infection

Infected Sore:

- Thick green or yellow drainage
- Foul odor
- Redness or warmth around sore
- Tenderness of surrounding area
- Swelling

Widespread Infection:

- Fever or chills
- Weakness
- Confusion or difficulty concentrating
- Rapid heart beat

Checking Your Progress

A health care professional should check your pressure sore regularly. How often depends on how well the sore is healing. Generally, a pressure sore should be checked weekly.

The easiest time to check pressure sores is after cleaning. Signs of healing include decreased size and depth of the sore and less drainage. You should see signs of healing in two to four weeks. Infected sores may take longer to heal.

Signs to Report

Tell your doctor or nurse if:

- The pressure sore is larger or deeper.
- More fluid drains from the sore.
- The sore does not begin to heal in two to four weeks.
- You see signs of infection (see earlier descriptions).

Also report if:

- You cannot eat a well-balanced diet.
- You have trouble following any part of the treatment plan.
- Your general health becomes worse.

Changing the Treatment Plan

If any of these signs exist, you and your health care professional may need to change the treatment plan. Depending on your needs, these factors may be changed:

- Support surfaces,
- How often you change how you sit or lie,
- Methods of cleaning and removing dead tissue,
- Type of dressing,
- Nutrition, and/or
- Infection treatment.

Other Treatment Choices

If sores do not heal, your doctor may recommend electrotherapy. A very small electrical current is used to stimulate healing in this procedure. This is a fairly new treatment for pressure sores. Proper equipment and trained personnel may not always be available.

If your pressure sore is large or deep, or if it does not heal, surgery may be needed to repair damaged tissue. You and your doctor can discuss possible surgery. Be active in your care

If you understand the basic ideas of pressure relief, sore care, and good nutrition, you can take the steps needed to heal pressure sores and prevent new ones. Not all steps apply to every person. The best program will be based on your needs and the condition of your sores. Be sure to:

- Ask questions,
- Explain your needs, wants, and concerns.
- Understand what is being done and why.
- Know what is best for you. Discuss what you can do to prevent and treat pressure sores: at home, in the hospital, or in the nursing home.

Being active in your care can mean better care.

Care of Healthy Skin

Having healthy skin is important to preventing future pressure sores. Healthy skin is less likely to be damaged and heals faster than skin in poor condition. You can help prevent new pressure sores while helping to heal the ones you have. To improve your skin's health:

- Bathe when needed for cleanliness and comfort.
- Use mild soap and warm (not hot) water.
- Apply moisturizers (such as skin lotions) to keep skin from becoming too dry.

Inspect your skin at least once a day for redness or color changes or for sores. Pay special attention to pressure points where pressure sores can form.

Skin problems can also result from bladder or bowel leakage (urinary or fecal incontinence). If you have these problems, ask your doctor or nurse for help. If the leakage cannot be controlled completely:

- Clean your skin as soon as it becomes soiled.
- Use a protective cream or ointment on the skin to protect it from wetness.
- Use incontinence pads and/or briefs to absorb wetness away from the skin.

For More Information

Information in this chapter is based on *Treatment of Pressure Ulcers. Clinical Practice Guideline, No. 15*. It was developed by a non-Federal panel sponsored by the Agency for Health Care Policy and Research (AHCPR), an agency of the Public Health Service. Other guidelines on common health problems are available, and more are being developed.

Four other patient guides are available from AHCPR that may be of interest to people at risk for or who have pressure sores:

Preventing Pressure Ulcers: Patient Guide gives detailed information about how to prevent pressure sores (AHCPR Publication No. 92-0048).

Urinary Incontinence in Adults: Patient Guide describes why people lose urine when they don't want to and how that can be treated. (AHCPR Publication No. 92-0040).

Pain Control After Surgery: Patient Guide explains different types of pain treatment and how to work with doctors and nurses to prevent or relieve pain (AHCPR Publication No. 92-0021).

Depression is a Treatable Illness: Patient Guide discusses major depressive disorder, which can be successfully treated with the help of a health professional (AHCPR Publication No. 93-0053).

For more information about these and other guidelines, write to:
AHCPR Publications Clearinghouse
P.O. Box 8547
Silver Spring, MD 20907

Additional Resources

The following organizations offer a variety of resources for people concerned about pressure sores.

Booklets and information for patients, caregivers, and families providing care at home:

National Pressure Ulcer Advisory Panel (NPUAP)
SUNY at Buffalo, Beck Hall
3435 Main Street
Buffalo, NY 14214
(716) 881-3558

Referrals to local Enterostomal Therapy Nurses:

Wound Ostomy and Continence Nurses Society (WOCN)
(Formerly the International Association of Enterostomal Therapy)
27241 La Paz Road
Suite 121
Laguna Niguel, CA 92656
(714) 476-0268

Information about nutrition:

National Center for Nutrition and Dietetics (NCND)
Consumer Hotline (toll-free): (800) 366-1655

Chapter 50

Dermatologic Surgery

What Does a Dermatologic Surgeon Do?

Using a variety of surgical techniques, dermatologic surgeons diagnose and treat conditions of the skin, hair, nails, mouth, mucous membranes and genitalia. Dermatologic surgeons are specialists in dermatology who are trained and experienced in the surgical removal of skin growths, as well as in a number of procedures to enhance a person's appearance.

What Types of Skin Problems Do Dermatologic Surgeons Treat?

Cancerous growths, such as basal cell cancer, squamous cell cancer and malignant melanoma, may be removed in a variety of ways. These include destruction of the tumor with an electric needle, scalpel excision laser surgery and Mohs micrographic surgery.
Mohs micrographic surgery involves microscopically tracing out the tumor as it is removed, layer by layer.

Warts and some precancerous lesions are treated by electrosurgical destruction, freezing with liquid nitrogen, or chemical peeling of the skin.

Cysts and moles are removed surgically and sometimes require suture repair of the wound.

© American Society for Dermatologic Surgery. Reprinted with permission.

Aging and sun damaged skin, including wrinkles and age spots, may be treated with liquid nitrogen, chemical peels, skin sanding (dermabrasion), face lifts or injections of filling materials, such as collagen, Fibrel or fatty tissue.

Baldness may be corrected by hair transplantation, surgical transfer of flaps of hair-bearing skin to the bald area, or by reducing the bald scalp by excision and suture. Sometimes balloon-like appliances are used to stretch the skin before scalp reduction surgery.

Fatty tumors and deposits of excess fat may be removed by liposuction.

Scars may be improved by scalpel surgery, dermabrasion or collagen injections.

Superficial spider veins and varicose veins may be treated by injecting sclerosing solutions or destroying the veins using an electric needle or laser.

Tattoos may be removed by dermabrasion surgical excision (if they are small enough), or with lasers.

Which Surgical Technique Is Best for Me?

Most of these techniques were originated and developed by dermatologic surgeons. The physician chooses the best procedure suited to each patient's condition. Although usually done in a doctor's office or in an outpatient surgical center, the dermatologic surgeon may occasionally use a hospital operating room.

Treatment of Acne Scars

Acne

Millions of people suffer the ravages of acne scars long after adolescence has passed, and the acne condition has faded. Acne in its most severe form can leave sufferers with deep permanent scars.

Acne can result in two types of scars—"icepick," or pitting scars, and "depressed," crater-like scars.

Removing Acne Scars

Due to the refinement of a variety of dermatologic surgical techniques, acne scars can be removed by a number of safe, effective procedures that

Dermatologic Surgery

improve the appearance of a patient's skin and subsequently the patient's self-esteem. The dermatologic surgeon will choose among several techniques based upon the nature of the scarring, the patient's medical history, and the status of recent experimental studies in this rapidly evolving area of research.

Dermabrasion: The dermatologic surgeon freezes the patient's skin and then removes or "abrades" the skin with a rotary instrument. A new layer of skin replaces the abraded skin during healing, resulting in a smoother skin appearance.

Excision and punch replacement graft: A depressed acne scar is surgically removed, and a patch of skin from elsewhere on the patient's body is transplanted onto the defect and/or closed with stitches.

Soft tissue augmentation: Bovine collagen, Fibrel, or a patient's own fat (taken from another part of the body) is injected in small quantities below the surface of the skin to elevate depressed scars.

- Collagen is injected to raise a scar up to the level of the surrounding skin. It is anticipated that the correction will last about one to one-and-a-half years. A series of injections may be given to correct the same scar.

- Fibrel is a form of gelatin matrix. It is implanted under the surface of the skin where it is activated by the patient's own blood products. A series of treatments may be given. The scar correction may last up to two years.

- Micro lipoinjection is an experimental procedure in which minute quantities of fat are extracted from another area of the patient's body. The material is then injected under the scar in order to raise it. The length of time that the correction may last is not clearly defined at this time.

- Liquid Silicone is injected to fill in depressed scars. However, the FDA has not ruled on its approval for this purpose.

Treatment of Aging Eyelids

Aging Skin

As a person ages, the skin surrounding the eyes tends to lose elasticity while the area under the eyes accumulates excess fat cells. This sometimes causes the face to appear bloated, giving it an older appearance. In severe cases, sagging skin can hinder normal eyesight.

What Is Blepharoplasty?

Blepharoplasty is a surgical procedure that can restore a youthful appearance to the eye area. The upper and lower eyelids are lifted and excess fat cells or loosened skin are removed from the eye area. The procedure is limited to the eyelids and does not attempt to improve other areas of the face.

How Is Blepharoplasty Performed?

There are three variations of the blepharoplasty procedure.

1. One removes excess skin from either the upper or lower lid as well as the underlying fat pad when indicated. The surgeon makes an incision along the crease in the eyelid, peels back the skin and punctures the underlying tissue to remove the fat pad. The pad is then cauterized (heat sealed). Loose skin is removed from the exterior, if necessary, and the incision is sutured. The procedure takes about two hours and can be performed with local anesthesia on an outpatient basis.

2. The second type of blepharoplasty procedure may benefit patients with protruding fat under the eye and not too much extra skin. This surgery is performed by entering just inside the lining of the lower eyelids. This approach eliminates the scar.

3. A third type of blepharoplasty may be performed with a laser instrument. The intense energy produced by the laser causes blood to coagulate, which may diminish bleeding and swelling during and after the operation. This is a relatively new procedure performed by a small number of physicians in a variety of specialties, including dermatologic surgeons, facial and reconstructive and plastic surgeons.

Dermatologic Surgery

What Are the Post-operative Effects?

The post-operative effects are minimal and temporary. Stitches are usually removed after five days. Minor swelling, bruising and discomfort should disappear within two weeks. Cold compresses will help alleviate these side effects.

What Are the Possible Complications?

Complications may arise from blepharoplasty. A "too tight" or uneven appearance can be caused by the removal of too much skin— or uneven amounts of fat. Further surgeries can usually reverse this problem. Bleeding behind the eye can cause blindness and may impose pressure on the eye, pushing it forward in the socket. These complications are rare.

Dry eyes may occur after belpharoplasty.

Liver Spots and Aging Hands

Time Leaves its Mark

As people age, unsightly blemishes, commonly called liver spots, can appear on the face and on the back of the hands. Another upsetting change for many is the loss of smoothly contoured hands. Dermatologic surgeons can remedy both of these distressing conditions.

What Are Liver Spots?

Liver spots, also called lentigines or lentigos, are sharply defined, rounded, brown or black, flat patches of skin. The epidermis is expanding with more pigment, developing what looks like a large freckle. One may appear by itself, or a few together. Many people have a hereditary predisposition to them. They may develop at an early age, even in childhood, but they are more common in older people especially those who have spent too much time in the sun.

Are Liver Spots Cancerous?

The spots are not cancerous, nor do they lead to cancer. On skin exposed to the sun, however, they may be accompanied by precancerous scaly, red elevations of the skin called actinic keratoses. Dark spots, which might be cancerous, may also appear on the lips. All of these blemishes should be evaluated by a dermatologic surgeon.

Can Liver Spots Be Prevented?

Although nothing can be done about the role heredity plays, excessive exposure to the sun should be avoided from childhood—a precaution that will also diminish the threat of skin cancer. To moderate exposure, the skin should be protected by a sunscreen having a minimum SPF (sun protective factor) of 15.

How Are Liver Spots Treated?

All treatment can be performed by the dermatologic surgeon in the office or other outpatient facility. Results can be permanent if a sunscreen is used continuously after removal.

Sunscreens: The simplest treatment is to protect the skin from further damage and worsening of the spots with a sunscreen. The sunscreen is important after therapy to remove the spots so they will not recur.

Bleaching Creams, Tretinoin, and Alpha-hydroxy Acids: These are prescribed by the physician to fade small spots. Treatment normally takes from two months to a year or longer.

Peeling: In one method, the dermatologic surgeon freezes the area of the spot which then peels away. An alternative is to use certain chemicals. The face takes about one week to heal; the hands usually heal in three to four weeks.

Dermabrasion: The skin is sanded lightly with a special instrument to remove the spot. Upon healing, which normally takes three to four weeks, the liver spot sloughs off.

Laser Surgery: New techniques with lasers are being developed by dermatologic surgeons to slough off the spots. Healing normally takes about one to two weeks.

How Are Youthful Contours Restored to the Hands?

The backs of the hands can be smoothed by a new procedure called micro lipoinjection, a form of soft tissue augmentation The dermatologic

Dermatologic Surgery

surgeon uses a syringe to remove a small amount of a patient's own fat from another part of the body, such as the buttocks or the thigh. The fat is then injected into the back of the hand and molded to restore a youthful contour. Since one's own tissue is used, there is little risk of the body's rejecting it, as can occur when a foreign substance is used. Some patients have permanent results; others need retreatment periodically.

Are There Any Side Effects or Complications?

Occasionally, when a liver spot is removed, a light but much less unsightly spot may appear in its place due to the corrective procedure necessary for more pronounced spots. Scarring does not usually occur.

Side effects from micro lipoinjection are temporary and minor, including minimal bruising and swelling that disappear within a week to 10 days.

Surgical Treatment of Aging and Sun-damaged Skin

The Ravages of Time and the Sun

Although it is not possible to turn back the hands of time, its effects on the skin can be slowed down. And there is help for those who have learned that bronze is not beautiful.

The aging process produces wrinkles and, often, other skin problems. A once-attractive mole may change into an unattractive protrusion, or a once-unnoticeable scar may become more apparent when wrinkles form around it.

Sun damage compounds the aging process. Ultraviolet light from the sun penetrates not only the outer layer of skin, but also those layers underneath which fortify the skin and lend it resilience. Anti-aging creams can treat only damage to the skin's uppermost layers.

Corrective Procedures

Chemical peels are now generally accepted as an effective treatment for sun damaged skin. The dermatologic surgeon applies chemical agents to the skin in a controlled manner. After healing, the new skin is noticeably smoother. A variety of peeling agents can be used to produce light, medium or deep chemical peels. The chemical peel appropriate for your amount of sun damage will be selected by your dermatologic surgeon.

The Facelift is a well-known procedure which removes sagging and redundant sin, particularly from the lower third of the face and under the chin. Uke the chemical peel, this technique has been refined over the years. Some dermatologic surgeons now perform both facelifts and eyelid tucks as in-office procedures under local anesthesia. Facelifts may last from five to seven years.

Dermabrasion is a technique in which a special instrument removes or abrades the upper layers of the skin and smoothes out irregularities in the skin surface. Although usually performed to correct scarring, some physicians prefer the technique to chemical peels for wrinkling.

Soft tissue augmentation involves injecting a substance under the skin. It is used to correct wrinkles, depressions and acne scarring. This relatively new form of treatment is finding increased acceptance and widespread use. There are several alternatives:

- **Collagen treatments:** Bovine collagen may be injected to soften wrinkles. **Zyderm collagen** is used for superficial to medium-depth wrinkling. **Zyplast collagen** is used to treat deeper scars, furrows, creases and wrinkles. The effects may last three to twelve months.

- **Fibrel:** Fibrel is a new form of soft tissue augmentation which has been tested in correcting scars. It is expected to be useful in treating aging skin. Fibrel is a gelatin matrix implant which is activated by the patient's own blood products. A series of treatments is normally necessary.

- **Micro lipoinjection:** In this new, experimental procedure, minute increments of fat are extracted from one part of a patient's body (the thigh, for example) and injected into the area of depression in another area of the skin. Evidence is being gathered to see how long the benefits last.

- **Liquid Silicone** is injected under the skin to fill in wrinkles and depression. However, the FDA has not approved silicone for this purpose.

Dermatologic Surgery

Treatment for Hair Loss

Hair Loss

Although an abundance of so-called "cures" for baldness is available, the only true way to restore a person's hairline is to seek treatment from a physician. As medical doctors specializing in problems of hair loss, dermatologic surgeons are uniquely qualified to diagnose the cause of hair loss and recommend a treatment plan.

Treatment Options

Because each case of baldness differs in severity and the position of the natural hairline, dermatologic surgeons have refined the range of anti-balding techniques in order to tailor treatment to suit each patient.

Techniques in the treatment of balding include:

Hair transplants: A section of hair-bearing skin is transplanted from the back of the head onto the balding area.

- **Punch transplanting** is performed using a round tool called a trephine. It is used to cut a piece of skin containing healthy hair from the donor site, usually from the back or side of the head on a patient with male pattern baldness. Next, a similar but smaller instrument is used to bore out and then discard a piece of skin in the balding area.

- **The hair-bearing graft** is carefully inserted into the site. Initially the donor hair falls out in a few weeks, but regrows about three months later. It continues to grow for as long as the hair would have in the site from which it was removed. For many years the basic size of the grafts were between four and five mm. Over the last few years smaller grafts, such as unigrafts, micro-grafts, bisected and quarter grafts, have also been successfully used.

- **Scalp reduction:** The area of baldness is reduced by surgical excision of the bald area, thus decreasing the size of the bald patch.

- **Skin flaps:** A "flap" of hair-bearing skin is created by making surgical cuts near the balding area. The flap is then pivoted onto the balding section.

- **Minoxidil (Rogaine):** This new anti-balding drug is applied directly to the scalp. Used in conjunction with surgical treatment, minoxidil can be effective in retaining hair which, combined with the transplanted hair, gives a fuller look. Minoxidil is not a cure for baldness, but it has been shown to retard hair loss and to stimulate new hair growth, particularly in the crown of the scalp, in certain, generally younger men.

Treatment of Skin Cancer

Skin Cancer

Skin cancer is the uncontrollable growth of cells in a layer of the skin. It attacks one out of every seven Americans each year, making it the most prevalent form of cancer. However, 90 percent of all skin cancers can be cured if detected and treated in time.

There are several different kinds of skin cancers, distinguished by the types of cells affected. The three most common forms of skin cancer are:

- **Basal cell carcinoma:** usually appears as raised, translucent lumps. This cancer develops in 300,000 to 400,000 persons each year. Although the disease does not usually spread to other parts of the body through the blood stream, it may cause considerable damage by direct growth and invasion.

- **Squamous cell carcinoma:** usually distinguished by raised reddish lumps or growths. This form of cancer develops in 80,000 to 100,000 persons per year. The disease can spread to other parts of the body. Approximately 2,000 deaths occur each year from this form of cancer.

- **Malignant melanoma:** first appears as a light brown to black irregularly shaped blemish. This serious form of cancer results in death if undetected and untreated. It can spread to other parts of the body through the bloodstream and the lymph drainage system.

Dermatologic Surgery

Treating Skin Cancer

A dermatologic surgeon selects the most appropriate treatment for a particular skin cancer or precancerous condition from among the following procedures and techniques:

Curettage, in which malignant tissue is scraped away with a sharp instrument. This method is most effective for small, superficial cancers that have not been treated previously. It is often followed by destruction of the cancerous tissue with an electric needle.

Surgical excision, or cutting into the skin and removing the growth. The skin is then closed with stitches.

Cryosurgery, in which liquid nitrogen is applied directly to the skin to freeze cancerous tissue.

Topical chemotherapy, or the application to the skin surface of chemicals capable of destroying precancerous growths.

Mohs micrographic surgery, or excision of a tumor and its surrounding skin with the aid of a microscope to trace with exceptional accuracy the outline of a cancerous growth.

Laser surgery, in which intense waves of light are beamed at affected skin to cut away or vaporize it.

Treatment of Genital Warts

What Are Genital Warts?

Genital warts are viral lesions which affect approximately eight million Americans per year. Lesser known but more common than herpes, genital warts are transmitted by sexual contact. The small growths, technically known as condylomata, are caused by the human papilloma virus (HPV).

What Are the Symptoms?

Genital warts have an average incubation period of three months, although they can develop anywhere within three weeks to eight months of exposure. The warts typically occur around the genital areas, the anus and the urinary passageways, appearing as single or multiple cauliflower-like pink or red swellings. They can be large and protruding, or flat. Other possible symptoms include itching, burning and tenderness around the affected area. Often, however, the warts may initially be painless and not cause any symptoms so patients may not be aware that they are infected.

Genital warts are most common among those aged 15 to 29. People who engage in frequent sexual activity with multiple partners have a higher risk of contracting the virus.

Why Should Genital Warts Be Treated?

Not only are genital warts highly contagious, but there is strong evidence that the HPV virus causes cervical cancer in women, cancer of the penis in men and anal cancer in both sexes. The HPV virus can also be transmitted from a pregnant woman to her child through the birth canal as she gives birth.

It is important that all sexual partners be treated for genital warts. If only one partner is treated, it is likely that he or she will easily be reinfected by the untreated partner.

In addition, the presence of other concomitant sexually transmitted diseases is much more likely in patients with existing genital warts. Early recognition and prompt treatment can prevent later complications.

What Treatments Are Available?

- **Cryosurgery:** Liquid nitrogen is applied directly to the wart in order to freeze the growth, destroying the infected tissue.

- **Electrosurgery:** A heated electric wire is applied to the growth, destroying the wart.

- **Laser Therapy:** A stream of laser light is directed at the infected site, burning the wart.

- **Surgical Excision:** The skin is cut, and the wart is removed.

- **Liquid Acid Application:** The wart is disintegrated by the application of either podophyllin or TCA (trichloracetic acid).

Dermatologic Surgery

- **Alpha-Interferon:** Patients with recurrent or extensive lesions who have previously been treated with other forms of therapy, as well as those with previously non-treated lesions, are prime candidates for interferon treatments.

    The drug alpha-interferon attacks the HPV virus instead of the infected cells. It may be used alone or in conjunction with chemical and surgical treatments of genital warts.

    Alpha-interferon is injected into the wart or infected area three times per week for up to three weeks. There is evidence that warts treated with the drug will not recur. Side effects are minimal and temporary. Some patients may feel slight chills and other flu-like symptoms.

Pregnant women should not be treated with alpha-interferon. Evidence suggests that the drug can harm an unborn fetus.

- **Condylox:** A prescription podophyllin now available for patient application at home (not to be used on perianal warts).

- **Bleomycin:** A medicine from the anti-cancer drug group. It is injected in a diluted form into the tissue at the base of the wart. This results in gradual death and sloughing of the infected wart.

Pregnant women should not be treated with bleomycin. Evidence suggests that the drug can harm an unborn fetus.

Genital warts can be very resistant. Many require more than one treatment. Close follow-up for a few months following complete clearing is necessary to ensure the absence of recurrences and new smaller warts within or near the treated area.

Tattoo Removal

Tattoos

A tattoo used to be a permanent and irreversible adornment to one's skin. However, in recent years physicians have developed safe and effective tattoo removal techniques which have proved successful in removing unwanted tattoos.

Patients request removal of a tattoo for a variety of reasons—social, cultural, or physical. Some patients develop an allergic reaction to a tattoo several years after the initial application.

Because each tattoo is unique, removal techniques must be tailored to suit each individual case.

Professionally applied tattoos penetrate the deeper layers of the skin at uniform levels. This uniformity allows dermatologic surgeons to use techniques which remove broader areas of inked skin at the same depth.

Homemade tattoos are often applied with an uneven hand and their removal may be more difficult. Blue and black colors are particularly difficult to remove.

Removing Tattoos

Tattoos can be removed by a dermatologic surgeon on an outpatient basis with local anesthesia. The most common techniques used are:

- **Dermabrasion:** The surgeon "sands" the skin, removing the surface and middle layers of the tattoo. Scabbing of the wound raises any residual ink from the deepest layers of the skin. The scabbing is a fundamental element of all tattoo removal techniques. This effect can also be achieved with chemicals, a process known as **chemabrasion,** or with salt, known as **salabrasion.**

- **Surgical excision:** The surgeon removes the tattoo with a scalpel and closes the wound with stitches. This technique proves highly effective in removing homemade tattoos and allows the surgeon to excise inked areas with great control.

- **Laser surgery:** The surgeon removes the tattoo by "vaporizing" it with a high-intensity laser beam. The procedure is virtually bloodless because the laser cauterizes the wound.

Are There Side Effects or Complications?

Side effects are generally minor, but they may include scarring, infection of the tattoo site, or lack of complete pigment removal. A raised or thickened scar may appear three to six months after the tattoo is removed. No procedure is "scarless," but your dermatologic surgeon will choose the best technique to minimize scarring.

Sclerotherapy for Spider and Varicose Veins

What Are Spider and Varicose Veins?

Spider veins are formed by the dilation of a small group of blood vessels located close to the surface of the skin. Although they can appear anywhere on the body, spider veins are most commonly found on the face and legs. They usually pose no health hazard but may produce a dull aching in the legs after prolonged standing.

Varicose veins are abnormally swollen or enlarged blood vessels caused by a weakening in the vein's wall. They can be harmful to a patient's health because they may be associated with the development of one or more of the following conditions:

- **Venous stasis ulcers** result when the enlarged vein does not provide adequate drainage of fluid from the skin. The waterlogged skin receives insufficient oxygen and an ulcer forms.

- **Phlebitis** is an inflammation of the vein.

- **Thrombosis** are blood clots forming in the enlarged vein.

Who Develops Spider and Varicose Veins?

The exact cause of spider and varicose veins is unknown, although heredity, pregnancy and hormonal changes are believed to be factors contributing to both conditions. More than 20 percent of women have some form of varicose condition. Four times more women than men have varicose veins.

What Is Sclerotherapy?

Sclerotherapy is relatively inexpensive, seldom leaves a scar, and can be performed by a dermatologic surgeon on an outpatient basis.
A concentrated saline or specially-developed chemical solution is injected with a very small needle into the spider or varicose vein. The solution washes over the tiny cells which line the inner wall of the

blood vessel. The solution dries out the cells, causing them to shrink and leaving them unable to carry blood. Eventually, the blood vessels disappear by a natural cleansing of the body. The work of carrying the blood is shifted to other healthy blood vessels nearby, consequently improving circulation.

Sclerotherapy generally requires multiple sessions with the surgeon. One to three injections are usually required to effectively treat any vein, and 10 to 40 veins may be treated in one session. The same area should not be injected for four to six weeks to allow for complete healing, although other areas may undergo treatment during this time.

When spider veins are interconnected, injection into one site may fade the entire network. Otherwise, individual treatments are necessary.

Post-treatment therapy includes wearing bandages and support hose for two days to two weeks following treatment. Walking and moderate exercise can also help speed recovery. The treated blood vessels disappear over a period of six months. Although sclerotherapy works for existing spider veins, it does not prevent new ones from developing.

Are There Any Side Effects Following Treatment?

Most patients report few, if any, minor side effects, which eventually disappear. Temporary reactions can include a slight swelling of the leg, or foot, minor bruising, itching, redness and moderate soreness.

What Are Other Treatments for Varicose Conditions?

Laser surgery: Most effective for facial blood vessels, laser surgery seals the blood vessel, thereby destroying it. The treatment may leave scars.

Electrodesiccation: The veins are sealed off with the application of a weak electrical current. The treatment may also leave scars.

Surgical ligation/stripping: Varicose veins may require an in-hospital procedure, usually performed by a vascular surgeon, that involves making an incision in the skin and either tying off or removing the blood vessel.

Dermabrasion Treatment

From the beginning of time, people suffering from the disfigurement of facial scarring have searched for ways to improve these imperfections. Thanks to refinements of a variety of dermatologic surgical techniques, there are several safe, effective procedures available today to improve facial scarring, including dermabrasion and scarabrasion.

What Is Dermabrasion?

While more than one hundred years old, dermabrasion has enjoyed a resurgence of popularity since the 1940s. The technique has been further perfected over the last few decades. Dermabrasion, or surgical skin planing, is a surgical procedure in which the dermatologic surgeon freezes the patient's skin, scarred from acne, pox or other causes, and then removes or "sands" the skin with a rotary abrasive instrument. This abrasive or planing action improves the contour as a new layer of skin replaces the abraded skin. The new-skin generally has a smoother appearance.

When Is Dermabrasion Indicated?

When dermabrasion was first developed, it was used predominantly to improve acne scars, pox marks and scars resulting from accidents or disease. Today, it is also used to treat other skin conditions, such as tattoos, age (liver) spots, wrinkles and certain types of skin lesions.

The conditions under which dermabrasion would not be effective include the presence of congenital skin defects, certain types of moles or pigmented birthmarks, and scars from burns.

What Happens Prior to Surgery?

Before surgery, a complete medical history is taken and a careful examination is conducted in order to evaluate the general health of the patient. During the consultation, the dermatologic surgeon describes the type of anesthesia to be used, the procedure, and what results might realistically be expected. The doctor also explains the possible risks and complications that may occur. Photographs are taken before and after surgery to help evaluate the amount of improvement.

Preoperative and postoperative instructions are given to the patient at this time.

How Does the Procedure Work?

Dermabrasion can be performed in the dermatologic surgeon's office or in an outpatient surgical facility. Medication to relax the patient may be given prior to surgery. The area is thoroughly cleansed with an antiseptic cleansing agent. The area to be "sanded" is treated with a spray that freezes the skin. A high-speed rotary instrument with an abrasive wheel or brush removes or abrades the upper layers of the skin and improves irregularities in the skin surface.

What Happens after the Surgery?

For a few days, the skin feels as though it has been severely "brush-burned." Medications may be prescribed to alleviate any discomfort the patient may have. Healing usually occurs within 7 to 10 days.

The newly formed skin, which is pink at first, gradually develops a normal appearance. In most cases, the pinkness has largely faded by six to eight weeks. Make-up can be used as a cover-up as soon as the crust is off. Generally, most people can resume their normal occupation in 7 to 14 days after dermabrasion. Patients are instructed to avoid unnecessary direct and indirect sunlight for three to six months after the procedure and to use a sunscreen on a regular basis when outdoors.

Liposuction Surgery and Micro Lipoinjection

Unwanted Fat

Both men and women can accumulate fat in areas of the body which cannot be removed by exercise and diet. Prior to the 1980s, extensive surgery was required to remove such fatty deposits, and was limited to a few areas, such as the abdomen and buttocks. There were substantial risks and a long convalescence. There were no generally available safe procedures for removal of fat from the knees, thighs, ankles and other body areas.

Liposuction Surgery

In the late 1970s, techniques were developed to safely and effectively remove undesired fat from nearly all body areas, including the face, neck, chin, breast, abdomen, hips, flanks (love handles), inner and outer thighs, buttocks, knees and ankles. Liposuction has also been used effectively to treat many non-cosmetic fat accumulations, such as lipomas (benign fatty tumors) and gynecomastia (fatty male breasts).

Liposuction is not generally intended for weight loss, but rather is a contouring procedure. It is best utilized in a program of exercise and optimal weight maintenance.

The procedure often first involves injecting a solution, such as saline, in the treatment area with local anesthesia and Adrenaline. This has been shown to increase the safety of the procedure by reducing bleeding. A small incision is made in the skin and a small tube connected to a vacuum is inserted into the fatty layer. Using to and fro movements, the fat is drawn through the tube into a collection system.

Liposuction can be performed in the office or in the hospital. If general anesthesia is not otherwise indicated, its potential complications can be avoided by the use of local anesthesia (often used with light sedation). There are other advantages. The patient is able to sit or stand for the surgeon to check the progress of the contouring. In addition, a costly hospital stay is not necessary.

Liposuction is a remarkably safe procedure with few significant side effects. A recent study in the *Journal of Dermatologic Surgery & Oncology* and similar studies by other specialists have demonstrated this finding.

Micro Lipoinjection

Micro lipoinjection (a form of soft tissue augmentation) was developed in the 1980s. Wrinkles, folds and other depressions resulting from injury or surgery, or resulting from aging or sun damage, can be safely and effectively filled with one's own fat.

Common conditions which can be treated are smile and frown lines. Used with other techniques, other problems like floppy jowls, double chins, drooping nasal tips, and wattles of the neck can be improved with the procedure.

Since one's own tissue is used, there is little risk of the body's rejecting it, which can occur when a foreign substance is used. The fat is taken with a syringe from areas, such as the buttocks or thighs, and then reinfected into the area to be filled.

Retinoids

Retinoids: the "Miracle Drugs" for the Skin

In recent years new synthetic derivatives of Vitamin A (retinoids) have been developed for the treatment of various skin conditions, such as severe acne, sun spots, wrinkles, and psoriasis. Some retinoids may help treat or prevent some forms of skin cancer. Because of their promise, there has been considerable public interest and demand for these drugs.

Some retinoids have been approved as safe and effective for certain conditions by the Federal Drug Administration (FDA). However, retinoids are powerful drugs which, if, not used correctly, can cause severe side effects. These drugs should only be used under the strict supervision of a physician. Also, people should have reasonable expectations of what these drugs can or might do to cure disease or make one look younger or healthier.

Acne and Retinoids

Tretinoin (Retin-A) is a drug approved in 1971 by the FDA for the topical treatment of some forms of acne. Applied to the skin, it can be very effective, but side effects are to be expected. A common side effect primarily associated with daily use is skin irritation, much like mild sunburn. Also, the skin is sensitized by Retin-A to ultraviolet rays. A person using Retin-A should use a sunscreen with a skin protection factor (SPF) of at least 15 and avoid unnecessary sun exposure. The use of tretinoin must be carefully monitored by a dermatologist.

Isotretinoin (Accutane) is taken orally for treatment of severe nodular, inflammatory or scarring acne. Approved by the FDA, it is the only known effective drug for this physically and psychologically disfiguring condition. However, it must be used with utmost caution, especially by women, because it can cause birth defects as well as other side effects.

There are several ways to treat acne. A dermatologist should be asked about appropriate treatment for acne before the use of accutane is considered. If appropriate treatment is started early enough, scarring can be prevented. For acne scars, dermatologic surgeons have a wide variety of treatments which can be tailored to the condition of the individual patient.

Aging and Sun-damaged Skin and Retinoids

Dermatologists have been doing considerable research to establish the effectiveness of topical tretinoin (Retin-A) for the treatment of wrinkles and sun spots caused by the natural aging process and the punishing effects of the sun. However, its use for these purposes has not yet been approved by the FDA.

At this point, it is clear that the drug is not the "fountain of youth," nor is it appropriate for everyone. There is no information regarding its long-term positive, negative or toxic effects. Improvement of wrinkles may disappear when use of the drug is discontinued, and the drug does not improve deeply-wrinkled skin. Dermatologists caution against the side effects of the drug, especially the increase in skin sensitivity to ultraviolet rays, one of the principal causes of the damaged skin patients hope to rejuvenate.

There are several treatment alternatives for aging and sun-damaged skin. Among them are chemical peeling, the facelift, dermabrasion, and soft tissue augmentation. In some cases, it has been found that tretinoin may be effective when used in conjunction with these procedures. A dermatologic surgeon should be consulted as to the appropriateness and effectiveness of different procedures, which will vary from patient to patient.

Skin Cancer

There is the possibility that tretinoin derivatives might one day prove to be a weapon against skin malignancies. Some initial studies have shown that the drug might inhibit, perhaps reverse, the development of sun spots which can develop into skin cancer. For the foreseeable future, however, avoiding tanning lights, moderating exposure to the sun, and wearing a sunscreen (SPF 15 or better) and protective clothing are the best preventative steps against skin cancer by ultraviolet rays.

Psoriasis and Other Scaling Skin Diseases

Etretinate is a retinoid taken orally. Approved by the FDA, the drug has brought good results in many cases of severe psoriasis, but it is usually reserved for use when the disease is not responsive to other therapy. It is not a drug for everyone. It is extremely potent and can have serious side effects, particularly in pregnant women. A dermatologist should be consulted for the treatment of psoriasis and other scaling diseases. Every case has to be considered individually.

Laser Applications in Dermatologic Surgery

What Is Laser?

Laser stands for Light Amplification by the Stimulated Emission of Radiation.

A laser is a device which supplies a powerful and highly focused beam of light whose energy can selectively eliminate tissue abnormalities.

What Are the Benefits of Laser Surgery?

Treatment of skin growths or conditions with lasers may offer the following advantages:

- Reduced risk of infection
- Relatively "bloodless" surgery
- Precisely controlled surgery which limits injury to normal skin
- An alternative to traditional scalpel surgery, in some cases
- Potentially less scarring, in some cases
- Safe and effective outpatient, same-day surgery

What Are the Common Laser Systems?

Argon Laser is used to treat blood vessel growths, port-wine stain birthmarks, malformations of skin blood vessels known as hemangiomas, enlarged blood vessels on the face known as telangiectasia, and the "red nose" syndrome that occurs as a result of acne, rosacea or nasal surgery.

Carbon-Dioxide Laser is one of the most frequently used surgical lasers for skin disease because it can be used in two different ways: "focused" for removing deeper skin cancers and growths, and "defocused" for superficially vaporizing skin in the treatment of warts or shallow tumors.

Argon-Pumped Tunable Dye Laser is used in the treatment of a wide variety of blood vessel conditions of the skin. In addition, this laser can be adjusted to produce the red light used in "photodynamic therapy," an experimental technique for the treatment of skin cancer.

Copper Vapor Laser heats copper to produce both yellow and green light. Yellow light is used for the treatment of blood vessel conditions like port-wine stain birthmarks and telangiectasia. **Green light** is used for the treatment of benign brown spot conditions.

Flashlamp-Pumped Pulsed Dye Laser produces a yellow light used to treat port-wine stain birthmarks, broken blood vessels and some types of hemangiomas. Like the other yellow light lasers, this system can be used to reduce the risk of scarring from treatment.

Ruby Laser has been approved for the treatment of tattoos. When applied in multiple sessions, it can effectively fade darkly colored pigments with little risk of scarring. It may be effective in the treatment of brown spots as well.

What Are the Common Clinical Applications?

There are many different types of lasers. Your dermatologic surgeon has the expertise to recommend the type of laser that can best treat a specific problem.

Are Lasers Effective in All Cases?

Not all conditions respond best to laser. Laser treatment of "spider veins" on the legs has not always been successful. The injection of sclerosing solutions (serotherapy) into these leg veins may be more successful in treating this condition. In addition, moles are best treated by surgical removal rather than laser therapy and deeper skin cancers or melanomas (malignant moles) are usually surgically removed.

Chemical Peeling Treatment

Chemical Peeling

Chemical peeling, also known as chemexfoliation or derma-peeling, is a technique used to improve the appearance of the skin. In this treatment, a chemical solution is applied to the skin which causes it to "blister" and eventually peel off. The new, regenerated skin is usually smoother and less wrinkled than the old skin. The new skin is also temporarily more sensitive to the sun. Dermatologic surgeons have used various peeling agents for the last 50 years and are experts in performing multiple types of chemical peels. A thorough evaluation by your dermatologist is imperative before embarking upon a chemical peel.

What Can a Chemical Peel Do?

Chemical peeling is often used to treat fine lines under the eyes and around the mouth. Wrinkles caused by sun damage, aging, and hereditary factors can often be reduced or even eliminated with this procedure. However, sags, bulges, and more severe wrinkles do not respond well to peeling and may require other kinds of cosmetic surgical procedures, such as a face lift, brow lift, eye lift or soft tissue filler. A dermatologic surgeon can help determine the most appropriate type of treatment for each individual case.

Mild scarring and certain types of acne can be treated with chemical peels. In addition, pigmentation of the skin in the form of sun spots, age spots, liver spots, freckles, and splotching due to taking birth control pills, as well as skin that is dull in texture and color may be improved with chemical peeling. The procedure can be performed on the face, neck, or hands.

Areas of sun-damaged, precancerous keratoses or scaling patches may improve after chemical peeling. Following treatment, new lesions or patches are less likely to appear.

Generally, fair skinned and light haired patients are ideal candidates for chemical peels. Darker skin types may also experience good results, depending upon the type of problem encountered.

How Are Chemical Peels Performed?

Prior to surgery, instructions may include the elimination of certain drugs and the preparation of the skin with topical preconditioning medications. The patient may be advised to clean the area with an antiseptic soap the day before surgery.

A chemical peel can be performed in a doctor's office or in a surgery center as an out-patient procedure. The skin is thoroughly cleansed with an agent that removes excess oils, and the eyes and hair are protected. One or more chemical solutions, such as glycolic acid, trichloroacetic acid, salicylic acid, lactic acid, or carbolic acid (phenol), are used. Dermatologic surgeons are well qualified to select the proper peeling agent based upon the type of skin damage present.

During a chemical peel, the physician applies the solution to small areas on the skin. These applications produce a controlled wound, enabling new, regenerated skin to appear.

During the procedure, most patients experience a warm to somewhat hot sensation which lasts about 5 to 10 minutes, followed by a stinging sensation. A deeper peel may require pain medication during or after the procedure.

What Should Be Expected after Treatment?

Depending upon the type of peel, a reaction similar to a sunburn occurs following a chemical peel. Superficial peeling usually involves redness, followed by scaling that ends within three to seven days.

Medium-depth and deep peeling may result in swelling and the presence of water blisters that may break, crust, turn brown, and peel off over a period of 7 to 14 days.

Some peels may require bandages to be placed on part or all of the skin that is treated. Bandages are usually removed in several days and may improve the effectiveness of the treatment.

It is important to avoid overexposure to the sun after a chemical peel since the new skin is fragile and more susceptible to complications. The dermatologic surgeon will prescribe the proper follow-up care to reduce the tendency to develop abnormal skin color after peeling.

What Are the Possible Complications?

In certain skin types, there is a risk of developing a temporary or permanent color change in the skin. Taking birth control pills, pregnancy, or a family history of brownish discoloration on the face may increase the possibility of developing abnormal pigmentation. Although low, there is a risk of scarring in certain areas of the face and certain individuals may be more prone to scarring. If scarring does occur, it can usually be treated with good results.

There is a small incidence of the reactivation of cold sores or herpes infection in patients with herpes. This problem is treated with medication as prescribed by the dermatologic surgeon. Prior to treatment, it is important for a patient to inform the physician of any past history of keloids, unusual scarring tendencies, extensive x-rays on the face, or recurring cold sores.

American Society for Dermatologic Surgery (ASDS)

The ASDS provides continuing training and education for its members in new dermatologic surgical techniques. Represented in the American Medical Association House of Delegates, the ASDS was formed in 1970 to promote the highest standards of patient care for the surgical treatment of the skin, hair, nails and mucous membranes.

Toll-Free Number: For more information on skin conditions and treatments, along with a referral list of dermatologic surgeons in specific geographic areas, please call the ASDS toll-free hotline, 1-800-441-2737, during weekday business hours (CST).

Chapter 51

Test-tube Skin and Other High-tech Treatments for Burns

When burns are so extensive that more skin is lost than is left, skin grafts become a matter of life or death. For more and more patients, even when burns cover 90 percent of the body, the verdict is "life," thanks to two new types of grafts: synthetic skin and skin actually grown in a laboratory.

These new grafting materials reflect improved knowledge about how burns heal. It has been learned, for instance, that severe burns cause less disfiguring scarring if surgeons remove the crust—called eschar—that forms over burns and close the wounds with skin grafts to keep fluids in and germs out. The earlier this is done, the lower the risk of organ failure and infection, which are the major causes of death from severe burn injury.

Ordinarily, the patient's unburned skin—from areas called "donor sites"—is "harvested," as they say, for the grafts. The harvested skin is stretched in a skin-expanding device and sewn over the wounds. (By perforating a skin graft in a lattice pattern, skin expanders can stretch it up to nine times the original size.)

If there isn't enough unburned skin for all the grafts, additional, temporary grafts can be taken from a source other than the patient: pigskin, cadavers, human donors, and the amniotic membrane surrounding the baby in the womb. Cadavers are the usual source, says Kenneth Palmer, Ph.D., of the Food and Drug Administration's Center for Devices and Radiological Health. Pigskin used for grafting is classified as a medical device, as are skin expanders and other surgical

FDA Consumer, June 1987.

tools. All are regulated by FDA. By the time the immune system rejects the transplanted skin, the patient's harvested skin areas, known as donor sites, are healed, and new skin can be reharvested for more permanent grafts. When many reharvests are needed, drugs that suppress the immune response can be given to buy extra time by delaying rejection of the temporarily transplanted tissue.

The threat of rejection posed by temporary grafts remains constant, pointing up the urgent need for a skin graft material with more permanence. One possibility is an artificial skin developed by plastic surgeon John Burke, M.D., of Harvard Medical School and Massachusetts General Hospital and Ioannis Yannas, Ph.D., of Massachusetts Institute of Technology. The experimental product has been used on about 80 severely burned patients and is undergoing clinical tests for safety and effectiveness.

The Burke-Yannas "skin" has two layers that closely simulate the layers of normal skin, the epidermis and the underlying dermis. (For more on skin anatomy, see chapter 1.) The artificial epidermis, a synthetic rubbery material called Silastic, is applied to the artificial dermis as a liquid, forming a tight bond as it hardens. The dermis is made of materials that appear naturally in human tissue: collagen and a derivative of cartilage. But this collagen comes not from humans but from cows; the cartilage derivative comes from sharks. The two-layer synthetic skin, which is generally not rejected, is sterile and can be stored at room temperature.

Severe burn wounds, then, are closed like this:

- The eschar is removed, the patient's available normal epidermis harvested for thin layers for grafting, and the grafts put through a skin expander and sewn over as many wounds as possible.

- The rest of the wounds are covered with the manufactured skin in 4-inch by 6-inch sheets for wide, flat areas and in narrow strips for limbs and joints.

- As healing allows, the patient's donor sites are reharvested for further epidermal grafts, and sections of the Silastic material are stripped away from the artificial dermis and replaced with permanent grafts.

- Meanwhile, the artificial dermis acts as a scaffolding on which tissue beneath the wound can grow. Fibroblasts move in to produce connective tissue, and blood vessels develop to supply oxygen and nutrients. As the growth increases, the cowhide collagen and shark substance are broken down and absorbed by the body.

Thus, the artificial dermis and epidermis are gradually replaced so that the final skin is, in fact, the patient's own. The skin isn't quite normal, having neither hair nor glands, but the color often matches the patient's normal skin.

A newer version of the Burke-Yannas skin is under development. It involves taking epithelial cells from the patient's own skin and seeding them into the dermis scaffolding at the edges of the Silastic material at the time of the initial grafting. This enables the epithelial cells to begin building a new epidermis while the fibroblasts and blood vessels rebuild the dermis. This Stage II version is still highly experimental, says a spokesman for Massachusetts General.

Other researchers report success with permanent grafts made of skin cells taken from sources other than the patient and then grown in culture in a laboratory.

Grafts of foreign skin are normally rejected because they have substances called Class II antigens that are unique to each individual; a person's immune system recognizes only its own as safe and considers foreign ones to be intruders and attacks them. But in some culture systems, explains Thomas Holohan, M.D., of FDA's Office of Health Affairs, the particular skin cells possessing the antigens die out, and only the cells without antigens continue to grow. "So, researchers can take epidermal cells from skin—from someone else or a cadaver—and grow them in culture. Then, when enough are produced, they're transplanted to the patient, and they grow and aren't rejected," says Holohan.

Success with grafting cultured cadaver skin onto three burn patients at New York Hospital-Cornell Medical Center in New York City was reported by John Hefton, Ph.D., and colleagues in 1983. Last November, Hefton, Michael Madden, M.D., and others reported in the *Journal of Trauma* about 26 patients treated with the cultured skin. Superficial wounds such as the patient's donor sites healed in six to eight days; deep wounds in which some dermis remained, in five to 18 days, though infection and damage to one grafting site interfered with healing." We have followed patients for up to three years after grafting and have not observed any acute episodes of rejections," they wrote. In wounds with no dermis, however, even several cultured skin grafts apparently contributed little, if any, to healing.

The Cornell skin is grown in culture until its surface area is 50 to 100 times the size of the original donor tissue. After 18 to 21 days, the skin is removed by hand from the container it grew in and is applied with the basal-cell side (the bottom layer) touching the wound. The cells adhere within 24 hours, and a stratum corneum develops in seven to 10 days. According to Hefton, "The cultured grafts produced by our culture process are sufficiently thick and pliable to permit manipulation with forceps and hands. No gauze supports are necessary with these grafts; they can be spread over a wound to conform to its shape and size." Not only can the cultured skin heal donor sites twice as fast as sites that heal naturally under gauze dressings, it also can be grown in large quantities and apparently isn't rejected. The Cornell team has now grafted more than 50 burn patients with the cultured skin, Hefton says.

Burn treatment continues to evolve as many research centers experiment with cultured skin and other wound coverings. Treatment with the patient's own cultured skin cells, for instance, was used by a research team led by G. Gregory Gallico, M.D., of Massachusetts General Hospital, to help two young boys survive burns that covered more than 95 percent of the body. The team reported in the Aug. 16, 1984, *New England Journal of Medicine,* "The smooth supple skin generated on the face and hands was particularly impressive."

(For information about other advances in burn treatment, see "Progress in Treating Burns" in the February 1985 *FDA Consumer.*)

—by Dixie Farley

Dixie Farley is a member of FDA's public affairs staff.

Part Seven

Hair, Scalp, and Nail Disorders

Chapter 52

Hair: From Personal Statement to Personal Problem

From the shaved heads of medieval monks, to the long-haired hippies of the 1960s, to the spiked hairdos of today's punk rockers, hair has always made a personal statement.

"It's one of the leading ways people can establish their individuality and express their style," says Jerome Shupack, M.D., professor of clinical dermatology at New York University Medical Center in New York City. "Hair has had sociological importance throughout the ages."

Because of its importance, anything that happens to our hair that we can't control, falling out or turning gray for instance, can be the source of much anxiety.

In the United States, some 35 million men are losing or have lost their hair from male-pattern baldness, according to the American Hair Loss Council. Approximately 20 million women have experienced a similar loss of hair (from female-pattern hair loss), and an estimated 2.5 million Americans have lost their hair due to other causes.

The Basics

Hair is produced by hair follicles—indentations of the epidermis (outer skin layer) that contain the hair root, the muscle attached to it, and sebaceous, or oil, glands. Hair is made up of dead cells filled with proteins, most of which are known as keratins. The cells are woven together like a rope to form the hair fiber. The hair fiber, in

---

FDA Consumer, December 1991.

turn, has three layers: the outer cuticle with its fish-scale like structure; the cortex, which contains the bulk of the fiber; and the center, or medulla. Hair color is determined by melanocytes, cells that produce pigment. When these cells stop producing pigment, hair turns gray.

Although it seems as if the hair on your head is always growing, hair actually has active and rest phases. The growth phase, known as anagen, lasts for two to six years. At any given time, about 90 percent of scalp hair is in the growth stage. The remainder is in the rest phase, known as telogen; this lasts from two to three months.

Once the rest phase is over, the hair strand falls out and a new one begins to grow. As a result, it's considered normal to lose from 20 to 100 hairs a day, says Diana Bihova, M.D., a dermatologist in private practice in New York City. Only a change in your regular pattern of loss is considered abnormal—but many things, including genetic factors, diet, stress, and medications, can change that pattern.

Baldness: Manifest Destiny?

The most common cause of hair loss in both men and women is rooted in genetic predisposition. Called androgenic alopecia, it is known as male-pattern baldness in men and female-pattern hair loss in women. (Alopecia is the scientific term for baldness.) According to the American Hair Loss Council, genetics accounts for 95 percent of all cases of hair loss in this country.

Baldness results from a combination of genetic factors and levels of testosterone (a hormone produced by the adrenal gland in both sexes and also by the testes in men). If hormone levels are right, then the hair follicles will express their genetic destiny by growing for shorter periods and producing finer hairs. In men, who have higher levels of testosterone than women, this eventually results in a bald scalp at the crown of the head and a horseshoe-shaped fringe of hair remaining on the sides. In women, the hair thins all over the scalp; the hairline does not recede. This type of hair loss doesn't usually show up in women until menopause; until then, estrogen tends to counteract the effects of testosterone.

One Approved Drug

The only drug approved by the Food and Drug Administration to treat pattern baldness or hair loss is minoxidil topical solution (Rogaine), which is rubbed into the scalp. Originally approved for hereditary male-pattern baldness in 1988, it was also approved for

Hair: From Personal Statement to Personal Problem

treating female-pattern hair loss in August 1991. However, it should not be used by pregnant or nursing women.

In his dermatological practice, Arthur P. Bertolino, M.D., Ph.D., director of the hair consultation unit at New York University, says that this lotion helps hair grow in 10 to 14 percent of the people who try it. He estimates that approximately 90 percent of the time, Rogaine at least slows down hair loss. (Minoxidil is also available in tablet form to treat severe high blood pressure. Oral minoxidil has a potential for serious side effects and is not approved to treat baldness.)

No one is certain yet just how topical minoxidil works to promote hair growth. "One theory is that it dilates the blood vessels, so it may stimulate nourishment of follicles," says Bihova. Alternatively, Rogaine may convert tiny hair follicles that produce peach fuzz into large hair follicles that produce normal-size hairs. Again, no one knows for sure.

What is certain is that, at least in men, Rogaine works better on patients who fit a certain profile: They've generally been bald for less than 10 years, have bald spots on top of the head that are less than 4 inches in diameter, and still have fine hairs in their balding areas. "The process begins very early," says Bihova. "I see 19-, 20-year-old males who have it."

The most common side effects with this medication are itching and skin irritation. Also, according to Bertolino, once you stop using it, any hair that grew as a result will fall out. Finally, the drug is expensive: In 1990 it cost about $600 a year to use it twice a day.

Transplants

Baldness can also be treated with hair transplants, in which plugs of "donor" follicles from the patient's scalp are used to fill the hairline. Although hair transplants work well in both men and women, the treatment tends to have a more dramatic effect on appearance in men with bald spots than it does on women with thinning hair.

"The less hair you have, the more drama in the change," says Robert Auerbach, M.D., associate professor of clinical dermatology at New York University School of Medicine. However, the American Hair Loss Council warns against attempting to replace lost hair with hair pieces sutured to the scalp. FDA has not approved any products specifically intended for this purpose; however, this does not preclude a physician from using sutures, which are approved devices, for this purpose. According to the council, although the procedure is legal, it can result in scars, infections, and even brain abscesses.

Another treatment for male-pattern baldness, hair implants made of high-density artificial fibers surgically implanted in the scalp was banned by FDA in 1984 because it causes infection. This is the only device FDA has ever banned.

Products That Don't Work

So-called "thinning hair supplements," "hair farming products," and "vasodilators" for the scalp will not promote hair growth, says Mike Mahoney, a spokesperson for the American Hair Loss Council.

Thinning hair supplements are nothing more than hair conditioners that temporarily make your hair feel or look a little thicker. The main ingredient in these products, polysorbate, is also found in many shampoos. Promotional materials for hair farming products claim that they will release hairs that are "trapped" in a bald scalp. Mahoney says these products, many of which are herbal preparations, can do no such thing. And so-called vasodilators do not increase the blood supply to the scalp and do not promote hair growth.

Everyday Hazards

While male- and female-pattern baldness results in permanent hair loss, other factors can cause temporary loss of hair. For instance, the drop in the level of estrogen at the end of pregnancy can cause a woman's hair to shed more readily. Two or three months after a woman stops taking birth control pills, she may experience the same effect, since birth control pills produce hormone changes that mimic pregnancy. A major physical stress, such as surgery, or a major emotional stress (positive or negative) can cause hair loss.

"I've seen women start losing their hair before getting married," says Bihova. Even jet lag can have a similar effect.

In most of these cases, the hormonal imbalance or stressful situation will correct itself, and the scalp will soon begin growing hair again. But, says Bihova, since most women are extremely upset by even a temporary hair loss, many dermatologists treat these conditions with either topical steroid preparations or localized injections of low doses of steroids. Bihova emphasizes that these are local, not systemic, injections of steroids; therefore, the shots do not have the same risk of dangerous side effects as systemic steroids. However, only a board-certified dermatologist should administer this treatment, she says.

The list of causes of temporary hair loss goes on: Pressure on the scalp from wigs or hairdos that pull too tightly can cause it. A fever of 103 degrees Fahrenheit or more often causes hair loss six weeks to three months later. And some medications can cause a temporary loss. These include vitamin A derivatives such as Accutane, cough medicines with iodides, anti-ulcer drugs, some antibiotics, beta blockers, antidepressants and amphetamines, anti-arthritis drugs, blood thinners, some cholesterol-lowering agents, aspirin taken over long periods, some thyroid medications, and chemotherapy.

You Hair What You Eat?

Although nutrition does play a role in hair loss and in the overall health of your hair, only extreme nutritional deficiencies or excesses will cause hair loss. For instance, people with anorexia and bulimia may temporarily lose hair. So will others suffering from malnutrition.

"It's pretty rare in the United States," says Bertolino. "If someone was on a real strange, restrictive diet, it could happen to them."

Megadoses of some vitamins (particularly A and E) and an iron deficiency may lead to hair loss. People who claim they can determine which vitamins are lacking in your diet by analyzing your hair, however, are not speaking from a scientifically sound basis. The test used with this type of hair analysis, atomic absorption spectrophotometry, is a legitimate analytical chemistry method; however, used on hair, the results of this test do not correlate with nutritional status, says Shupack. "Because of the sociological importance of hair, a lot of people try to cash in on it," he says. "[Hair analysis] is all witchcraft as far as I'm concerned."

There are, however, a few legitimate hair tests for substances such as arsenic and lead.

For Beauty's Sake

Every time you shampoo, blow dry, perm, straighten, or dye your hair, you damage it slightly, says Bertolino. For the most part, hair can withstand this type of treatment. But overzealous beautifying can damage the hair fiber, resulting in many broken strands, and a frizzy, split-end look. For instance, if you bleach your hair and then have a bunch of perms done in a short time, you're heading for trouble.

Misuse of hair cosmetics can cause the hair to break as it comes out of the scalp, says Frances Storrs, M.D., professor of dermatology at the Oregon Health Sciences University. Permanent wave solutions break the bonds that hold hair together and then re-form them. But with a perm that is not diluted right or not rinsed off properly, for instance, those bonds may not re-form and the hair would soon fall out as a result. Fortunately, most professional hair dressers know how to use perms correctly, says Storrs.

Most hair dyes are not as irritating as permanent solutions, mostly because they do not break the bonds between hair fibers and are therefore not likely to cause a hair loss, she says. However, a severe allergic reaction to hair dye could cause hair loss. "The allergy is pretty common, actually," says Storrs. Permanent solutions can also cause allergic reactions, though that's a rare side effect.

Other beauty-related manipulations of the hair can cause problems, too: Hot irons, corn rows, and braids may bring on temporary or permanent hair loss. If the hair breaks often enough, the follicles may eventually not be able to produce normal hair, says Bihova. "If someone has a problem with thinning and excessive loss, we advise being gentle," she says. "Don't use rollers; don't use blow dryers on a hot setting; don't wear tight hair styles." Rough shampooing may accelerate any loss, though it's usually not a problem in people with healthy hair.

The Medical Side

Some hair loss is the result of a type of immune disorder known as alopecia areata. Some 2.5 million people suffer from this condition in which antibodies attack the hair follicle, causing the hair to fall out. Alopecia areata often causes small, oval or circular areas of hair loss. However, in some forms of the condition, all the scalp hair falls out; in other forms, all body hair is lost. Although the loss is usually temporary, the condition can recur. Treatments include topical steroids or the use of chemicals to produce an allergic reaction to start the hair growing again.

Finally, chronic, systemic conditions—including one form of lupus, abnormal kidney and liver function, and hypothyroidism or hyperthyroidism—can affect the hair. If you're experiencing hair loss, see a doctor. He or she will want to order some basic blood tests to rule out any medical cause of the condition.

—by Devera Pine

Devera Pine is a freelance writer in New York City who frequently writes about health and science.

Chapter 53

Controlling Dandruff: Over-the-Counter Options

If you're troubled by dandruff, that snowy, dust-like stuff that falls from scalp to shoulders, you're not alone: Nearly everyone has dandruff to some degree.

Dandruff is treatable with over-the-counter (OTC) products and causes no general health problems or permanent damage. But care must be taken not to confuse simple dandruff with other conditions that also cause flaking of the scalp, such as seborrheic dermatitis or psoriasis.

What Is Dandruff?

Dandruff occurs when the scalp sheds dead epidermal (skin) cells in large clumps. Dandruff scales appear dry, white or grayish, appearing as small, unsightly patches, especially on top of the head.

Scalp cells replenish themselves in a pattern similar to that of hair, but more rapidly: The skin of the head renews itself about once a month. Dead scalp cells are constantly being pushed from the deepest layer of the epidermis to the skin's surface, where they gradually die. Usually the scalp sheds them in a nearly invisible way. But for reasons that are still unclear, cell turnover sometimes becomes unusually rapid, and dead cells are shed as the visible flakes called dandruff.

FDA Consumer, October 1994.

Dandruff Shampoos

In 1990, FDA banned 27 ingredients in dandruff shampoos because they were not proven safe and effective. Today dandruff can be treated with OTC drug products containing five ingredients FDA has verified as safe and effective: salicylic acid, pyrithione zinc, sulfur, selenium sulfide, and coal tar. FDA allows drug products to be sold without a prescription if they are safe for consumer use without a doctor's supervision and provide adequate detailed information for use on their labels.

Approved OTC ingredients for dandruff treatment are available in shampoos, rinses, or in products that users apply and leave on the scalp. Each works in different ways to control dandruff symptoms like scaling or itching.

OTC drug products are available in an estimated 750,000 outlets nationwide, including pharmacies and supermarkets, according to the Nonprescription Drug Manufacturers Association (NDMA). NDMA also reports that dandruff is among the top 10 problems consumers are most likely to treat with OTC drug products: 59 percent of the time dandruff sufferers use OTC drug products.

Coal-tar preparations and salicylic acid are approved for treating dandruff, seborrheic dermatitis, and psoriasis; pyrithione zinc and selenium sulfide for dandruff and seborrheic dermatitis; sulfur for dandruff; and salicylic acid and sulfur in combination for dandruff treatment. On Jan. 28, 1994, FDA published a final rule amending the monograph published in the Dec. 4, 1991, Federal Register allowing micronized selenium sulfide in a concentration of 0.6 percent to be included as an active ingredient to control dandruff.

According to Ida I. Yoder, a chemist in FDA's Office of OTC Drug Evaluation and a member of its drug policy staff, micronized selenium sulfide is a very finely ground form of selenium sulfide, with a particle size of approximately five micrometers. Because the selenium sulfide is more finely ground, it can be used at lower concentration levels.

"A drug is intended for use in the diagnosis, cure, mitigation, treatment, or prevention of disease, or intended to affect the structure or function of the body," says Yoder. Shampoos classified as cosmetics cannot make such medical claims. They are marketed for cleansing, beautifying, or promoting attractiveness.

If a product only claims to wash off dandruff flakes, it could be considered a cosmetic, Yoder says. But if it claims to prevent or treat the condition, it's considered a drug.

Controlling Dandruff: Over-the-Counter Options

What Makes the Flake?

Although most people assume dandruff comes from a dry scalp, the opposite is true: People with oily scalps tend to suffer most from dandruff.

"This may be due to an oily scalp supporting the growth of yeast in the scalp, which is thought to be instrumental in the development of scaling and scalp irritation," says Joseph P. Bark, M.D., chairman of dermatology at St. Joseph's Hospital in Lexington, Ky. "A large preponderance of males have dandruff, which may suggest some role of androgen hormones in dandruff."

Children under 10 rarely have dandruff but it is common in adolescents. While some experts say it tends to decrease in middle and old age, Bark disputes this.

"It really is a post-pubescent disease, but I don't believe it diminishes in old age. We see a lot of dandruff and seborrheic dermatitis in stroke patients and in older people," he explains.

Bark says that dandruff has its bright side: If the scalp doesn't shed its dead skin cells, the human scalp would be tremendously thick. "But when the cell turnover goes too far and increases, then you get not only visible excess scaling, but redness and itching," he says. "Redness and itching is actually seborrheic dermatitis, and it frequently occurs around the folds of the nose and the eyebrow areas, not just the scalp."

Although seborrheic dermatitis mimics dandruff with its flaky scales, the inflammation and itching that accompanies it sets it apart from simple dandruff. OTC preparations are available to help mild cases, but seborrheic dermatitis often is best treated by prescription medications.

"All the evidence points strongly to this yeast, known as Pityrosporum ovale, as a causation of seborrheic dermatitis, in that when you treat it with anti-fungal shampoos [such as Nizoral (ketaconazole) a prescription shampoo], you destroy the organism and the condition stops," Bark says.

What do you do if you have dandruff but suspect your problem may be a more severe disorder like seborrheic dermatitis?

"If you have mild scaling, you can usually take care of it with an OTC dandruff shampoo containing salicylic acid," Bark advises. "Use it for several weeks, and if you don't see a clear-cut improvement in the scaling, consult a dermatologist. A dermatologist can diagnose whether you have a fungus infection of the scalp, seborrheic dermatitis, or some other disorder."

A form of seborrheic dermatitis that sometimes alarms new parents is known as "cradle cap." The scaly scalp inflammation is common in newborn babies, although it can occur anytime in infancy. Rubbing warm olive or mineral oil into the baby's scalp and leaving it on overnight can loosen and soften scales, which can be washed off the next day with a mild shampoo. It usually clears up quickly and does not recur.

Psoriasis

Psoriasis is an inflammatory skin disease in which skin cells replicate at a rapid rate. Although the symptoms of psoriasis—silvery scales covering reddened areas of the scalp—seem similar to dandruff, psoriasis is very different. New skin cells are produced about 10 times faster than normal, but the rate at which old cells are shed is unchanged. Live cells then accumulate and form the thick patches covered with flaking skin.

The scales are heaped-up, and the disorder may involve other areas of the body besides the scalp, most commonly the knees, elbows, back, or buttocks. It can also affect legs, arms, and just about any other part of the body. Psoriasis can be chronic or it may have periods of flare-ups and remission periods.

Psoriasis is annoying mainly because of its tendency to return again and again, and because of its unsightly, blotchy appearance. It is more common in whites than in blacks and Asians.

If you think you may have psoriasis, consult a doctor about treatment

Coal tar

Coal tar, one ingredient in OTC dandruff products, is a byproduct of treated bituminous coal. In constant exposure to concentrated solutions in industrial settings over long periods (20 to 25 years), coal tar has been associated with skin cancer. But coal-tar products are considered safe for topical use in shampoos because contact with the scalp is only for a short duration.

For body seborrheic dermatitis and psoriasis, however, products containing coal tar remain on the skin for longer periods. There are no well-defined, long-term studies that demonstrate how long coal-tar products can be used safely. FDA has noted that prolonged use of

Controlling Dandruff: Over-the-Counter Options

such products may not be completely risk free due to possible cancer-causing effects.

Coal tar also produces photosensitivity reactions (reactions that occur with exposure to sunlight). Residual amounts of coal tar may remain on the scalp, hair, or surrounding areas after using. So if you're going out in the sun after shampooing with these products, you may want to take extra precautions.

FDA requires OTC dandruff products that contain coal tar to state on their labels, "Do not use for prolonged periods without consulting a doctor. Use caution in exposing skin to sunlight after applying this product. It may increase your tendency to sunburn for up to 24 hours after application."

Coal-tar shampoos also tend to give an orange tinge to light-colored hair.

Dave Bostwick, a reviewer in FDA's division of anti-infective drugs, Office of Drug Evaluation II, says one alternative to using OTC products to control dandruff is mechanical.

"Washing your hair more often means you remove dandruff flakes that otherwise would remain on the head," he says.

Other than washing your hair more frequently, there is really no way to control dandruff without treatment. So if you find you're flakier than you'd like to be, OTC drug products may solve your problem.

—by Audrey T. Hingley

Audrey T. Hingley is a writer in Mechanicsville, VA.

Chapter 54

Hair Dye Dilemmas

Many graying baby-boomers find themselves lingering in the hair dye aisles of drugstores, wistfully eyeing boxes displaying the colors their hair once was.

Members of the 40-plus generation are not the only ones who change their hair color. The Cosmetic, Toiletry, and Fragrance Association estimates that close to two out of every five American women and a smaller number of men dye their hair.

The decision to change hair color has recently become more complicated because some recent studies have linked hair coloring with an increased risk of contacting certain cancers. To make matters more confusing, other studies do not support those findings. Most hair dyes also don't have to go through pre-market testing for safety that other cosmetic color additives do before hitting store shelves. Consumers are often on their own, consequently, when deciding whether hair dyes are safe.

Coloring Choices

Consumers considering changing their hair color have a choice of four main types of coloring agents to use. What distinguishes them is how long they last and how they color hair. Coal-tar ingredients are found in some products in all categories except gradual dyes.

NIH Publication Number (FDA) 94-5014. Reprint of *FDA Consumer*, April 1993.

Temporary hair colors are applied in the form of rinses, gels, mousses, and sprays. These products merely sit on the surface of the hair and are usually washed out with the next shampoo, although some may last two to three washings. If the hair gets wet during a rainstorm, for example, the color can run from the hair onto clothing or the face.

Semi-permanent dyes penetrate into the hair shaft and do not rinse off with water like temporary colorings. They do wash out of the hair, however, after about five to ten shampoos. Semi-permanent dyes usually come in liquid, gel or aerosol foam forms. After applying the product to the hair, the user waits 20 to 40 minutes before working it in like a shampoo and then thoroughly rinsing with water.

Permanent dyes require a bit more work, but the pay-off is hair color that lasts until the new hair roots grow in. Because permanent dyes contain hydrogen peroxide, they cover gray hair more effectively and can be used to lighten hair color, unlike other dyes.

To apply permanent dyes, the user mixes together a hydrogen peroxide liquid with another liquid, works the mixture into the hair, and after about half an hour rinses the dye out with water. Permanent dyes not only penetrate deeply into the hair shaft, but get locked within it due to a series of chemical reactions that occur while the dye is applied. Consequently, permanent dyes can't be washed out with shampoo.

A fourth type of hair dye is known as a **gradual or progressive dye**. This dye, in the form of a rinse, slightly darkens hair by binding to compounds on the hair's surface. Gradual dyes are usually applied daily until a dark-enough shade is achieved, after which it may be used less often to maintain the color. Unlike temporary dyes, gradual dyes don't wash off readily or run when the hair gets wet.

Compounds suspected of causing cancer are found in temporary, semi-permanent and permanent dyes.

The Link to Cancer

FDA is responsible for overseeing the safety of cosmetics sold in this country and can prohibit the sale of any cosmetics found harmful except most hair dyes. Although the adulteration provision of the Food, Drug, and Cosmetic Act enables FDA to seek removal of a cosmetic from the market if it is shown to be harmful under conditions of use, hair colorings made from coal tar were given special exemption from such bans when the act was passed in 1938.

Hair Dye Dilemmas

The main ingredient in the coal-tar hair dyes manufactured at the time prompted an allergic reaction in some susceptible individuals. Fearing FDA would ban the sale of the hair dyes because some users might develop a rash or have other allergic reactions, the industry successfully lobbied before the act passed to get coal-tar hair dyes exempted from the adulteration provision. Manufacturers were required, however, to include a warning in the labels that the products can cause skin irritation in certain allergic individuals. Most hair dyes in use today derive their ingredients from petroleum sources, but have been considered coal-tar hair dyes by FDA because they contain some of the same compounds found in these older dyes.

Cancer in Animals

In 1978, FDA proposed to require a warning on the labels of hair dyes containing the compounds 4-methoxy-m-phenylenediamine (4MMPD) or 4-methoxy-m-phenylenediamine sulfate (4MMPD sulfate), two coal-tar ingredients. This followed findings by researchers at the National Cancer Institute in Bethesda, Md., that rodents fed either of the chemicals were more likely to develop cancer than animals not fed the substances.

The researchers put the compounds in the animals' feed rather than on the animals' skin because they were trying to assess the effects of hair dye ingredients inside the body. (Other studies have shown that a small percentage of hair dye is absorbed from the scalp and passed into the bloodstream, where it can travel to other organs and tissues.) To detect a cancer-causing effect of the compounds in a short period in a limited number of animals, researchers fed the animals large doses of the hair dye ingredients.

Some researchers say that extrapolating results from ingested hair dye studies to absorbed hair dye use cannot accurately assess cancer risk because the compounds being tested are altered or are absorbed differently in the gut than they are when applied to the scalp. Moreover, tests of individual hair dye ingredients don't measure the health hazards of the highly reactive compounds that are formed when the various ingredients in a specific hair dye are mixed together and applied to hair.

In other studies, when investigators painted 4MMPD on the skin of rodents, there was no evidence that the compounds caused cancer in the animals. But critics claim that not enough of the chemical penetrates the skin from the small areas on which it is applied to accurately assess the compound's ability to prompt cancers in a limited number of animals.

After FDA adopted the requirement of a warning about 4MMPD and 4MMPD sulfate, manufacturers stopped using the chemicals in their hair dyes. In addition, the hair dye industry has stopped using several other ingredients found to cause cancer in animals. But some of the cancer-causing compounds have been replaced by similarly structured chemicals. However, some scientists feel that the similar structure of these ingredients makes it likely that their cancer-causing potential won't differ much from the chemicals they are replacing. The agency continues to monitor the situation and review studies as they are completed.

Cancer in People

Several studies have tried to pinpoint the risk of various cancers to hair dye users by calculating the difference in frequency of cancer in people who color their hair and those who don't.

Some of these studies found an increased risk of cancer associated with hair dye use, but failed to consider the effects of other cancer-causing agents, such as cigarette smoke, when comparing the two groups. In other studies, the numbers of people included were too small to lend much statistical credence to the findings. Several studies found no risk of cancer. Few studies looked at long-term use of hair dyes (greater than 20 years).

The findings so far are inconclusive, according to chemist John Bailey, Ph.D., who directs FDA's colors and cosmetics program. "The studies raise some questions about the safety of hair dyes," he says, "but at this point, there's no basis for us to say that hair dyes pose a definitive risk of cancer. In the final analysis, consumers will need to consider the lack of demonstrated safety when they choose to use hair dyes."

Hair Dye Precautions

The less hair dye used over a lifetime, the less likely a person will be exposed to enough dye to cause cancer, according to Bailey. "My personal recommendation is that consumers use good judgment and exercise moderation," he says. "You may reduce the risk of cancer by exposing yourself to less hair dye—you probably shouldn't change your

Hair Dye Dilemmas

hair color every week, for example." People can also reduce their risk by delaying dyeing their hair until later in life when it starts to turn gray, he adds.

Consumers might also want to consider using henna, which is largely plant-derived, or hair dyes that are lead-acetate-based. These colorings don't fall into the coal-tar dye category and therefore any additive ingredients they contain have been tested for safety before marketing, in accordance with FDA requirements. Henna products on the market can give a range of colors, from dark brown through various reddish-brown and lighter red to reddish-blond shades. They cannot, however, lighten hair. Lead acetate dyes gradually darken hair and are commonly used in progressive type hair colorings, such as those advertised as being for men. None of these colors may be used on eyelashes or eyebrows.

People who dye their hair should follow these safety precautions:

- Don't leave the dye on your head any longer than necessary.
- Rinse your scalp thoroughly with water after use.
- Wear gloves when applying hair dye.
- Carefully follow the directions in the hair dye package.
- Never mix different hair dye products, because you can induce potentially harmful reactions (if not an unappealing hair color).

Be sure to do a patch test for allergic reactions before applying the dye to your hair. Almost all hair dye products include instructions for conducting a patch test. and it's important to perform the test each time you dye your hair. (Salons should also perform the patch test before dyeing the hair of their patrons.) To test, put a dab of hair dye behind your ear and don't wash it off for two days. If no itching, burning, redness, or other signs of allergic reaction develop at the test spot during this time, you can be relatively sure that you won't develop a reaction to the dye applied to your hair. If you do react to the patch test, do the same test with different brands or colors until you find one to which you're not allergic.

Never dye your eyebrows or eyelashes. An allergic reaction to the dye could prompt swelling, inflammation, and susceptibility to infection in the eye area. These reactions can severely harm the eye and even cause blindness. (Inadvertently spilling dye into the eye could also cause permanent damage.) FDA prohibits the use of hair dyes for eyelash and eyebrow tinting or dyeing, even in beauty salons or other establishments.

Permanent Eyeliner

The attempt to achieve a socially determined level of cosmetic perfection is not limited to changing hair color. Women who want their eyes to be enhanced by eyeliner, but don't have the time to put it on every day or are allergic to make-up, are having permanent eyeliner tattooed onto their eyelids.

Introduced to this country from the Orient more than 10 years ago, permanent eyelining is now offered in many beauty salons. Using disposable needles, pigment is implanted into the skin at the base of the upper or lower eyelashes. The pigments used are derived from vegetable products. A local anesthetic is often given to relieve pain during the tattooing, which takes from 20 minutes to an hour. Some swelling may follow the procedure. Scabs that form in the treated area fall off within a week.

But "we can't vouch for the safety of permanent eyelining," points out chemist John Bailey, Ph.D., director of FDA's colors and cosmetics program, because the procedure hasn't undergone any formal safety testing. FDA is currently considering requiring safety testing for tattooed eyeliner. If such testing finds permanent eyelining unsafe, FDA could ban the procedure because it uses colors that are under the agency's jurisdiction.

Although FDA has received no reports that this permanent make-up causes harm, there's concern that tattooed eyelining could induce an allergic reaction that might permanently damage the eyes and eyelids. If such a reaction did occur, it would be difficult to treat, and surgery might be required to remove the pigment in the tattoo. Such surgery might harm the eye or cause unsightly scarring.

"There's a misperception on the part of the public that tattooed eyelining is a risk-free procedure," says Bailey.

Researchers continue to study the cancer-causing potential of hair dye ingredients, and FDA continues to keep abreast of such findings. Until definitive evidence comes in, consumers may want to proceed with caution when selecting a hair dye.

—by Margie Patlak

Margie Patlak is a freelance writer in Elkins Park, PA.

Chapter 55

Alopecia Areata and Other Hair-Loss Disorders

Alopecia areata is a condition in which hair is lost from the head (scalp) and sometimes from other parts of the body. In alopecia areata, a malfunction of the hair follicle results in hair loss. The follicle consists of cells and tissue that surround the root of a hair and normally give rise to the hair in a manner similar to a flower stem growing out of a bulb. Alopecia areata occurs in 1 to 2 percent of the population (more than two million people) and has several forms: patchy alopecia areata (AA), which is patchy hair loss on the scalp or elsewhere; alopecia totalis (AT), which is loss of all hair on the scalp; and alopecia universalis (AU), which is loss of all hair on the scalp and body. (Hereafter, the term "alopecia areata" will be used to refer to all three forms unless otherwise specified.)

Biology of the Hair Follicle

The hair follicle is made up of several types of cells. These include cells called keratinocytes, which produce the major hair proteins, and melanocytes (pigment-producing cells), which determine hair color. The hair follicle cells interact with fibroblasts, nerve cells, blood vessels,

The National Alopecia Areata Foundation and the National Institute of Arthritis and Musculoskeletal and Skin Diseases (NIAMS) sponsored a workshop on alopecia areata and its related forms in November 1994. The workshop, held at the National Institutes of Health, assessed current knowledge and future research directions. The presenters focused on hair follicle biology, causes of alopecia areata, the role of the immune system, treatment, current experimental approaches, and research directions.

and connective tissues. Scientists are studying the cells, proteins, and genes that control the growth, death, and regeneration of hair. For example, they are investigating how the hair follicle cells, particularly keratinocytes, communicate with cells surrounding the follicle and what happens when this communication is interrupted.

The hair follicle is a complicated biological structure. Scalp hair follicles, of which there are normally about 100,000, grow for four to six years. Not all follicles are at the same stage of development at the same time. After growth, the hair follicle withers at its base over a period of two to three weeks, then rests for two to three months. After this resting phase, cells located in a little bulge extending from the old follicle rapidly multiply and move downwards to form a new growing follicle.

Once the follicle has reached its full length, dividing cells at its base are pushed upward to create a sheath, which helps mold the new hair strand that eventually grows up from the root. As the hair grows inside the sheath, it is pressed into shape and becomes stiff and strong before it emerges onto the surface of the scalp. At the end of the growth cycle, the hair falls out as the follicle withers. Scientists believe hair growth is controlled by cells called dermal papilla cells that form in a cluster outside the bottom of the follicle and are embraced by the hair bulb. In turn, growth proteins in the blood supply surrounding a follicle seem to activate the dermal papilla cells into a growth phase.

Genetic and Environmental Causes and the Role of the Immune System

Scientists are unravelling the causes of alopecia. Some people appear to have a genetic (hereditary) susceptibility to the disorder. The earlier the age of onset, the more severe the disease and the more likely someone else in the family will have the disease. In one study, 45 percent of patients who had long-standing AT or AU experienced their first patch of hair loss by age 10; 37 percent of these patients had alopecia areata in the family, compared with only 7 percent in a late-onset group. Research has shown that identical twins may develop alopecia areata at the same time, sometimes in the same part of the scalp. Two or three generations in one family may be affected.

Scientists have identified genes which may increase the susceptibility to develop alopecia areata. Research is also revealing that there may be environmental triggers (for example, infection, injury, stress) for the disease. These findings hold promise of possible therapies that

Alopecia Areata and Other Hair-Loss Disorders

will strengthen the body's immune system and block triggers of the disease. Most cells in the body have markers on their surface, some of which correlate with specific autoimmune diseases. These markers, called HLA (human leucocyte antigen), help the body distinguish its own cells from foreign invaders. Studying HLA markers in people with alopecia areata may help scientists understand the susceptibility, outlook, and potential treatments for the disease. One study showed an increased prevalence of one type of HLA marker in a group of patients who had AT or AU for more than two years. Patients with patchy alopecia areata did not show an increased prevalence of these HLA markers. These findings suggest that HLA markers could be used to identify patients who are likely to develop more severe, long-lasting disease.

Treatment of Alopecia

Treatments for alopecia do not cure the disorder. They may stimulate hair growth, but they do not prevent new patches from developing. Most current treatments have been in use for a number of years. For patients with less than 50-percent hair loss, treatments include injection of a corticosteroid into the area of hair loss, topical anthralin, minoxidil alone or with anthralin, topical corticosteroid creams, or tretinoin cream.

For those with more than 50 percent hair loss, systemic (oral or injected) corticosteroids may be used under a doctor's supervision. Phototherapy and minoxidil solution with topical corticosteroids are also treatment options. Applying a sensitizing substance (such as diphenylcyclopropenone or DCPP) to the scalp to cause an allergic or immune response is being studied abroad but this treatment is not widely available in the United States. Treatments involving cyclosporin, thymopentin, inosiplex, nitrogen mustard, and calcipotriol have been tried on only a very limited basis and are still considered experimental.

Even without treatment, hair regrowth may occur spontaneously. In patients with less than 50-percent hair loss, there is a 60-percent chance of spontaneous recovery within two years.

New Experimental Approaches

One of the difficulties scientists have in conducting research on alopecia areata is that the AA cells are difficult to grow in a laboratory and, therefore, it may take months to get a specimen to study. However, researchers have made technological advances in growing hair follicles, grafting hair follicles onto laboratory mice, conducting research on a single hair, and reconstructing hair follicles in the laboratory. Until recently, there were no reliable animals for the study of alopecia areata. Scientists have been seeking both a type of mouse and rat to use in research because these animals have many more follicles than humans and could thus speed up the process of research.

Research Directions

In the workshop wrap-up session, participants noted research advances since the first alopecia workshop, which was held in 1990. These include progress toward identification of appropriate animals for research, HLA findings, greater understanding of the antigen/antibody response and the role of cytokines, and advances in methods to grow hair in the laboratory.

Future research may concentrate on identifying triggering events for alopecia (for example, viral, bacterial, toxic, or psychological) and ways to control or reduce the body's immune response. Investigators hope to make progress in identifying factors that make people susceptible to AA, signals that interrupt the normal hair follicle cycle, and ways to reverse the disease or control its severity.

Other sources of information include:

National Alopecia Areata Foundation
710 C St., #11
P.O. Box 15070
San Rafael, CA 94901
(415) 456-4644

This is the main voluntary organization for alopecia areata. It provides information to patients and physicians and supports research related to alopecia areata. It offers free pamphlets on the disorder, including one on parenting a child with alopecia; produces a monthly newsletter; and makes physician referrals. The Foundation also has video- and audiotapes for distribution. A special support group network has been formed. For information about a support group in your area contact Rose Kozar, National Support Group Coordinator, phone: (404) 816-6803.

Alopecia Areata and Other Hair-Loss Disorders

American Academy of Dermatology
930 Meacham Road
P.O. Box 4014
Schaumburg, IL 60168-4014
(708) 330-0230

This is a major, national professional association for dermatologists. Single publications on hair loss and permanent hair replacement are available free from the Academy. Physician referral is another service provided.

American Hair Loss Council
100 Independence Place
Suite 315A
Tyler, TX 75703
(214) 561-1107

This non-profit organization provides information on hair loss and safe replacement products, including cosmetic and pharmaceutical products, surgical and non-surgical alternatives, and wigs and hair pieces. It publishes a quarterly newsletter, which is available by subscription.

Information Center for Rogaine (minoxidil) (800) 635-0655
Upjohn Company, the manufacturer of Rogaine, has a consumer information number to answer general questions about Rogaine, such as the drug's capabilities, ingredients, and long-term effects.

Chapter 56

Hair Loss in Men, Women, and Children

Androgenetic Alopecia

Androgenetic Alopecia. The modern medical term for either male or female pattern hair loss can be broken down in two parts.

First, Androgenetic, consisting of ANDROGEN (Any of the various hormones that control the appearance and development of masculine characteristics such as testosterone). And GENETIC—the inheritance of genes from either the mother or the father's side of the family. Add age, which when coupled with genetics, represents a time clock that will signal the hair follicle to produce an enzyme named 5 alpha reductase. When the testosterone present in the follicle combines with the enzyme 5 alpha reductase, it produces dihydrotestosterone (DHT). Hair follicle receptors are sensitive to DHT and thereby start the process of male or female pattern hair loss.

Second, Alopecia meaning hair loss, of which there are many types.

Put simply, scientists are working against aging, hormones and genetics. This is no easy task. Add the fact that male or female pattern hair loss is not life threatening, and it is easy to see why many physicians do not view hair loss as a priority in scientific research.

What is working for you in terms of research is that large pharmaceutical firms now know that a cure for hair loss could mean a

---

©1994 American Hair Loss Council. Reprinted with permission. All rights reserved. Material may not be reproduced in any manner without the express written permission of the AHLC.

fortune in revenue for their companies and stockholders. This is fuel enough and the race HAS begun.

Although we may not see a cure in our lifetime, it is possible. Science is closer to understanding hair loss due to many recent advancements. To say the cure is around the comer would only be speculation but hope certainly is alive.

Until then, since there are other causes of hair loss, it is advisable to consult with a dermatologist who is competent and experienced with diagnosing hair loss. Confirming the type of hair loss you have will make it possible for you to know which treatment options may be best for you.

MALE PATTERN HAIR LOSS

Dating as far back as history will take us, baldness has been a part of the aging process that many men fear the most. Before Rogaine, hair transplants and hair additions, men coped in various ways from

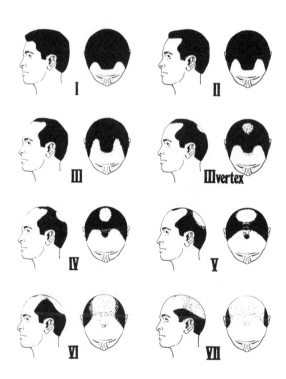

Figure 56.1. The Norwood Classifications of Hair Loss

Hair Loss in Men, Women, and Children

magic ointments to the styling of their hair. Julius Caesar grew his hair long in the back and combed it all forward. Napoleon did the same thing. Somehow we often disregard history and the fact that this has been an age old condition. We can't imagine or accept the fact that there is not a cure.

Understanding the cause of male pattern hair loss may better indicate exactly why it presently has no cure.

Other Causes

Alopecia areata: Generally thought to be an autoimmune disorder. Causes "patchy" hair loss, often in small circular areas in different areas of the scalp.

Alopecia totalis: Total hair loss of the scalp, (an advanced form of alopecia areata).

Alopecia universalis: Hair loss of the entire body, (also an advanced form of alopecia areata).

Traction alopecia: Hair loss caused by physical stress and tension on the hair such as prolonged use of hair weaving, corn rows etc. Done too tightly on weak hair these can cause permanent hair loss.

Telogen effluvium: (usually temporary hair loss) CAUSES: Physical stress, emotional stress, thyroid abnormalities, medications and hormonal causes normally associated with females.

Anagen effluvium: Generally due to internally administered medications, such as chemotherapy agents, that poison the growing hair follicle.

All of these represent only a few of the different types of hair loss. Androgenetic alopecia represents close to 95 percent of all hair loss however.

FEMALE PATTERN HAIR LOSS

The most common type of hair loss seen in women is androgenetic alopecia, also known as female pattern alopecia or baldness. This is seen as hair thinning predominantly over the top and sides of the head. It affects approximately one-third of all susceptible women, but is most commonly seen after menopause, although it may begin as early as puberty. Normal hair fall is approximately 100-125 hairs per day. Fortunately, these hairs are replaced. True hair loss occurs when lost hairs are not regrown or when the daily hair shed exceeds 125 hairs. Genetically, hair loss can come from either parent's side of the family.

There are two different types of hair loss, medically known as **Anagen effluvium** and **Telogen effluvium**. Anagen effluvium is generally due to internally administered medications, such as chemotherapy agents, that poison the growing hair follicle. Telogen effluvium, is due to an increased number of hair follicles entering the resting stage.

The most common causes of telogen effluvium are:

- **Physical stress:** surgery, illness, anemia, rapid weight change.

- **Emotional stress:** mental illness, death of a family member.

- **Thyroid abnormalities.**

- **Medications:** High doses of Vitamin A, Blood pressure medications, Gout medications.

- **Hormonal causes:** pregnancy, birth control pills, menopause.

When the above causes of telogen effluvium are reversed or altered you should see the return of normal hair growth.

Diet Considerations

Hair loss may also occur due to dieting. Franchised diet programs which are designed or administered under the direction of a physician with prescribed meals, dietary supplements and vitamin ingestion have become popular. Sometimes the client is told that vitamins are a necessary part of the program to prevent hair loss associated with dieting. From a dermatologists's standpoint, however, the vitamins cannot prevent hair loss associated with rapid, significant weight loss. Furthermore, many of these supplements are high in vitamin A which can magnify the hair loss.

Hair Loss in Men, Women, and Children

Physical and Emotional Stress

Surgeries, severe illnesses and emotional stress can cause hair loss. The body simply shuts down production of hair during periods of stress since it is not necessary for survival and instead devotes its energies toward repairing vital body structures. In many cases there is a three month delay between the actual event and the onset of hair loss. Furthermore, there may be another three-month delay prior to the return of noticeable hair regrowth. This then means that the total hair loss and regrowth cycle can last six months or possibly longer when induced by physical or emotional stress. There are some health conditions which may go undetected that can contribute to hair loss. These include anemia or low blood count and thyroid abnormalities. Both of these conditions can be detected by a simple, inexpensive blood test.

Hormonal Considerations

Hormonal changes are a common cause of female hair loss. Many women do not realize that hair loss can occur after pregnancy or following discontinuation of birth control pills. It is important to remember that the hair loss may be delayed by three months following the hormonal change and another three months will be required for new growth to be fully achieved.

TREATMENT OPTIONS AVAILABLE FOR ANDROGENETIC ALOPECIA

- Learning to live with hair loss. Often the assistance of a professional counselor can be helpful in coping with hair loss.

- Hair styling and cosmetic techniques such as permanent waves and hair colors. The proper haircut alone can make a vast difference in diffusing hair

- Rogaine, the only FDA approved topical treatment for male or female pattern hair loss. Although Rogaine is not effective in stimulating new hair growth in many males, it appears to be more effective in retarding hair loss in a substantial amount of both male and females.

- Hair Additions have made many advances in both simulation of natural appearance and more secure attachment methods.

- Hair Replacement Surgery has also made many advances towards more natural appearing results. Modern surgical techniques have made transplantation for females a viable treatment option providing they are qualified candidates and have realistic expectations.

- A combination of Hair Additions with Hair Replacement Surgery.

To find out more about these options contact the American Hair Loss Council for consumer's guidelines to finding qualified specialists.

MYTHS RELATED TO HAIR LOSS

- Frequent shampooing contributes to hair loss.
- Hats and wigs cause hair loss.
- 100 strokes of the hair brush daily will create healthier hair.
- Permanent hair loss is caused by perms, colors and other cosmetic treatments.
- Women are expected to develop significant hair loss if they are healthy.
- Shaving one's head will cause the hair to grow back thicker.
- Standing on one's head will cause increased circulation and thereby stimulate hair growth.
- Dandruff causes permanent hair loss.
- There are cosmetic products that will cause the hair to grow thicker and faster.
- Stress causes permanent hair loss.
- Hair loss does not occur in the late teens or early twenties.
- Hair loss affects only intellectuals.
- There is a cure for androgenetic Alopecia.

These are only a few of the common myths heard by physicians and other hair loss specialists on a daily basis. The AHLC suggests that you first have your hair loss diagnosed by a competent dermatologist who sees hair loss patients on a regular basis. Once you know the diagnosis, you will have a better understanding of exactly which treatment option may be best for you.

Chemotherapy-Related Hair Loss

Chemotherapy consists of the administration of drugs that destroy rapidly reproducing cancer cells. Cancer cells are some of the most rapidly reproducing cells in the body, but other cells, such as those which contribute to the formation of hair shafts and nails, are also rapidly reproducing. Unfortunately, while chemotherapy drugs preferentially destroy cancer cells, the drugs also can destroy those cells responsible for normal growth of hair and nails. Cancer patients sometimes shed the hair and nails during treatment. Chemotherapy drugs are poisonous to the cells of the hair root responsible for hair shaft formation. Usually, the hair is lost rapidly in large quantities during treatment. No hair growth stimulants, shampoos, conditioners or other cosmetic treatments can prevent or retard the hair loss. The good news, however, is that once chemotherapy is completed, the hair usually grows back.

How and When Hair Growth Occurs

Adequate hair growth may take six months to one year.

Returning hair may be different from the hair that was lost. Due to the absence or alteration of pigment the hair may grow back white, gray or a different color. Eventually, as the pigment cells return to normal, the original color should return.

It is common for the new hair returning to be finer in texture initially, but like color, the texture should return to its original thickness. It is sometimes difficult to be patient, but as the body is returning to normal and getting over the significant insult, time is a necessary ingredient.

Hair Care Tips for New Hair Growth

- Shampoo hair twice weekly with a mild shampoo such as those intended for dry or damaged hair.

- The scalp should also be thoroughly massaged to remove any scale.

- Follow shampoo with a conditioner for fine or limp hair.

- Avoid high heat from blow dryers to the hair and skin.

- Keep hairstyling to a minimum due to the new hair being prone to breakage. Brushing, combing, hair pins and curling should all be minimized. Curling appliances should be avoided as the scalp is very tender following chemotherapy.

- Hair styling aids such as mousse, hair spray, hair spritz, styling gel and sculpturing gel may be used in moderation. It is best to select products with normal to light holding ability as the high hold products may not be completely removed with mild shampoos. Hair styling aids can build up on the hair shaft resulting in dullness and possibly scalp disease.

Chemical Curling or Permanent Waving

Chemical curling or permanent waving of the hair is best avoided until the hair is at least three inches long. It is difficult to get nice curls if the hair is much shorter even with a healthy head of hair. For best results use a mild body wave with short processing time. The hair should be wrapped loosely on the largest size curling rod possible. Looser curls will be less damaging to the recovering hair shaft, and will thus minimize hair shaft breakage.

WARNING: Many patients cannot tolerate the permanent wave solution on their scalp for some times up to one year following chemotherapy. This extreme sensitivity of the scalp is not unusual during the regrowth period. In such cases permanents should not be attempted.

Hair Coloring: Hair coloring may also be irritating to the sensitive scalp and should be avoided until the scalp sensation returns to normal. Once the scalp is healed, the hair may be colored.

Permanent hair colorings are the most damaging to the hair shaft and should be minimized in favor of semi-permanent hair colorings which are gradually washed away with four to six shampooings.

Bleaching: Bleaching to lighten the hair color should not be attempted at this time. Additionally, the hair should be altered only 3 shades from its regrowth color as more drastic color changes could increase hair shaft breakage.

Hair Loss in Men, Women, and Children

The period of time following chemotherapy treatment is a time of healing and rebuilding for the body. Hair growth will gradually return, and with time most patients regain a healthy head of hair. Following some of the enclosed hair care tips will insure that the regrown hair looks and feels its very best.

Children

A word of caution to parents with children undergoing chemotherapy. The absence of hair can be used in a positive manner. It can signal to others "handle with care." While undergoing chemotherapy the child has a low blood count and can be bruised easily.

The insistence of parents, although well meaning, for a child to wear a wig or prosthesis can signal the message "YOU'RE NOT O.K. THE WAY YOU ARE." A child should have all of the options but the choice should be his or hers. Hugs and tender loving care along with your physician's suggestions for care are all that is necessary from the parents.

Treatment Options

At the onset of hair loss, (the very first hair fall), some patients choose to shave the total scalp.

Their reasons are the following:

- The elimination of uncontrolled hair fall and embarrassing shedding.

- Some feel that total baldness is more attractive than the spotty hair loss (especially males). Many believe that after 25-50 percent hair loss, males or females look healthier with no hair at all.

- Shaving facilitates prosthetic hair security and comfort (i.e., vacuum bases, two way tape and other adhesives for hair prostheses. What may seem extreme to some, may not be for others.

- Attractive head coverings are available from a variety of manufacturers as an alternative to wigs.

Hair Prosthesis

- Insurance sometimes covers a wig or hair prosthesis.

- Assume you will lose all of your hair when you begin chemotherapy treatment. By doing so your advance planning will assist you considerably. (Custom made wigs and hair prosthetics may take from six weeks to four months to be delivered and made for you.)

- Your first wig or hair prosthesis should duplicate your hair as closely as possible. (Be conservative in color, length, thickness and style.)

- In chemotherapy related hair loss avoid the following: weaves, hair extensions, hair integration and hair intensifiers. You will require a full prosthesis and not a partial hairpiece.

The American Hair Loss Council is a nonprofit organization and does not endorse individual physicians or business firms. It is advisable to consult with several specialists in order to be a well informed patient/consumer.

Prepared for the American Hair Loss Council by Zoe Draelos, M.D. and Mike Mahoney, AHLC Executive Director.

Chapter 57

Minoxidil: Hair Apparent? For Some, a New Solution to Baldness

Samson's hair made him the strongest man alive, according to the Bible. He killed a lion with his bare hands, wreaked havoc on his enemy's cornfields, vineyards and orchards, and slaughtered a thousand Philistines with the jawbone of an ass.

Eager to capture Samson, the Philistines sent the beautiful seductress Delilah, who asked Samson to prove his love to her by revealing the source of his strength. Eager to please the woman, Samson told her his secret, his hair was cut while he slept, and he was captured by the Philistines.

Samson's story notwithstanding, hair serves no vital human function. Its psychological impact, however, is immeasurable. In an age where narcissism reigns supreme, Americans spent $24 billion in 1987 to cut, curl, color, tint, perm, style, wash, condition, mousse, gel, and blow-dry their hair. A musical has been written about it, people have been fired over how they styled it, kids have been expelled from school over its length, and millions of men agonize over its loss.

But at last this agony has now been tempered. A new hair product has arrived on the scene. Called Rogaine (also known as minoxidil, the generic name of its active ingredient) it is manufactured by the Upjohn Company of Kalamazoo, Mich. For an estimated 50 million to 55 million balding Americans this product holds the promise of restoring lost locks.

FDA Consumer, January 1989.

But that promise won't be fulfilled for everyone. While minoxidil helps grow hair for some men, for many it won't work. Nonetheless, it is a worthy beginning to solving the problem of hair loss.

The battle against baldness goes back at least to Julius Caesar. When he was pursuing Cleopatra up and down the Nile, he carefully combed his thinning hair across the bald spot on the top of his head.

In the 1800s, hair strengtheners, baldness cures, and hair restorers were a major staple of the traveling medicine show. If the balding man missed the show, he could purchase a nostrum at his pharmacy, through a catalog, or from a traveling salesman. These hucksters sold men elixirs whose ingredients included cantharides (more commonly known as Spanish fly) that could blister the skin, olive oil, borax, sulfur, bone marrow, and lead acetate.

Even today, the willingness of balding men to fork over hundreds of dollars for remedies that don't work is testimony to mankind's vanity. FDA estimates that approximately $100 million is spent annually on fraudulent balding remedies, whose advertisements grace the pages of even reputable magazines.

But now comes minoxidil, the first product to be medically proven to remedy hair loss in some patients. And in August of 1989, it became the first, and only, FDA-approved treatment for hair loss.

Minoxidil's hair-growing properties were discovered accidentally. It was originally marketed as a high blood pressure medicine known as Loniten. Doctors noticed that many who took Loniten (about 80 percent) grew hair, not only on their heads but often on their foreheads and upper cheeks. Understandably, patients weren't crazy about these results, but it didn't take long to figure that a topical solution of minoxidil—rubbed on the scalp—might help balding men.

Just how minoxidil works remains a mystery, although, according to an Upjohn spokesperson, "minoxidil somehow reverses the genetic instructions which tell the hair follicle to stop growing hair."

In 1982 and 1983, Upjohn tested minoxidil in clinical trials at 27 medical centers across the country. The 2,300 participants (mostly males, although a few women were included) were young (18-49) and healthy with typical male pattern baldness (androgenetic alopecia)—a pattern of baldness in which hair thins out at the crown while the frontal hairline recedes.

Participants in the study were split into two groups: One group applied minoxidil twice a day, while the control group applied a placebo (inactive) solution. At the end of four months, some in the minoxidil group began showing some hair growth. Since it was obvious the drug had an effect, the placebo participants were switched over to the minoxidil group. At the end of a year, 39 percent of the men had experienced moderate or dense hair growth on their balding spots, while the remaining 61 percent experienced little or no hair growth.

Closer examination of Rogaine and the design of the study, however, shows that this 39 percent figure needs qualification.

There was no definition of "dense" or "moderate" hair growth. Beauty, or, in this case, hair growth, was in the eyes of the researchers; no objective criteria guided their judgment.

A more accurate figure for the percentage of men who had moderate or dense hair growth is 10 percent to 20 percent, say a number of dermatologists. An article in the May 2, 1987, British medical journal *Lancet* concurs. Drs. Anton C. De Groot, Johan P. Nater, and Andrew Herxheimer of the Willem-Alexander Hospital in the Netherlands and Westminster Medical School in London, state that after reviewing a number of studies (including Upjohn's) "less than 10 percent of men treated obtain a result that a neutral observer would find cosmetically acceptable." (Minoxidil is already marketed in some 40 other countries.)

In reviewing one study, the *Lancet* authors found that "moderate" hair growth meant that "mean hair density increased from 72 to 110 hairs per square centimeter—an increase of 38 hairs." A more accurate description of "moderate growth," concluded the authors, might be "mostly fluff."

Dr. Elise Olsen, a dermatologist at Duke University who's done extensive research with Rogaine, is slightly more optimistic. She says that on the average, the number of non-vellus hairs (hairs that are thick and dark enough to be readily seen) doubled in her studies, although what this means to individual users varies—there's a big difference between going from 10 to 20 hairs compared to from 50 to 100 hairs.

Findings varied widely among the 27 centers in the Upjohn studies, and "statistical significance could not be shown in 19 centers for the mean terminal hair [hair that can be readily seen] count" concluded *Lancet*.

Nonetheless, "patients' subjective evaluations of new hair growth should also be valued," says Dr. Raymond Lipicky, director of FDA's division of cardio-renal drug products. In reviewing Upjohn's study data, he noted that many of the patients assessed their new hair growth more positively than their physicians.

In the Upjohn studies, researchers selected men who were more likely to benefit from minoxidil—younger men who were just beginning to lose hair on the crown. Older men and men with a longer history or greater amount of baldness are poor candidates for minoxidil's course of treatment. And while minoxidil helps hair growth on the crown of the head, it rarely grows hair on the receding hairline and doesn't grow hair at the temples. Ironically, doctors reported that some of the men in the placebo group of the Upjohn studies appeared to be growing new hair. What was going on?

Most dermatologists don't think that rubbing the scalp with the placebo nurtured hair growth. Instead, a number of dermatologists suggest that doctors in the study had such high expectations of minoxidil that their appraisal of the hair growth was unconsciously biased. (The doctors didn't know which group was getting minoxidil and which the placebo.)

"There was a strong clear bias on the part of the researcher which made it very difficult to assess hair growth," says Dr. Robert Stern, a dermatologist with Harvard University and chief of FDA's minoxidil review committee.

Counting hairs is very difficult, says Stern, who likens it to counting the number of weeds on your lawn. (Researchers concentrate on a section of the balding scalp and literally count the exact number of hairs under some magnifying device.)

Although taking minoxidil orally for hypertension can have serious side effects, including difficulty breathing, rapid heart beat, fainting and vomiting, spreading the lotion all over the scalp seems to be safe for most men for very little of the drug is absorbed through the skin.

The most common complaint among the study participants: 3 percent said Rogaine made their scalps feel itchy and dry. This side effect could be due to the solution itself (it includes alcohol and propylene glycol, which tends to dry the skin) or to possible allergic reactions to minoxidil.

Some study participants complained of lightheadedness, nausea, chest pain, pulse rate changes, and backaches, but the frequency of these complaints was no greater than complaints in the placebo group. In one study, two men complained of impotence, which disappeared a few days after they stopped using the lotion. Twelve people have died while using minoxidil, but there is no suggestion that these deaths were related to the drug.

To get a better grip on the long-term health effects of Rogaine, Upjohn has started a follow-up study that will follow 10,000 users for one year, comparing them with a group of individuals who do not use Rogaine. Study participants will be interviewed over the course of a

Minoxidil: Hair Apparent? For Some, a New Solution

year regarding their use of drugs other than Rogaine, their use of medical facilities, and whether any major medical events occur.

Minoxidil's cost may make it too expensive for some wallets. A month's supply costs between $50 and $85, an expense that must be borne over a lifetime because if treatment is stopped the new hair will fall out in three or four months. Add to this the cost of periodic visits to a dermatologist and many men may choose the balding look over the hirsute look. And because treatment with Rogaine is considered a cosmetic service most health insurance companies will not reimburse the expense.

Another question arises. Just how easily can one maintain this bothersome grooming ritual over a lifetime? (Minoxidil must be used twice a day on a dry scalp.)

"People get tired of using it and it becomes difficult to use judiciously day after day," says Duke University's Olsen. New hair growth reaches a plateau after approximately one year of use, so psychologically it becomes more difficult to use a product that just maintains hair growth rather than adding new hair, she adds.

Nevertheless, in a study on long-term use, out of 156 patients 46 percent were still using minoxidil at the end of 33 months, says Olsen.

Dr. Thomas Nigra, a dermatologist at the Washington Hospital Center in Washington, D.C., says that 65 percent of his 500 study participants were still using Rogaine at the end of five years. Those who had stopped complained of expense or felt that the lotion didn't work for them.

A couple of issues were not addressed in the Upjohn studies. No one knows if minoxidil might prevent the loss of hair. And the sample of women in the studies was too small to draw hard and fast conclusions about how well minoxidil works on females who are losing hair. (Women's hair generally thins out all over the head rather than following a male pattern of baldness.) Currently, controlled studies at 10 centers are under way to test minoxidil on women. Anecdotally, Washington Hospital Center's Nigra says, based on the few women in his studies and conversations with colleagues, minoxidil seems to aid hair growth in women better than in men.

Although a number of mysteries still surround hair loss, one piece of the puzzle has been found. In the spring of this year, scientists discovered what may be the cause of balding. Researchers have known for years that the male hormone testosterone influences baldness. But they didn't know how the hormone caused hair to fall out. Now, dermatologists led by Dr. Marty Sawaya at the University of Miami School of Medicine think they might have an answer.

They examined plugs of hair from 60 men who had undergone scalp reduction surgery. After analyzing the hair shaft, the follicles and sebaceous glands, Sawaya discovered that the hair root cells have two proteins, a large one and a small one, that bind to testosterone. These proteins regulate the input of testosterone to the hair cells.

Sawaya found that when testosterone binds to the smaller protein it is carried to the hair cells, shutting down hair production. If testosterone binds to the larger protein, the hormone remains outside the hair cells, causing no damage. When Sawaya compared cells from the balding part of a man's scalp to the hairy parts, she found that the small protein was more prevalent in the balding root cells than in the hair-growing cells. Balding men have a genetic propensity to the smaller protein, says Sawaya.

"If too much testosterone reaches the hair follicles," says Sawaya, "it short-circuits the system, and hair production shuts down." The obvious solution to this problem is to prevent testosterone from attaching to the smaller protein and turning off hair production.

That possibility lurks in the future. Sawaya and her colleagues have discovered an inhibitor protein in healthy root cells that keeps testosterone from binding to the smaller proteins. "If we can somehow get these inhibitors into the scalp, we may be able to prevent baldness," says Sawaya.

Another possibility is to manufacture antibodies to the small hair-destroying proteins to prevent them from reaching the root cells.

Meanwhile, those already facing approaching baldness in the mirror must rely on whatever minoxidil has to offer. While minoxidil might not work for you, the truth is that it does work for some. And chances are that if you're just beginning to lose hair, if you're under 30, and if you're only losing hair on the crown of your head then minoxidil might be the solution.

—by Judy Folkenberg

Judy Folkenberg is a member of FDA's public affairs staff.

Chapter 58

Hair Replacement Surgery

What Is Hair Replacement Surgery?

Modern techniques in hair grafting (the most frequently performed method of transplanting hair) are performed by taking small pieces of hair bearing scalp from the back and sides of the head and moving them into holes and slits on the top of the head. This technique is commonly called hair grafting, punch grafting, plug grafting or hair transplantation. This procedure is performed by many physicians and in many clinics throughout the world. No new hair is added—hair and skin are relocated.

Grafting techniques include the following types of grafts:

- Micrograft: 1 to 2 hair grafts into needle holes.
- Small slit grafts: 3 to 4 hairs into a slit recipient site.
- Large slit grafts: 5 to 7 hairs into a slit recipient site.
- Small minigraft: 3 to 4 hairs into a small recipient site.
- Large minigraft: 5 to 8 hairs into a small round recipient site.
- Standard round or square grafting: Approximately 9 to 18 hairs in a 3-4.5 mm size graft placed into a slightly smaller round recipient site.

©1994 American Hair Loss Council, Inc. All rights reserved. Material may not be reproduced in any manner without the express written permission of the AHLC. Reprinted with permission.

(Marketing terms used by different physicians and businesses may be confusing. In hair transplants all grafting procedures will be one of the above or a combination.)

How Many Grafts Does it Take to Get Adequate Coverage?

A square of paper 3.3 inches long will give you a realistic idea of the area that would require approximately 500-600 standard grafts. This will indicate the importance of strategic planning and precise placement of grafts to give the illusion of more hair.

The Future

Instead of basing your decision on the immediate results, keep in mind androgenetic alopecia (male or female pattern hair loss) is progressive. Outstanding results may be obtained today that may not be there in the future. Plan your hairline and density conservatively as though you were already in the future.

Flaps

Although flaps transfer the greatest amount of hair in the shortest amount of time, the surgery is more extensive and specific skill and experience is required by the doctor.

A much larger portion of hair bearing skin (a flap) is transferred from sides and back to the balding area. The flap remains attached at one end through which it maintains nourishment. Therefore the hair in the flap can grow continuously unlike grafted hair which falls out before regrowing.

Scalp Reduction

The surgical removal of bald areas of the top of the scalp. Usually multiple scalp reductions are done, with success dependent on the laxity of the scalp and the limited degree of hair loss as well as the age of the patient. Almost all scalp reductions are done with a combination of either flaps or grafts.

Hair Replacement Surgery

Scalp Expansion and Scalp Extension

These are done to accommodate scalp reductions when the laxity of the scalp is too tight. Expansion is also used to prepare individuals for flap surgeries.

The Essential Ingredients Needed to Achieve Superior Results

The Patient: Qualified in respect to age; degree of hair loss, type and color of hair, cause of hair loss, his expectations as well as the ability to afford and endure the multi-sessions often required to obtain excellent results.

The Physician: Credentials, experience, aesthetic vision, honesty and the ability to educate you before surgery are all important elements necessary for successful hair transplantation. The experienced, qualified physician will be able to inform you as to being properly qualified for hair replacement surgery. It is best to consult with several physicians offering hair replacement surgery before choosing one. Prepare your questions prior to the consultation.

To insure the that the physician is capable of offering the results you desire, ask to meet a patient or two that he/she has recently completed. Seeing the results firsthand helps to insure you are in capable hands. This is far superior to photos or advertising.

Check the Following for References

- Your city, county and state medical societies.

- Your family physician or any physician you see professionally or socially.

- Your local medical library

- Your hairstylist

- The Better Business Bureau

American Academy of Cosmetic Surgery
401 N. Michigan Ave.
Chicago, IL 60611-4267
(312) 527-6713

American Society for Dermatologic Surgery
1567 Maple Ave.
Evanston, IL 60201
(708)-869-3954

American Academy of Facial and Reconstructive Surgery
1101 Vermont Avenue N.W. #404
Washington, D.C. 20005
800-332-FACE

American Hair Loss Council
100 Independence Place Suite. #207
Tyler, TX 75703
800-274-8717
Fax: 903-561-8603

How Much Will it Cost?

Cost will vary with the individual's degree of hair loss and the individual physician. Cost can vary from $4,000.00 for a lesser degree of hair loss to over $20,000.00 for more extensive hair loss.

Whom Do I Consult with Prior to Hair Transplantation?

Although there are knowledgeable consultants, the AHLC recommends that you do not start any type of surgery without consulting with the physician who will be performing the surgery.

Preferably the surgeon should be a resident of the community. It is normally beneficial to continue sessions with the same surgeon and to have him or her available throughout the entire period of surgical procedures.

Chapter 59

Of Lice and Children: Going to the Head of the Class

"Oh, honey, another note from the school nurse," you sigh. What is it this time, a vaccine shot, toothache, ear infection? What on earth could be wrong with you now! ... Will you please sit down, honey, and stop that scratching!"

You open the tightly sealed envelope and read:

Dear Parent/Guardian:

Upon inspecting your child's head today it was discovered that he/she has a lice infestation. It is necessary to exclude him/her from school until adequately treated.

YOUR CHILD MAY RETURN TO SCHOOL AFTER SHE/HE HAS BEEN TREATED.

Sincerely,
Principal & School Nurse

The head louse, technically known as *Pediculus capitis humanus*, is by no means a new nuisance. The insect has been an unwelcome companion to humans probably from the beginning, as have its close relatives, the body louse and the pubic or crab louse. But head lice infestations seem to be on the rise in recent years as almost any parent of an elementary school-aged child can tell you.

FDA Consumer, November 1989.

A parent's first reaction to head lice is often revulsion, sometimes accompanied by a sense of shame due to the misperception that head lice only live on "dirty" people. In truth, the only thing that the presence of head lice tells about children is that they've been around other kids with head lice.

Head lice are parasites about the size of a small ant. They get their nourishment by sucking small amounts of blood from humans. Their favorite feeding area is the scalp behind the ears and at the nape of the neck. Their feeding and sucking activity is responsible for the itching that is so frequently the first hint of infestation. Left untreated, rash and infection can occur. In severe cases, the lymph glands in the neck may swell. Although usually confined to the head, head lice sometimes also set up shop in beards, eyebrows and, rarely, eyelashes.

Though they don't fly, lice are quite adept at getting from head to head, especially when those heads are close together. Good hygiene is always an admirable goal, but a clean head of hair is no guarantee that they won't invade. Because children play so closely together, often in large groups, lice have an easy time traveling from child to child. Cases of lice seem to increase in the winter, possibly because kids are inside and close together, sometimes sharing hats, combs and, consequently, "cooties," as kids sometimes call them. The creepy critters can live up to two to three days apart from the body and, in closets where clothes hang close together, may hop from hat to scarf. They also may be lurking on the headrest of a school bus seat, just waiting to get aboard an attractive head. (The stitchings of those upholstered headrests can hide the tiny gray-white lice eggs called nits.)

How to Spot Lice

It's easier to spot the nits than the lice themselves. And, because nits are "dandruffy" in appearance, they are easier to see on people with darker hair. To distinguish them from dandruff or hair spray, pick up a strand of hair close to the scalp and pull your fingernail across the area where the whitish substance appears. Dandruff (or hair spray) will come off easily, but nits will stay firmly attached to the hair. If you look carefully, you may be able to see the bugs themselves on the back of the head and around the ears.

Once you have discovered head lice on one family member, all other members of the family, as well as close friends, should be checked. Also, look for lice or their nits in fabrics of stuffed toys, upholstered furniture, and bedding.

Of Lice and Children: Going to the Head of the Class

Routing the Louse

Both over-the-counter (OTC) and prescription shampoos are available to get rid of head lice. OTC anti-lice shampoos, which are not to be confused with medicated shampoos to treat dandruff and similar problems, contain two pesticides: pyrethrums, derived from chrysanthemum plants, and the chemical piperonyl butoxide. These shampoos should be left on the hair 10 minutes. The hair should be towel-dried, and nits should be removed using a special comb or tweezers (included in some OTC product packages). Remember to give the hair a second application after seven to ten days, even if you see no signs of lice. People who are allergic to ragweed should only take these products under a physician's direction. Pyrethrums can cause asthma, allergy symptoms, and even severe, potentially life-threatening allergic reactions in sensitive individuals.

There are two types of prescription products to help rout lice. One is a shampoo containing the chemical lindane. The other is a cream rinse that contains permethrin, a chemical form of the pyrethrums found in the OTC products.

Lindane shampoos must be applied to the hair for four minutes. The nits are then removed in the same way as for OTC products. A second application is usually not required. Though it's good at getting rid of the varmints, lindane in large doses can be toxic to the human central nervous system so that care—and the guidance of a physician—is especially important when treating babies. It should not be used for premature infants or by people who have had seizures. Pregnant women should seek the advice of their physicians before using lindane products on themselves and should wear rubber gloves if they must apply them to others' hair.

The cream rinse containing permethrin is applied after shampooing with a regular shampoo and towel-drying the hair. It should be left on the hair 10 minutes before rinsing off. Usually, only one application is necessary. Combing the nits out is not required, although some parents may prefer to do this anyway for aesthetic reasons. Like the OTC products, the cream rinse should not be by anyone allergic to chrysanthemums or pyrethrums.

With either the OTC or the prescription products, directions for the specific shampoo or cream rinse you're using should be carefully followed. It's a good idea to place a clean towel across the forehead to keep the medication from dripping into the eyes. (If accidental contact with eyes occurs, flush with water. If irritation develops, discontinue use and consult your physician.) Be sure to apply a generous amount, sufficient to thoroughly cover all the hair. With the shampoos, wet the hair thoroughly, until a good lather forms.

In the rare case of lice infestation of eyebrows and lashes, a physician should be consulted. Shampoo should not be used around the eyes. Petrolatum products may help get the lice out of these areas, or the physician may have to remove them with forceps.

Beyond Shampooing

Now that you've gotten rid of them, you don't want the nasty nuisances to come back, do you? To prevent re-infestation, the following may be helpful:

- Make sure all family members and friends of the infested person have been closely scrutinized for signs of lice. If any of them appear to have lice, make sure they are treated.

- Wash all clothing and bed linens used by the infested members of your family in hot water and place in a hot dryer for at least 20 minutes. If this cannot be done, place the linens and clothing into an airtight bag for two weeks. Dry cleaning also kills lice and nits.

- Vacuum backs of chairs, pillows in living and bedroom areas, mattresses, car seats and headrests, and rugs that might be in contact with infested hair. Empty the vacuum bag (if it is the paper disposable sort, discard the bag). There are some OTC sprays for disinfecting furniture and bedding. They contain insecticides that are not suitable for humans or animals, so be careful not to confuse them with the products that are for human use.

- Disinfect combs, brushes, sports helmets, and other objects that come in contact with the head by soaking in medicated shampoo or very hot soapy water.

- Recheck all family members and friends 7 to 14 days and 21 to 28 days after initial treatment to be sure lice have not reappeared (eggs that remain after treatment will hatch in 7 to 14 days).

Of Lice and Children: Going to the Head of the Class

Though discovering that your child has head lice is no picnic, is it not cause for panic or shame. The problem is shared by a good portion of the American school population and can be controlled by vigilance and appropriate treatment.

You Say You Itch Somewhere Else?

Body lice (*Pediculus humanus corporis*) and pubic lice (*Phthirius pubis*) are pesky parasites closely related to the head louse.

Fortunately, the body louse is relatively rare in this country. It thrives in unsanitary, overcrowded living conditions and historically has been common in military, refugee and concentration camps, prisons, and overcrowded city dwellings. It can carry organisms that cause diseases such as epidemic typhoid fever. This critter lives and deposits its eggs in clothes, bedding, and other personal articles and then hops aboard a human when it needs a feed.

The body louse has figured in a number of history's main events. The story goes that after Archbishop Thomas à Becket was assassinated at Canterbury Cathedral in 1170, the penitential hair shirt he never removed was found to be swarming with lice. And the term "cootie" is said to have originated in the trenches of World War I as a nickname for the body louse that was all-too-familiar to so many of the soldiers.

Body lice usually go their own way when living conditions are improved. Thus, today they are a rarity in most developed areas of the world.

Pubic lice are transmitted by close— usually sexual—contact. Also called crab lice, or simply "crabs," pubic lice seen close up resemble a crab, with two grasping "arms" in front. They live on the human body where the hair is coarse—mostly in the pubic area and armpits. The infested area frequently becomes itchy and, as with head lice, a rash often results. Like head lice nits, the whitish eggs of the pubic louse are firmly attached to the hair shaft. The lice may look like small scabby crusts, or they may appear as small bluish spots on the skin. Sometimes infested people may notice louse excretions—minute brown specks—on their underwear.

Along with other sexually transmitted diseases (STDs), "crabs" seems to be enjoying a resurgence, especially among those in their teens and 20s. Therefore, people who find they have pubic lice would be wise to be examined for other STDs.

The same products that get rid of head lice will also do away with crab lice.

—by Theresa A. Young and Judith Levine Willis.

Theresa A. Young is an FDA consumer affairs officer with the Philadelphia district. Judith Levine Willis is editor of *FDA Consumer*.

Chapter 60

Fingernails: Looking Good While Playing Safe

With the ease that comes from years of practice, Julie Le, of Nails R Us in Alexandria, Va., sets out to remake customer Natalie Harris' nails. She buffs, files, snips, clips, smoothes, and then, with a nod from Harris, paints on ruby red polish.

It's a process repeated every day throughout the country as thousands of women like Harris—and men, too— strive for beautiful nails. They seek the services of nail and beauty salons or manicure their nails themselves with a host of nail products available on the market.

The reason, said Kim Siridavong, owner of Nails R Us, is simple: "Everybody wants to look good."

But achieving that look is not without potential hazard. Infections and allergic reactions can occur with some nail services and products. Some chemicals in nail products, if ingested, are poisonous. Many are flammable.

Relying on nail and beauty salons is not risk free, either. They use the same products, and they may present a greater risk for disease transmission.

Federal and state regulations help reduce the risks, but consumers also need to take care that their pursuit of beautiful nails ensures healthy nails.

FDA Consumer, December 1995.

Growth of an Industry

With the increased use of nail services and products in recent years has come growing concern about safety. According to *Nail 1995 Fact Book*, U.S. consumers will spend an estimated $5.2 billion on nail services in 1995, half a billion more than in 1994. They can choose from 34,852 freestanding nail salons across the country—nearly 2,000 more than a year ago—or hundreds of thousands of beauty salons that offer nail services.

The most requested service, according to the *Fact Book* is artificial nails. Manicures are No. 2. Other popular services include nail jewelry and nail art.

Because of the variety of nail services, the preferred term for a person who provides nail services is "nail technician" rather than manicurist said Suzette Hill, managing editor for *Nails*, a magazine for professionals and students.

"Twenty years ago, they mainly did manicures," she said. "Now, they're doing so much more."

They use a range of products, including polishes, paints, artificial nails, glues, and laminates, many of which are available for home use, too.

Nail Products as Cosmetics

Nail products for both home and salon use are regulated by the Food and Drug Administration. Under the Federal Food, Drug, and Cosmetic Act, these products are considered cosmetics because they are "articles other than soap which are applied to the human body for cleansing, beautifying, promoting attractiveness, or altering the appearance."

By law, nail products sold as cosmetics in the United States must be free of poisonous or deleterious substances that might injure users under the usual or customary conditions of use intended by the manufacturer. These uses are printed on the package or on a package insert. Many nail products contain poisonous substances, such as acetonitrile in glue removers, but are allowed on the market because they are not harmful when used as directed. They are poisonous only when ingested, which is not their intended use.

Products sold for home use also must be labeled properly, with the names of the ingredients listed in descending order of predominance. (See "Decoding the Cosmetic Label" in the May 1994 *FDA Consumer*.)

Fingernails: Looking Good While Playing Safe

FDA does not review or approve nail products and other cosmetics before they go on the market. However, the agency inspects cosmetic manufacturers and samples and analyzes cosmetics as needed. If a safety problem arises, the agency can take legal action against the product.

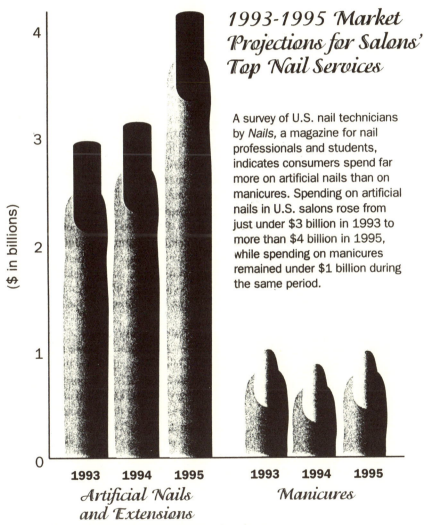

1993-1995 Market Projections for Salons' Top Nail Services

A survey of U.S. nail technicians by *Nails*, a magazine for nail professionals and students, indicates consumers spend far more on artificial nails than on manicures. Spending on artificial nails in U.S. salons rose from just under $3 billion in 1993 to more than $4 billion in 1995, while spending on manicures remained under $1 billion during the same period.

(Sources: *Nails 1994 Fact Book* and *Nails 1995 Fact Book*)

Figure 60.1.

FDA also tracks safety problems through its Cosmetic Voluntary Registration Program, in which cosmetic manufacturers voluntarily report to FDA the types of adverse reactions their customers have reported to them. FDA uses this information to determine a baseline reaction rate for specific product categories, such as cuticle softeners, nail extenders (artificial nail ends), and nail polishes. The agency gives this information to participating companies so they can compare their adverse reaction rates to FDA's determined baseline.

FDA also learns about potentially harmful products from manufacturers' competitors, consumers, doctors, and nail technicians, who report adverse reactions directly to the agency.

Salon Safety

The salons and their technicians are regulated by the states, usually their cosmetology boards. Lois Wiskur, past president of the National Interstate Council of State Cosmetology Boards, said that as far as she knows, every state has some licensing requirements for nail salons, nail technicians, or both.

Under these requirements, salons providing nail services usually must meet certain requirements, such as:

- Employing nail technicians who have had a minimum number of hours of classroom and practical training.
- Properly sterilizing manicure implements. The preferred methods are autoclaving (heat sterilization) or chemical sterilization.
- Undergoing a state inspection periodically.
- Maintaining sufficient equipment, such as at least one manicure table and one sink that runs hot and cold water.
- Making sure that employees wash their hands before beginning work on a customer.

To prevent blood-borne infections, such as HIV and hepatitis, the national Centers for Disease Control and Prevention recommended similar sanitary practices for salon employees in guidelines issued in 1985. The guidelines targeted, among others, personal-service workers, such as manicurists and pedicurists. To date, there have been no reports of transmission of blood-borne diseases to or from a personal service worker, according to CDC.

Fingernails: Looking Good While Playing Safe

Nail Infections

More common nail problems, dermatologists report, are infections from bacteria, such as Staphylococcus; fungi, such as Candida (also known as yeast); and skin viruses, such as warts.

Bacterial and fungal infections frequently result from artificial nails, whether applied at home or in a salon. A bump or knock to a long artificial nail may cause it to lift from the natural nail at the base, leaving an opening for dirt to get in. If the nail is reglued without proper cleaning (with rubbing alcohol, for example), bacteria or fungi may grow between the nails and spread into the natural nail.

Also, as the natural nail grows, an opening develops between the natural nail and artificial nail. If this space is not filled in regularly, it can increase the chances for infection.

A fungal infection can take hold when an acrylic nail is left in place too long—such as three months or more—and moisture accumulates under the nail.

Bacterial, fungal and viral infections also can occur from using insanitary nail implements, especially in a salon, where the same implements are used on many people.

Unclean implements are especially dangerous if the skin around the nail is broken. This can occur with overzealous manicuring—if, for example, too much of the cuticle is cut or pushed back too far. If the cuticle is cut or separated from the fingernail, infectious agents can get into the exposed area. This is why dermatologists recommend leaving cuticles intact.

Symptoms of an infection include pain, redness, itching, and pus in or around the nail area. Yellow-green, green, and green-black nail discolorations are signs of a Pseudomonas bacterial infection. A blue-green discoloration signals a fungal infection.

If an infection appears while wearing artificial nails, they should be removed and the area cleaned thoroughly with soap and water. If symptoms persist, the person should consult a doctor, who may prescribe a topical or oral anti-infective medicine.

There are no approved nonprescription products to treat fungal nail infections, and over-the-counter products to treat other types of fungal infections should not be used for nail infections. In a review of OTC antifungal products, FDA found that fungal infections of the nails respond poorly to topical therapy, partly because of the nail's thickness. So, in 1993, the agency ruled that any OTC product labeled, represented or promoted as a topical antifungal to treat fungal infections of the nail is a new drug and must be approved by FDA before marketing. This rule, which went into effect in 1994, does not include prescription antifungal products.

Despite the rule, some companies continue to sell unapproved OTC nail products, such as nail glues, with antifungal claims. FDA has warned these companies it might take legal action if they don't stop selling the products.

Allergies and Other Hazards

Other common problems associated with nail products are allergic reactions, such as contact dermatitis, a skin rash characterized by redness and itching and sometimes tiny blisters that ooze. (See "Contact Dermatitis: Solutions to Rash Mysteries" in the May 1990 *FDA Consumer* and Omnigraphics' *Allergies Sourcebook*.)

Certain nail ingredients are known for their tendency to cause allergic reactions. Residual traces of the basic building blocks of acrylic resins ("acrylics") used in artificial nails, for example, can cause redness, swelling and pain in the nail bed. In some cases, the reaction is so severe that the natural nail separates from the nail bed, and although a new nail usually grows in, it may be imperfect if the nail root has been damaged.

Nail strengtheners that contain "free formaldehyde" may cause an irritation or reaction, as can certain other chemicals in nail glues and polishes.

In the late 1970s, use of methyl methacrylate, then a common ingredient in artificial nail products, resulted in FDA receiving a number of reports of injuries and allergic reactions, including damage and deformity of fingernails and contact dermatitis. The ingredient now is rarely used because of legal action against a former manufacturer of methyl methacrylate-containing products and numerous seizures and recalls of such products. Methyl methacrylate has since been replaced with other chemicals, such as ethyl methacrylate. However, according to John Bailey, Ph.D., acting director of FDA's office of cosmetics and colors, the replacement chemicals have never been fully studied for safety, and they may be as harmful as methyl methacrylate.

"Our current guidance is that products containing ethyl methacrylate should be used only by trained nail technicians under conditions that minimize exposure and skin contact because of their potential to cause allergies," he said.

Fingernails: Looking Good While Playing Safe

Whatever the cause, allergic reactions usually take place where the product has been applied or where it has inadvertently come in contact with other skin surfaces, such as the face, eyelids and neck.

When the offending agent is no longer used, reactions clear up. Sometimes, the user can identify the chemical causing the allergic reaction and avoid it.

Though rare, some nail products can cause illness and even death, particularly if ingested by children. In 1987, a 16-month-old toddler died of cyanide poisoning after swallowing a mouthful of solvent used to remove sculptured artificial fingernails. At least one other youngster was rushed to the emergency room for intensive care after swallowing a similar product. These products contained acetonitrile, a chemical that breaks down into cyanide when swallowed. Since 1990, the Consumer Product Safety Commission has required household glue removers containing more than 500 milligrams of acetonitrile in a single container to carry child-resistant packaging. This includes glue removers for artificial nails.

Nail products also can be dangerous if they get in the eyes. And they can easily catch on fire if exposed to the free flame of the pilot light of a stove, a lit cigarette, or even the heating element of a curling iron.

Consumers should read labels of nail products carefully and heed any warnings.

Precautions for Artificial Nails

- If there is any question about sensitivity to the materials in artificial nails, have one nail done as a test and wait a few days to see if a reaction develops.

- Never apply an artificial nail if the natural nail or skin around it is infected or irritated. Let the infection heal first.

- Read the directions for do-it-yourself nails before applying them, and follow the directions carefully. Save the ingredient list for your doctor in case you have an allergic reaction or other injury.

- Treat your artificial nails with care. They may be stronger than your own, but they still can break and separate. Try not to bump or knock them. Find new ways to do ordinary tasks, like using a pencil to dial or depress the numbers on the phone.

- If an artificial nail separates, dip the fingertip into rubbing alcohol to clean the space between the natural and artificial nails before reattaching the artificial nail. This will help prevent infection.

- Never use household glues for nail repairs. Use only products intended for nail use, and follow directions.

- Don't wear artificial nails for longer than three months at a time. Remove them for one month to give nails a rest.

- Keep nail glues and other poisonous substances out of the reach of children.

Reporting Adverse Nail Product Reactions

Doctors, nail technicians, and consumers should report adverse reactions from nail products to the nearest FDA office, listed in the blue section of the telephone hook. Or, write to:

Food and Drug Administration Center for Food Safety and Applied Nutrition Office of Cosmetics and Colors (HFS-100)
200 C St., S.W.
Washington, D.C. 20204

Selecting a Safe Nail Salon

To help you decide if a salon provides sanitary nail services, nail and public health experts suggest considering the following:

- Is the salon licensed? Licenses often are posted. If you don't see one, ask.

- Are the nail technicians licensed? These licenses also are usually posted. Ask if you don't see one for your technician.

- How are nail implements sanitized? Autoclaving (heat sterilization) is best, says Ralph Daniel, M.D., a dermatologist in Jackson, Miss. But most states allow chemical sterilizing as long as the implements are immersed in the solution for at least 10 minutes between customers. Ask the technician what the salon's practices are. If they're using a chemical solution, check the

Fingernails: Looking Good While Playing Safe

product's label for words like "germicidal" to indicate that it is strong enough to kill bacteria. If in doubt, bring your own implements, Daniel suggests.

- Is there a pre-service scrub? Both the nail technician and the client should wash their hands with an antimicrobial soap before nail work begins.

- Is each customer given a fresh bowl of soapy water to soak their nails in and is a new nail file used for each customer? Both practices should be followed.

- Is the facility neat and clean? Paul Kechijian, M.D., a clinical associate professor of dermatology and chief of the nail section at New York University, compares selecting a salon to selecting a restaurant. "Ask yourself when you walk in: Would you want to eat there?" he says.

- Is there a strong smell of fumes? If there is, it's a sign that the facility is poorly ventilated, says John Bailey, Ph.D., acting director of FDA's office of cosmetics and colors. Inhaling the fumes from nail products can make you sick.

If you have a complaint about a salon providing nail services, contact your state board of cosmetology.

Healthy Nails

From current consumer habits, one might surmise that the main function of nails is to look good. But nails serve several physiological purposes: They enhance fine touch and fine motor skills and protect the fingers and toes. Doctors also may examine them for indications of serious underlying diseases; for example, clubbed nails (a condition in which fingers or toes thicken and the nails wrap around them) is a classic sign of chronic lung and heart disorders. For those reasons, it's important to keep nails healthy.

With proper care and precautions, nails can be both healthy and attractive.

— by Paula Kurtzweil

Paula Kurtzweil is a member of FDA's public affairs staff.

Part Eight

Cosmetics and the Skin

Chapter 61

Cosmetic Ingredients: Understanding the Puffery

The lotion contained bovine albumin and the label claimed it would give a "face lift without surgery." The Food and Drug Administration said the claims caused the product to be a misbranded drug. In 1968, the court said no. "If lifting and firming products are deemed intended to affect the structure of the body, girdles and brassieres must be devices within the meaning of the law."

In 1969 an appellate court overturned this decision, but the issues persist today. "Most cosmetics contain ingredients that are promoted with exaggerated claims of beauty or long-lasting effects to create an image," says John E. Bailey, Ph.D., director of FDA's division of color and cosmetics. "Image is what the cosmetic industry sells through its products, and it's up to the consumer to believe it or not," Bailey says.

In the past, cosmetic manufacturers have depended upon mysterious "gimmick" additives, such as turtle oil to promote skin rejuvenation or tighten chin muscles, shark oil, queen bee royal jelly, chick embryo extract, horse blood serum, and pigskin extracts.

Promotion of these "gimmick" additives, combined with today's more sophisticated cosmetic ingredients, is what Bailey and the cosmetic industry call "puffery."

The argument is sometimes made that while Congress intended to safeguard the health and economic interests of consumers with the Federal Food, Drug, and Cosmetic Act, it also meant to protect a manufacturer's right to market a product free of excessive government regulation. And, in an industry that sells personal image, especially

DHHS Publication No. (FDA) 93-5013. Reprint of *FDA Consumer*, May 1992.

images of beauty and sex appeal, not allowing the puffery claims would certainly hurt the marketing, says Bailey.

But there's hope for credibility in claims for cosmetic ingredients. Some of the more responsible cosmetic firms are rethinking their claims that push believability to its outside edge. Linda Allen Schoen of Neutrogena says that today's more knowledgeable consumer wants "facts versus puffery: products based on skin care realities, promises banked on achievable benefits." Besides, says Schoen, limited recession dollars tend to be spent on products consumers can trust.

Still, with the exception of colors and certain prohibited ingredients, a cosmetic manufacturer may use essentially any raw material in a product and market it without prior FDA approval. The prohibited ingredients are biothionol, hexachlorophene, mercury compounds (except as preservatives in eye cosmetics), vinyl chloride and zirconium salts in aerosol products, halogenated salicylanilides, chloroform, and methylene chloride.

Federal regulations require ingredients to be listed on product labels in descending order by quantity, but often the list is not user-friendly. Because cosmetic ingredients are often complex chemical substances, the list may be incomprehensible to the product's average user. (See "Cosmetic Safety: More Complex Than at First Blush" in the November 1991 *FDA Consumer* and reprinted later in this sourcebook.) However, if the same name is used by all manufacturers, consumers can compare different products and make reasonable value judgments.

Although cosmetic claims, even those considered "puffery," are allowed without scientific substantiation, if a cosmetic makes a medical claim, such as removing dandruff, the product is regulated as an over-the-counter drug for which scientific studies demonstrating safety and effectiveness must be submitted to FDA.

Baffling Names

Because of the unusual and sometimes bewildering nature of some ingredients in cosmetics, consumers often ask FDA for explanations. "My night cream contains liposomes—what is that?" "Why is placenta used in cosmetics—is it human placenta, and could I get a disease from it?" "What are cerebrosides and ceremides?"

FDA cosmetic scientists can explain the nature of an ingredient when it is identified by its chemical name. But when an ingredient is listed by its trade name, FDA usually must consult the manufacturer's

Cosmetic Ingredients: Understanding the Puffery

trade literature or the International Cosmetic Ingredient Dictionary (CIR), published by the Cosmetic, Toiletry, and Fragrance Association, Inc., the industry's major trade association. The dictionary, now in its fourth edition, provides a uniform system for assigning ingredient names. FDA currently recognizes the second edition as a primary reference.

Here is what FDA knows about some currently marketed ingredients:

- Liposomes are microscopic sacs, or spheres, manufactured from a variety of fatty substances, including phospholipids. While phospholipids are natural components of cell membranes, the material actually used in cosmetics may be obtained either from natural or synthetic sources. When properly mixed with water, phospholipids form liposome spheres, which can "trap" any substance that will dissolve in water or oil.

    Manufacturers say that liposomes act like a delivery system. They claim that, when present in a cream or lotion, liposomes can more easily penetrate the surface skin to underlying layers, "melt," and deposit other ingredients of the product.

- Nayad is a trade name for yeast extract. The manufacturer's literature describes Nayad as a "new system that takes yeast cells and refines them hundreds of times . . . . What results is a highly concentrated, odor-free, unusually potent yeast extract...." The same literature reports that "no one really knows how Nayad is working in the skin; all we know for certain is the way it makes the skin look and feel. Test subjects report a noticeable smoothing of lines and wrinkles." FDA has no data to either substantiate or refute these claims.

- Vitamins are added to cosmetics by manufacturers because foods containing vitamins A, D, E, K, and some of the B complex group are necessary in diets to maintain healthy skin and hair. Using these vitamins in cosmetics that are applied to the skin surface implies that skin will be nourished by them.

    But Stanley R. Milstein, Ph.D., associate director for FDA's cosmetics division, says the notion that skin can be nourished by a vitamin applied to its surface has not been proven clinically. For that reason, says Milstein, a vitamin added to a cosmetic product must be listed in the ingredient label by its chemical name so that it doesn't convey a misleading message. However, FDA does not prohibit listing vitamins by their common names on the principal display panel of a cosmetic as long as the consumer is not misled and no therapeutic claims are made.

Some leaders in the cosmetic industry, such as Neutrogena's Schoen, agree with the FDA position on vitamins in skin care products. Others, such as Chris Vaughn of Sun Pharmaceuticals, Ltd., cite clinical studies done by Hoffmann-La Roche and others that show that vitamins can penetrate layers of skin and have beneficial effects. This, however, would make it a drug use, and manufacturers who use vitamins in their products don't usually make claims that would cause their products to be classified as drugs. Vaughn says that getting a drug classification is time-consuming and expensive, and in his opinion not justifiable because the informed consumer understands the beneficial properties of vitamins.

Although the debate about the value of vitamins in skin care products continues, it is generally accepted that a sufficient quantity of vitamin E (shown on ingredient lists as tocopherol), an antioxidant, preserves the fatty components in cosmetic creams and lotions to prevent off-color and off-odors.

- Aloe vera is a plant from the lily family whose anti-irritant properties have been recognized since before the days of Cleopatra. It is listed as an ingredient in many skin lotions, but it would take much more aloe vera than most products contain for the anti-irritant properties to work.

    Milstein explains that aloe vera, as a cosmetic ingredient, is expensive because it requires delicate processing and handling. A product that contains the 5 to 10 percent aloe vera necessary for the anti-irritant properties to be effective would send the price out of range for many consumers.

What about Biological Ingredients?

A number of biological products in cosmetics have raised consumer concern:

- Human placenta is the nourishing lining of the womb (uterus), which is expelled after birth. When placental materials were

Cosmetic Ingredients: Understanding the Puffery

first used as cosmetic ingredients in the 1940s, manufacturers promoted the products as providing beneficial hormonal effects such as stimulating tissue growth and removing wrinkles. (Although newborn infants emerge from the womb with wrinkled skin.) The hormone content and the tissue-growth and wrinkle-removing claims classified the placenta-containing products as drugs, and FDA declared them to be ineffective and therefore misbranded.

FDA's challenge caused placenta suppliers to change marketing strategies by claiming that hormones in their placenta ingredients had been extracted and were no longer in the product. They then offered placental raw materials without medical claims—only as a source of protein.

Can you get a disease from placental cosmetic ingredients? Bailey says no. Placenta used in cosmetics is washed and processed many times to destroy any harmful bacteria or viruses. Besides that, says Bailey, the cosmetic matrix (components that bind the ingredients in products) is made from a wide variety of substances, such as alcohol and preservatives, that would present a hostile environment to any viruses or bacteria the placenta might have carried.

- Amniotic liquid (from cow or ox) is the fluid that surrounds the developing fetus and protects it from physical injury. It is promoted for benefits similar to those of human placenta and has limited use in moisturizers, hair lotions, scalp treatments, and shampoos.

- Collagen (from young cows) is the protein substance found in connective tissue. (Connective tissue binds together and supports organs and other body structures.) A great deal of research has been done on the different types and uses for collagen. In cosmetics, collagen has a moisturizing effect. It is not water soluble, but it holds water. FDA says there is no convincing evidence that collagen can penetrate the skin and have an effect below the surface.

- Cerebrosides (from animals or plants) are a type of glycolipid (a chemically combined form of fatty substance and carbohydrate) produced naturally in basal epidermal cells—the deepest layer of skin. After cerebrosides are formed, they are secreted to the outside of the cells and serve as a protective coating. As new cells form in lower layers of skin, the older skin cells move closer to surface layers and start to dry out. During this process, the cerebrosides are chemically changed and form ceremides, part of a network of membranes between cells. Skin moisture and suppleness comes from this network.

The raw material for cerebrosides in cosmetics comes from cattle, oxen or swine brain cells or other nervous system tissues. Alteratively, the raw material may be isolated from plant sources. Industry cosmetic scientists claim that the use of cerebrosides in skin products results in a smoother skin surface and better moisture retention, effects that translate into marketing claims such as luminosity and ever-improving hydration. FDA has not evaluated the studies on which these claims are based.

Industry Self-regulation

"The cosmetic industry is sensitive to the image of an uncontrolled market where anything goes," says Bailey. "They counter this image with well-established self-regulation programs. Part of the incentive for such industry policy is to avoid increased regulatory authority."

The most well-known of industry-sponsored self-regulation is the Cosmetic Ingredient Review, sponsored by the Cosmetic Toiletry and Fragrance Association. The CIR is accomplished by a panel of scientific and medical experts who evaluate cosmetic ingredients for safety and publish detailed reviews of available safety data. "A finding of safety by the CIR provides a degree of confidence that the ingredient can safely be used in cosmetics," Bailey says. "In the absence of the CIR program, there would be no systematic examination of the safety of individual cosmetic ingredients." FDA has no statutory authority to require that the data be submitted to the agency.

FDA encourages industry cooperation through its cosmetic voluntary reporting program. Cosmetic firms registered in the program voluntarily report manufacturing and formulation information, along with product experience data, to FDA. Adverse reactions such as skin irritations are also reported. Using this information, FDA can determine a baseline reaction rate for specific product categories such as hair coloring or eye makeup preparations. The agency gives participating companies this baseline information so they can compare their own adverse reaction rates to the FDA-established baseline.

Cosmetic Ingredients: Understanding the Puffery

"Registration in this voluntary program does not mean that FDA approves or endorses a firm, raw material, or product," says Mary Lipien, chief of the cosmetic registration program. "But it does provide for an interaction between the industry and government for exchange of information."

FDA would like to see wider industry participation. "Based on the number of companies we think are eligible to participate, only about 35 percent do," Lipien says. There are also other problems. "Sometimes the information a firm submits is incomplete," Lipien says. "And if a firm does not update its submissions with additions or deletions, the information in the registration files could accumulate as inaccurate information."

FDA continues to explore ways to make the program more useful for both industry and government, says Bailey. "We compare product information available to the agency with registered data, and now we're considering periodic field surveys of products on the shelves. Such a review would include comparison of label ingredient declarations with information reported to FDA."

The quest for sustained youth and beauty that sells cosmetics is age-old, though ingredients used to achieve that image may change. Shakespeare noted the same concern that keeps the cosmetic industry going when he said:

*Time doth transfix the flourish set on youth
And delves the parallels in beauty's brow.*

But he gave voice to another standard when he wrote,

*To me, fair friend, you never can be old,
For as you were when first your eye I eyed,
Such seems your beauty still.*

—*by Judith E. Foulke*

Judith Foulke is a staff writer for *FDA Consumer*.

Chapter 62

The Collagen Connection

It is the chief constituent of skin and body connective tissue. It is the living component of bone. It gets its name from the Greek words *kolla* (glue) and *gennan* (to produce). It is collagen, according to Dr. Christopher Lovell of St. John's Hospital in London, "the most important structural protein in the entire animal kingdom."

Collagen makes up 25 percent of all protein in the human body. Its primary function is to act as a connecting structure and give mechanical stability to the entire body.

Collagen is essential for maintaining both durability and flexibility. It performs this role by arranging itself in various patterns according to function. For example, in the tendons, which connect bone to muscle, the collagen fibers are arranged in parallel bundles to permit a twisting, turning and stretching effect. In the skin, that protective blanket that envelopes the body, the fibers form a flat crisscross pattern that provides strength and flexibility in all directions.

Collagen has other useful features, and probably the most important is its ability to slow and halt bleeding in body tissues. It does this by providing a fibrous mesh in which blood platelets can coagulate and form a clot.

According to Lovell, there was little medical interest in collagen until well into this century, although its commercial uses have long been understood. Leather, for example, has been manufactured for centuries by removing the gluey collagen from animal skins and then soaking the hide in a tanning solution. The leftover collagen can be

FDA Consumer, June 1985.

processed into glue or, if further treated and purified, can become medical collagen, food gelatin, and numerous other products.

Collagen molecules originate in the various body cells, then move out through the cell membrane to help form the bones, tendons and other structural body parts. The supply of collagen is continuously being replenished to meet the needs of healing, growth and replacement.

Several disorders, generally inherited and all quite rare, can hinder or prevent the proper formation of collagen. One of these is Marfan's syndrome, characterized by long, thin arms, legs, fingers and toes, excessive height, overly flexible joints, and subtle eye and blood vessel changes. Lovell speculates that Abraham Lincoln may have had this condition and might have died of one of the associated blood vessel problems, an aortic aneurysm ballooning out of a weakened wall of the aorta, had he not been assassinated. Lovell notes that the painter El Greco seems to have Marfan-like subjects in his works. He also notes that some persons with a similar disorder (Ehlers-Danlos syndrome) have such extreme elasticity of their bodies and such mobility of their joints that they become contortionists.

Brittle-bone disease (osteogenesis imperfecta) is another inherited collagen disorder, which is marked by soft-skin changes, easy bruising, and abnormal fragility of bone. Persons with this condition also suffer from dwarfism and often have deformed limbs where broken bones have not healed properly. Lovell places the painter Toulouse-Lautrec in this group.

Much more common than these conditions is fibrosis, the excessive or inappropriate deposit of collagen in body organs and tissue. This can result in scarring, contracture and other changes that interfere with the function of the organ. It is seen in cirrhosis of the liver, where the cell structure of a healthy organ is gradually replaced by scar tissue that cannot do the work of the original cells and so the liver fails. The same process occurs in pulmonary fibrosis, where functioning lung cells that provide oxygen to the blood are replaced by non-functioning collagen scar tissue that blocks oxygen transfer.

Collagen disorders can be triggered by alcohol, as in cirrhosis of the liver; by asbestos and silica, as in fibrotic lung disease; by inflammatory illnesses such as rheumatoid synovitis, a joint disease that damages the collagen-based cartilage; and by injury and trauma in almost any part of the body that results in scar formation.

Animal collagen, usually bovine (i.e., from cattle) is processed and purified for a number of medical uses. Because it absorbs blood and encourages coagulation, this collagen can be formed into surgical

The Collagen Connection

sponges for use in operating procedures where control of bleeding by tying or other means is not practical. When Food and Drug Administration approval was sought for one such sponge, the manufacturer tested the product by placing collagen disks over skin-graft sites. The disks effectively stopped the bleeding and could be removed without the bleeding starting up again. Tests in other surgical procedures showed much the same results.

A much different use for collagen was approved by FDA in 1981. In this procedure, the collagen material is injected into the skin to minimize or eliminate wrinkles, frown lines, and other appearance "flaws" and to build up and fill defects such as acne scars.

The physician, usually a dermatologist, injects tiny amounts of bovine skin collagen with a very fine hypodermic needle just beneath the patient's skin where the repair is needed. From two to six visits over a period of several weeks may be needed to get the desired effect of filling in and plumping up the skin to get rid of the wrinkle, scar or indentation. The cost per visit can be $200 or more, and the entire course of treatment can become quite expensive.

Collagen injection has been promoted as a simple office procedure—which, in a way, it is. It has also been described as "lunch hour" and "two-minute" surgery, but it is not that casual a treatment.

Patients must be selected with care, since collagen therapy is not intended for those with a personal or family history of autoimmune disease such as rheumatoid arthritis, psoriatic arthritis, lupus erythematosus, scleroderma, or various other connective tissue diseases. Those who pass this initial screening are injected with a minute amount of the collagen and then observed for four weeks to see if any allergic reactions occur. If there are none, they can go on to treatment. In one group of 650 patients only 21 showed allergic reactions and were eliminated after this test.

The bovine collagen used is type I protein, like that of human skin, that has been processed to remove any traces of type III protein, which might make the human body reject it. However, there have been skin and other reactions, usually mild, and some patients show bruising and swelling that can last for a week or more. Occasionally there will be a granulous buildup of tissue, much like that of a scar, at the injection site. There have also been accidental injections of the collagen into blood vessels, where it can cause clots. This caused blindness in one woman's eye when the collagen put into a blood vessel near her eye was carried to the eye itself.

Although initial results may be excellent, there are no guarantees as to how long the cosmetic effect will last. The collagen will, within two years, be broken down by enzymes in the patient's body. Then a new series of touch-up injections are needed or the skin site will return to its original condition.

Despite its cost of several hundred dollars for a course of treatment (probably not covered by insurance) and despite the need to repeat that treatment within a year or so, collagen therapy has become a very popular method of correcting certain skin cosmetic flaws. One Manhattan dermatologist now devotes his entire practice to it.

As for collagen in cosmetics to be rubbed onto, and supposedly into, the skin to help rejuvenate it, Dr. Lovell has strong opinions. "It has no scientific basis," he says flatly. "Apart from anything else, it would be totally impossible for anything the size of a collagen molecule to penetrate the skin. Even if it did so, it would be immediately gobbled up by a reception committee of enzymes waiting there for it." Despite their popularity, collagen-based cosmetics offer no benefits beyond that of softening and moisturizing the skin, and that can be accomplished with any moisturizing cream or lotion.

FDA Finds No Use of Fetal Collagen in Cosmetics

There have been pamphlets and letters to newspapers in recent years claiming that human fetuses are being used as a source of collagen by the cosmetic industry. The charges were renewed in 1984 by a French book called *The Traffic in Unborn Babies*. The book led to a Vatican newspaper editorial, which gave the charges even greater exposure.

Some of the allegations in the United States are traceable to a 1981 article by a syndicated columnist who suggested that fetal remains might be a source of protein in cosmetics. The Moral Majority organization investigated and said in its July 1984 Moral Majority Report that it had found nothing to substantiate the charges. The protein used was animal (bovine) collagen, which is inexpensive and plentiful. The columnist also disowned his earlier remarks.

The allegations may arise from a misunderstanding. Human placenta, the afterbirth of normal delivery, has for many years been collected for its plasma, protein and other substances, which are purified and processed into medically useful products. It is used in some cosmetics, notably hair shampoos and conditioners. But it is not fetal tissue.

FDA does not believe that fetal collagen is used in cosmetics in the United States and is not aware that any such use occurs in Europe,

The Collagen Connection

as some have claimed. To be more certain, the agency asked its inspectors last year to check U.S. cosmetic firms for any indication that human fetal materials were being used. The inspectors found none.

— by Richard Thompson

Richard Thompson is a member of FDA's communications staff.

Chapter 63

Cosmetic Safety: More Complex than at First Blush

The European cosmetic known as ceruse was used faithfully—and fatally, because it was mainly white lead—by wealthy women from the second century until well into the 19th century to make their faces look fashionably pale.

Nothing on the market today approaches ceruse's deadliness. But many consumers wonder about the eye makeup, lipsticks, foundations, and nail products that are on the shelves. Are there any risks in using these cosmetics? Are long lashes, even skin tone, and brightly colored nails worth any risk at all?

Serious injury from makeup is a "pretty rare event," says John E. Bailey, Ph.D., director of FDA's division of colors and cosmetics. "We don't see it happen that often."

Even one of the most serious problems, eye infections from a scratch on the eyeball with a contaminated mascara wand, has become rare. January 1989 was the last time an infection of this type was reported to FDA.

In 1990, FDA headquarters received approximately 100 reports of adverse reactions to cosmetics. Less than 25 were about makeup and, of those, most were either allergic reactions or skin irritation. (The other complaints were about hair products, soaps, fragrances, and lotions.)

Although industry probably received about 50 reports for every one made to FDA, says Bailey, the problems reported to the companies are along the same lines—allergies and skin irritation.

DHHS Publication No. (FDA) 93-5012. Reprinted from *FDA Consumer*, November 1991.

The agency can't do much about isolated allergic reactions or irritation problems. It's up to the individual to avoid the product that caused the reaction and any other products that contain the offending ingredient. (See "Contact Dermatitis: Solutions to Rash Mysteries" in the May 1990 *FDA Consumer*.)

But that doesn't mean reporting the problem isn't important.

"We look for clusters," says Bailey. "If we see we're getting a number of complaints for the same product, then that is cause for concern."

Unlike reports of allergic or irritation reactions, even one report of an acute injury, usually caused by a contaminated product, results in quick action by the agency. "We'll inspect the establishment, talk to the consumer, talk to the doctor, collect samples, and analyze them to determine the extent of contamination," says Bailey.

Moldy Oldies

Contaminated makeup is the result of either inadequate preservatives or product misuse. But contamination doesn't necessarily translate into serious injury for the user.

"Cosmetics are not expected to be totally free of microorganisms when first used or to remain free during consumer use," according to a 1989 FDA report on contamination of makeup counter samples in department stores. The report was based on a survey which found that over 5 percent of samples collected were seriously contaminated with such things as molds, other fungi, and pathogenic organisms.

Every time you open a bottle of foundation or case of eye shadow, microorganisms in the air have an opportunity to rush in. But adequately preserved products can kill off enough of the little bugs to keep the product safe.

Occasionally, however, a product will be seriously contaminated. According to FDA data, most cases of contamination are due to manufacturers using poorly designed, ineffective preservative systems and not testing the stability of the preservatives during the product's customary shelf life and under normal use conditions.

Driving and Making-up Don't Mix

Consumers must take an active role in keeping product contamination and potential infection to a minimum once they take a product home, says Gerald McEwen, Ph.D., vice president for science for

Cosmetic Safety: More Complex than at First Blush

one of the cosmetic industry's trade associations, The Cosmetic, Toiletry and Fragrance Association (CTFA).

"You need [to follow] good personal hygiene—clean hands, clean face," he says. "And common sense."

One of the riskiest things a woman can do is put on mascara while she's driving, says McEwen. "You hit a bump and you scratch your eyeball," he explains. "Once you've scratched your eyeball, you have all kinds of possibilities of contamination. We're not talking about disease germs here. We're talking about normal bacteria that are all over the air. Those get into that kind of cut, and without proper medical attention you can go blind."

Testing the Testers

There's something else that is definitely taboo when using makeup: sharing.

"Never share, not even with your best friend," says Irene Malbin, CTFA's vice president of public relations. Sharing cosmetics means sharing germs, and the risk, though small, isn't worth it, says Malbin.

Shared-use cosmetics—the testers commonly found at department store cosmetic counters—are even more likely to become contaminated than the same products in an individual's home, according to the 1989 FDA report.

FDA followed its 1989 report on makeup testers with a survey of corresponding unopened retail packages. The survey found only negligible contamination, and the agency concluded that the preservatives couldn't handle the challenge of constant use.

"At home, the preservatives have time—usually a whole day—to kill the bacteria that is inevitably introduced after each use," says Bailey. "But in a store, there may be only minutes between each use. The preservatives can't handle it."

If you really want to test a cosmetic before you buy, "you should insist—must insist—on a new, unused applicator," says CTFA's Malbin. She says that some companies use cotton swabs for that purpose.

Allergic Reactions

Do the preservatives themselves pose any safety risk?

According to a study of cosmetic reactions conducted by the North American Contact Dermatitis Group, preservatives are the second most common cause of allergic and irritant reactions to cosmetics. Fragrances are number one. Although the study is more than 10 years old, the results can still be considered valid today, says Harold R. Minus, M.D. an associate professor of dermatology at Howard University Hospital. (For more information on this study, see "Cosmetic Allergies" in the November 1986 *FDA Consumer*.)

People who have had allergic reactions to cosmetics may try hypoallergenic or allergy-tested products. These are, however, only a partial solution for some and no solution at all for others.

"Hypoallergenic can mean almost anything to anybody," says Bailey.

"Hypo" means "less than," and hypoallergenic means only that the manufacturer feels that the product is less likely than others to cause an allergic reaction. Although some manufacturers do clinical testing, others may simply omit perfumes or other common problem-causing ingredients. But there are no regulatory standards on what constitutes hypoallergenic.

Likewise, label claims that a product is "dermatologist-tested," "sensitivity tested," "allergy tested," or "non-irritating" carry no guarantee that it won't cause reactions.

"FDA tried to publish regulations [in 1975] defining hypoallergenic to mean a lower potential for causing an allergic reaction," says Bailey. "In addition, we were going to require that companies submit information to FDA establishing that in fact their products were hypoallergenic." However, two cosmetic manufacturers, Almay and Clinique, challenged the proposed regulations in court, claiming that consumers already understood that hypoallergenic products were no panacea against allergic reactions. In July 1975, the U.S. District Court for the District of Columbia upheld FDA's regulations, but the two companies appealed. On Dec. 21, 1977, the U.S. Court of Appeals for the District of Columbia reversed the district court's ruling.

What's "Natural"?

Like hypoallergenic, "natural" can mean anything to anybody. "There are no standards for what natural means," says Bailey. "They could wave a tube [of plant extract] over the bottle and declare it natural. Who's to say what they're actually using?"

Revlon, Inc., uses natural plant extracts in its New Age Naturals cosmetics line, says Dan Moriarity, Revlon's director of public relations. "But the base formulas are the same as our conventional products," he

Cosmetic Safety: More Complex than at First Blush

says. In addition, because these products contain fragrances, they don't fit Revlon's definition of hypoallergenic, he explains.

Anyone who has ever had poison ivy knows that "natural" and "hypoallergenic" are not necessarily interchangeable terms. For example, some manufacturers of cosmetics marketed as natural products use naturally occurring vitamins E and C as preservatives. But, according to Alexander Fischer, M.D., author of Contact Dermatitis, "Topical vitamin E is a potent sensitizer which can produce both delayed allergic contact dermatitis and immediate allergic hives."

In addition, natural doesn't mean pure or clean or perfect either. According to the cosmetic trade journal Drug and Cosmetic Industry, "all plants [including those used in cosmetics] can be heavily contaminated with bacteria, and pesticides and chemical fertilizers are widely used to improve crop yields."

Safety Testing

Whether driven by altruism, liability, or the bottom line, most companies see the need for safety testing. But safety testing can rarely be mentioned without bringing up the controversy surrounding the use of animals for those tests.

Many companies have begun to label their products with statements indicating that no animals have been used in testing.

"As far as we know," says Neil Wilcox, D.V.M., director of FDA's Office of Animal Care and Use, "what these companies do is use, for the most part, old reliable ingredients that have been proven safe [based on past animal data and a history of safe use] and then test the final product on people."

"There's kind of a fine point here," says CTFA's McEwen. "These companies that say they don't test on animals are skirting the issue. Practically every ingredient that's used in cosmetics was at some point tested on animals. Probably a statement like 'no new animal testing' would be more accurate."

But what if a company wants to use a new ingredient?

Unlike drugs, FDA does not require pre-market approval for cosmetics. However if a safety problem with a cosmetic product arises after it's been marketed, FDA can take legal action to obtain the manufacturer's safety data on the product. Because there is not yet enough information on alternatives to animal testing to validate their use in ensuring human safety, FDA, at this point, would only accept animal safety data.

The most widely used, and possibly most controversial, animal test, the Draize Eye Irritancy Test, involves putting drops of the substance in question into the eye of an albino rabbit. Investigators then note if any redness, swelling, cloudiness of the iris, or corneal opacity occurs. In addition, the ability of the eye to repair any damage is noted.

"Draize may be impossible to replace with a single alternative test," says Sidney Green, Ph.D., a toxicologist with FDA's Center for Food Safety and Applied Nutrition.

He explains that because the Draize test measures three different areas of the eye, replacing Draize will probably take a combination of alternative tests, "but we've not seen that combination yet."

Wilcox explains that for FDA to approve other methods, those methods will have to produce test results that can be reproduced in other labs. In addition, databases will have to correlate historical animal test results with newer lab results.

"Database development and cooperation [between industry and FDA] are pivotal to the validation process," says Wilcox.

The cosmetics industry has taken one step towards database development: the Cosmetic Ingredient Review. The basic purpose of the review is to gather information from the scientific literature and from company files on the safety of cosmetic ingredients and make that information publicly available.

FDA's division of toxicological review and evaluation is currently evaluating two alternatives for the Draize eye test. One is Eytex, manufactured by Ropak Corp., Irvine, Calif., a chemical assay that produces opacity similar to that of an animal cornea upon exposure to irritants. The other is vertebrate cell cultures from humans and mice.

But until alternatives have been scientifically verified, the option for animal testing must be available for new ingredients and new products, says Wilcox. "No one wants to think of animals being used for anything other than kindness and human companionship," he says. "But it's important that we continue to recognize the risk to human health if unreliable tests are used."

Consumers and their dermatologists should report cosmetic adverse reactions to:

Food and Drug Administration
Center for Food Safety and Applied Nutrition
Division of Colors and Cosmetics
200 C St., S.W.
Washington, D.C. 20204

Cosmetic Safety: More Complex than at First Blush

Regulating Cosmetics

The U.S. Food, Drug, and Cosmetic Act defines cosmetics as "articles other than soap which are applied to the human body for cleansing, beautifying, promoting attractiveness, or altering the appearance."

FDA has classified cosmetics into 13 categories:

- skin care (creams, lotions, powders, and sprays)
- fragrances
- eye makeup
- manicure products
- makeup other than eye (e.g., lipstick, foundation and blush)
- hair coloring preparations
- shampoos, permanent waves, and other hair products
- deodorants
- shaving products
- baby products (e.g., shampoos, lotions and powders)
- bath oils and bubble baths
- mouthwashes
- sunscreens

It is against the law to distribute cosmetics that contain poisonous or harmful substances that might injure users under normal conditions. Manufacturing or holding cosmetics under insanitary conditions, using non-permitted colors, or including any filthy, putrid or decomposed substance is also illegal.

Except for color additives and a few prohibited ingredients, a cosmetic manufacturer may use any ingredient or raw material and market the final product without government approval. The prohibited ingredients are:

- biothionol
- hexachlorophene
- mercury compounds (except as preservatives in eye cosmetics)
- vinyl chloride and zirconium salts in aerosol products
- halogenated salicylanilides
- chloroform
- methylene chloride

Manufacturers must test color additives for safety and gain FDA approval for their intended use.

Cosmetic firms may voluntarily register their manufacturing plants with FDA, file cosmetic formulas, and report adverse reactions.

Cosmetic labels must list ingredients in descending order of predominance. Trade secrets (as defined by FDA) and the ingredients of flavors and fragrances do not have to be specifically listed.

Beauty on the Safe Side

Besides never putting on makeup while driving, consumers should follow other precautions to protect themselves and the quality of their cosmetics:

- Keep makeup containers tightly closed except when in use.

- Keep makeup out of sunlight; light can degrade preservatives.

- Don't use eye cosmetics if you have an eye infection, such as conjunctivitis, and throw away all products you were using when you first discovered the infection.

- Never add any liquid to bring the product back to its original consistency. Adding water or, even worse, saliva could introduce bacteria that could easily grow out of control. "If it has lost its original texture and consistency," says McEwen, "the preservatives have probably broken down."

- Never share

- Throw makeup away if the color changes or an odor develops. Preservatives can degrade over time and may no longer be able to fight bacteria.

"We don't have a hard and fast rule [on when to throw cosmetics out]," says McEwen. McEwen says makeup can be kept indefinitely as long as it looks and smells all right and the consistency doesn't change. "It would be difficult to have any kind of bacterial growth and not have it be noticeable," he explains. However, Janice Teal, a microbiologist who heads the product and package safety division of Avon Products, Inc., disagrees. "Even after the preservatives have stopped working, you may not be able to see or smell anything different," she says.

Cosmetic Safety: More Complex than at First Blush

She agrees with McEwen that there is no absolute date for discarding various products, but says Avon recommends that consumers throw mascara away after three months. They can keep other makeup products a few months longer.

"Mascara is our biggest concern because of the wand," she says. "Normally, the eye is a good barrier to bacteria, but one slip and that wand can scratch the cornea and introduce all kinds of bacteria."

— by Dori Stehlin

Dori Stehlin is a staff writer for *FDA Consumer*.

Chapter 64

Decoding the Cosmetic Label

How can you be sure your shampoo that claims to have all natural ingredients does not also contain some synthetic chemicals? Or that your hand lotion actually does contain the vitamin E it claims? The logical response should be. "Read the ingredient label on the back of the product." Logical, if you happen to be a chemist or a cosmetic scientist. Perplexing, if you are the average cosmetic consumer.

A quick glance at the back of the cosmetic label is all it takes to see that the ingredients are written in the language of chemistry. (See Chemical Translations below.)

Unless you know that one of the shampoo ingredients—methyl paraben—is a synthetic preservative derived from a petroleum base, or that tocopherol is vitamin E, you may never be able to check the claims against the contents.

John Bailey, Ph.D., director of the Food and Drug Administration's Office of Cosmetics and Colors, understands such consumer dilemmas. He and the scientists on his staff admit that most of us don't recognize the names of the ingredients listed. But there's no way to change that and still accurately identify the ingredients.

Chemical names are the only way ingredients can be listed because that's what they are. Most are cosmetic formulations, but in some products, such as an underarm deodorant that also claims to stop perspiration, the first chemical listed may be a drug ingredient and FDA would classify the product as a drug as well as a cosmetic.

FDA Consumer, May 1994.

Many ingredients are marketed with trade names, but these often provide few clues to the identity and intended use of the material. Trade names in the ingredient list could be confusing to consumers purchasing a cosmetic because they would have no way to compare similar ingredients in similar products. Also, some trade names include mixtures of raw materials—for example, an ingredient could be combined with a preservative.

Despite the highly technical language of the ingredient list, Bailey says it's entirely possible for consumers to get valuable information about a product by checking the label—front and back. To decode the cosmetic label, here's what you need to know.

Image vs. Reality

Don't be fooled by claims made for certain cosmetic ingredients. Their presence in the products could be pure puffery because the law does not require cosmetic manufacturers to substantiate performance claims.

"Image is what the cosmetic industry sells through its products," Bailey says, "and it's up to the consumer to believe it or not." (See "Cosmetic Ingredients: Understanding the Puffery" in the May 1992 *FDA Consumer* and reprinted as an earlier chapter in this sourcebook.)

FDA considers the labeling of vitamins in cosmetics a separate issue, however, and does not recognize health claims for them in cosmetics. A product that features a vitamin—for example, vitamin E—must list it by its chemical name—tocopherol—on the ingredient list. Listing it as a vitamin in the ingredient statement would give the misleading impression that vitamin E in the product offers a nutrient or health benefit. (Vitamin E is usually added as an antioxidant to prevent chemical deterioration of the product.)

Consumers can get important health and value information by checking the ingredient list. For example, if you need fragrance-free hair spray because you have a sensitivity, a product containing a fragrance—even one that just masks the chemical odors of the raw materials—could be a waste of money if you can't use it.

Ingredient statements on cosmetics were first required in 1973 under the Fair Packaging and Labeling Act, enforced by FDA. Before then, consumers could only guess what was in a cosmetic product or if the product contained what it claimed. That requirement is especially valuable today with the industry competition for new ingredients.

Decoding the Cosmetic Label

The law allows a manufacturer to ask FDA to grant "trade secret" status for a particular ingredient. FDA grants this status under very limited circumstances and after careful review of the manufacturer's data. The manufacturer must prove that the ingredient imparts some unique property to a product and that the ingredient is not well known in the industry. If trade secret status is granted, the ingredient does not have to be listed on the label, but the list must end with the phrase "and other ingredients."

Consumers can also check value by comparing ingredient lists of similar products. Ingredients are listed in descending order, starting with the greatest amount in the product. A lotion with a featured ingredient close to the beginning of the list, for example, would have more of that ingredient than any other ingredient. A featured ingredient listed close to the end suggests that not much of that ingredient is present.

Anyone curious about an ingredient in a cosmetic can find answers in the International Cosmetic Ingredient Dictionary, published by the Cosmetic, Toiletries, and Fragrance Association. The dictionary provides a complete list of the most widely known cosmetic ingredients and their definitions and trade names. The dictionary, and all other compendia FDA recognizes to name ingredients, are available for reference at many public libraries, or at the Office of the Federal Register, 1100 L St., N.W., Washington, DC 20408.

Cosmetic ingredient declaration regulations apply only to retail products intended for home use. Products used exclusively by beauticians in beauty salons or cosmetic studios, and cosmetic samples such as those distributed free at hotels, are not subject to the ingredient labeling rules. They must, however, state the name and address of the manufacturer, packer or distributor, and give an accurate statement of quantity and all necessary warning statements, as do all other cosmetics that weigh over one-fourth ounce or one-eighth fluid ounce.

Cosmetics That Are Also Drugs

Cosmetics making therapeutic claims—that they may affect the structure or function of the body—are regulated as drugs and cosmetics and must meet the labeling requirements for both. One way you can tell if you're dealing with such a product is if the first entry in the ingredient list says "Active Ingredient." (The active ingredient is the chemical that makes the product effective, and it must be safe for its intended use.) However, active ingredients are not legally required to be identified by this term. The law does require the active ingredient(s) to be listed first, followed by a list of all inactive cosmetic ingredients.

Examples of products that are both cosmetics and drugs are shampoos that treat dandruff, fluoride toothpastes to prevent dental decay, and sunscreens and sunblocking cosmetics, including foundations that contain sunscreens. (See "Dodging the Rays" in the July-August 1993 *FDA Consumer*.)

A product with a drug and cosmetic classification must be scientifically proven safe and effective for its therapeutic claims before it is marketed. If the product is not, FDA considers it to be a misbranded drug and can take regulatory action.

Preventing Problems

Under FDA's good manufacturing practice guidelines, even cosmetic products that are not regulated as drugs should be thoroughly tested for safety and subject to quality control during manufacture. But the law does not require the agency to review these tests before the cosmetics are marketed. Nevertheless, FDA does require safety warnings when problems become apparent.

Misuse of some cosmetic products can cause problems that range in severity from a mild rash to skin burns, or from burning eyes to blindness.

Look for warnings about the consequences of misuse required on products that could be hazardous, in addition to the detailed directions for use that appear on almost all cosmetics.

For example, products containing halocarbon or hydrocarbon propellants, such as aerosol hair sprays or deodorants, must bear the exact wording: *"Warning – Use only as directed. Intentional misuse by deliberately concentrating and inhaling the contents can be harmful or fatal."*

All cosmetics in self-pressurized containers, such as shaving creams, must have specifically worded warnings against spraying near the eyes, puncturing, incinerating, storing, and intentionally misusing.

"Keep out of the reach of children" is also required for all products in pressurized containers. In the case of products intended for use by children, such as foaming soap, the phrase *"except under adult supervision"* may be added.

Other products requiring specific wording include:

Decoding the Cosmetic Label

- **Detergent bubble bath products:** may irritate skin and the urinary tract through excessive use or prolonged exposure. The labeling instructs users to discontinue the product if rash, redness or itching occur, to consult a physician if irritation persists, and to keep out of reach of children. These adverse reactions reportedly occur mostly with prolonged soaks. According to some studies, the adverse reactions either subside or disappear with discontinued use. In 1987, FDA started requiring all foaming detergent bath products not labeled as intended for exclusive adult use to display the caution statement in addition to directions for use.

- **Feminine deodorant sprays intended for use in the genital area**: are for external use only and should not be applied to broken, irritated or itching skin. A physician should be consulted if persistent, unusual odor or discharge occurs. The statement instructs users to discontinue immediately if rash, irritation or discomfort develops. Labeling on self-pressurized containers must state that the product should be sprayed at least 8 inches from the skin.

- **Coal-tar color-containing hair-dye products:** contain ingredients that may cause skin irritation on certain individuals, and a preliminary test according to the product's accompanying directions should first be made. Users are cautioned not to dye eyelashes or eyebrows because doing so may cause blindness. In addition, the ammonia, soaps, detergents, conditioning agents, and dyes in hair-dye products are all strong eye irritants and could also cause allergic reactions in other areas. (See "Hair Dye Dilemmas" in the April 1993 *FDA Consumer* and reprinted as an earlier chapter in this sourcebook.)

The following products require explicit warnings, though not with specific wording:

- **Depilatories and hair straighteners:** are highly alkaline; if they are used incorrectly, they may cause serious skin irritation.

- **Shampoos, rinses and conditioners:** can cause eye problems that range from irritation to permanent damage. If the eye's cornea is scratched or otherwise damaged, a contaminated product could cause infection. These cosmetics, as well as others that contain water, usually have antimicrobials that discourage growth of bacteria.

- **Nail builders (elongators, extenders, hardeners, and enamels):** can cause irritation, inflammation and infection of the nail bed and nail fold (where the nail meets the finger) due to residual traces of the methacrylate monomers. Also, nail hardeners and enamels often contain formaldehyde and formaldehyde-releasing preservatives, which may cause allergic reactions in people who are sensitive to them. In addition, the solvents or plasticizers may be irritating. Nail enamels that are also nail hardeners cause the most problems. Their high resin content or low concentration of plasticizer seals the nail surface to air and makes the nail too brittle. Another frequent problem is flammability during and shortly after application. These products require a flammability caution.

- **Flammable products such as aerosol hair sprays containing alcohol and an isobutane propellant:** include caution statements on the label. Also, the label usually cautions about avoiding heat, fire and smoking during use until the product is fully dry. Last year, FDA received reports of a fatality that occurred from burns suffered when a woman's hair ignited. Apparently, she tried to light a cigarette before her hair spray had completely dried.

Manufacturers often use warning statements on labels when there is even a small chance of a problem. Baby products often contain such warnings. Baby powder, for example, if used carelessly and accidentally inhaled by the baby in large amounts, can block the infant's bronchial and lung passages and cause suffocation. (For more about cosmetic safety, see "Cosmetic Safety: More Complex Than at First Blush" in the November 1991 *FDA Consumer* and reprinted in this sourcebook.)

Cosmetic labels are more than product advertising. They connect cosmetic science with consumer protection by providing a means for consumers to know what's in a product and how to safely use it. A wise consumer will take the time to read the label to get the best value and results without incurring any of the possible harmful effects.

Decoding the Cosmetic Label

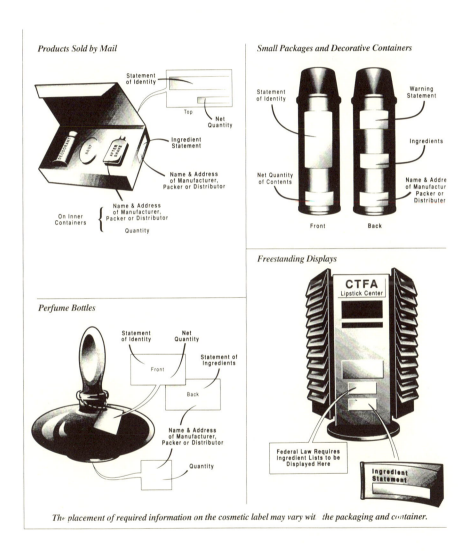

Figure 64.1. Where's the Label Information?

Chemical Translations

At present, the cosmetic industry selects from more than 5,000 different ingredients. It's no wonder consumers can be perplexed when they see the list. Here are some common cosmetic ingredients and their usual functions (active drug ingredients are not included):

Moisturizers function as a moisture barrier or to attract moisture from the environment:

- cetyl alcohol (fatty alcohol): keeps oil and water from separating, also a foam booster
- dimethicone: silicone skin conditioner and anti-foam ingredient
- isopropyl lanolate, myristate, and palmitate
- Lanolin and lanolin alcohols and oil (used in skin and hair conditioners)
- octyl dodecanol: skin conditioner
- oleic acid (olive oil)
- panthenol (vitamin B-complex derivative): hair conditioner
- stearic acid and stearyl alcohol

Preservatives and antioxidants (including vitamins) prevent product deterioration:

- trisodium and tetrasodium edetate (EDTA)
- tocopherol (vitamin E)

Antimicrobials fight bacteria:

- butyl, propyl, ethyl, and methyl parabens
- DMDM hydantoin
- methylisothiazolinone
- phenoxyethanol (also rose ether fragrance component)
- quaternium-15

Thickeners and waxes used in stick products such as lipsticks and blushers:

- candelilla, carnauba, and microcrystalline waxes
- carbomer and polyethylene: thickeners

Decoding the Cosmetic Label

Solvents used to dilute:

- butylene glycol and propylene glycol
- cyclomethicone (volatile silicone)
- ethanol (alcohol)
- glycerin

Emulsifiers break up and refine:

- glyceryl monostearate (also pearlescent agent)
- lauramide DEA (also foam booster)
- polysorbates

Color additives: synthetic organic colors derived from coal and petroleum sources (not permitted for use around the eye):

- D&C Red No. 7 Calcium Lake (lakes are dyes that do not dissolve in water)

Inorganic pigments—approved for general use in cosmetics, including for the area of the eye:

- iron oxides
- mica (iridescent)

Hair dyes—phenol derivatives used in combination with other chemicals in permanent (two-step) hair dyes:

- aminophenols

pH adjusters stabilize or adjust acids and bases:

- ammonium hydroxide: in skin peels and hair waving and straightening
- citric acid: adjusts pH
- triethanolamine: pH adjuster used mostly in transparent soap

Others:

- magnesium aluminum silicate: absorbent, anti-caking agent
- silica (silicon dioxide): absorbent, anti-caking, abrasive
- sodium lauryl sulfate: detergent

- stearic acid cleansing, emulsifier
- talc (powdered magnesium silicate): absorbent, anti-caking
- zinc stearate: used in powder to improve texture, lubricates.

—by Judith E. Foulke

Judith E. Foulke is a staff writer for *FDA Consumer*.

Chapter 65

Tattooing in the '90s

Ancient Art Requires Care and Caution

Tatooing, a technique of marking the skin with colors, has been practiced since antiquity. Now this ancient art form appears to be enjoying a renaissance. Movie and television stars have begun sporting small tattoos on unobtrusive parts of the body, and others are following their lead.

Tattooing also has cosmetic medical applications, including covering "port wine stains," coloring skin of people with vitiligo (a disorder that gives the skin a "mottled" appearance because areas have become depigmented), and obscuring color defects in the lips after facial surgery. It is also promoted for "permanent" eyeliner; however, there are safety concerns about this procedure (see "Permanent Eyeliner," which accompanies "Hair Dye Dilemmas" in the April 1993 *FDA Consumer* and reprinted in this sourcebook).

Although there are no firm statistics, an unpublished 1990 random survey of 10,000 U.S. households revealed that 3 percent of the population as a whole, and 5 percent of men, had tattoos. Brisk sales of tattoo inks also suggest that the number of people receiving tattoos is increasing rapidly, according to a letter in the January 16, 1992, *New England Journal of Medicine*.

Today's tattoos are applied in one of two ways. "Permanent" tattoos are applied by tattooists using a machine that pierces the skin

---

FDA Consumer, October 1993.

with needles. "Temporary" tattoos can be applied by anyone by pressing a color-permeated design against the skin with a moistened wad of cotton.

Permanent tattooing is generally safe when done by an experienced tattooist who sterilizes the equipment and follows appropriate sanitation procedures, according to Kris Sperry, M.D., co-founder with tattooist Mick Michieli-Beasley of the Alliance of Professional Tattooists (APT), a nonprofit organization that educates tattooists in proper infection control practices. However, medical complications may occur if the tattooist is careless about cleanliness, or if the person receiving the tattoo doesn't care for the tattooed area properly in the first week or so after it is applied.

Tattooing is illegal in some cities and states, largely because, historically, tattoo parlors often operated without a concern for health and safety, Beasley says. In New York City, for example, tattooing was banned in the mid-1960s after an outbreak of hepatitis B was traced to unsterilized equipment in tattoo parlors. To improve safety, APT organizes seminars for tattooists throughout the country to instruct them in cleanliness and sterilization techniques.

Selecting a Tattooist

The first step when getting a permanent tattoo is to select a good tattooist, according to Beasley. "Tattooing in unsanitary conditions can set the stage for infection of the customer or the tattooist," says Beasley, who is also co-owner of a tattoo parlor.

"Scratchers" who work out of their kitchen or the back of a van should be scrupulously avoided," adds Sperry, a forensic pathologist in Atlanta, Ga., who has several tattoos. "A tattooist who is genuinely concerned with both his and his customer's health will not risk his livelihood and reputation by failing to follow appropriate health measures."

Beasley and Sperry decided to form APT after meeting with Cathy Backinger, Ph.D., a public health analyst in the Food and Drug Administration's Office of Training and Assistance. In 1988, Backinger developed a resource curriculum for personal service workers—people other than health-care workers whose work puts them in close personal contact with clients, and who may be exposed to a client's blood or risk transmitting blood from client to client. These include people who perform ear piercing, electrolysis, acupuncture, and tattooing.

"Our primary concern was prevention of the transmission of blood-borne pathogens such as human immunodeficiency virus and hepatitis B," Backinger explains. "The curriculum is designed to help state health departments set up courses to educate personal service workers in the techniques of infection control." The curriculum was distributed in 1989 to all state health departments, but not all states have used it as yet, Backinger says.

To help ensure that tattooists were appropriately trained, Beasley and Sperry worked with Backinger to customize the curriculum for tattooists that is presented by APT at national tattoo conventions.

"Our APT guidelines are often more rigorous than those imposed by local health departments," Beasley notes. "Thus, the fact that a tattoo parlor is operating and has not been closed down by the health department does not necessarily mean that the tattooists are following stringent health practices."

Tattooists who complete the course receive a certificate. When selecting a tattooist, a consumer can ask whether the tattooist has taken the infection control course and ask to see the certificate.

According to the APT guidelines, these practices should be followed:

- The tattooist should have an autoclave (a heat sterilization machine regulated by FDA) on the premises.

- Consent forms (which the customer must fill out) should be handled before tattooing.

- Immediately before tattooing, the tattooist should wash and dry his or her hands thoroughly and don medical latex gloves, which should be worn at all times during application of the tattoo.

- Needle bars and tubes should be autoclaved after each customer. Non-autoclavable surfaces such as pigment bottles, drawer pulls, chairs, tables, sinks, and the immediate floor area should be cleaned with a disinfectant such as a bleach solution.

- Used absorbent tissues should be placed in a trash can lined with a plastic bag.

- Used needles and razor blades should be placed in a special puncture-resistant, leak-proof container for disposal.

Beasley advises visiting several tattoo parlors to see whether the tattooists follow these recommended safety guidelines, and asking questions about cleanliness and sterilization. "If a tattooist refuses to discuss cleanliness and attempts to minimize your concerns, go elsewhere," she says.

Applying Permanent Tattoos

Permanent tattoos are applied using a small electric machine with a needle bar that holds from 1 to 14 needles, each in its own tube. Tattoo needles are regulated by FDA.

The tattooing machine operates like a mini-sewing machine: The needle bar moves up and down as it penetrates the superficial (epidermis) and middle layer (dermis) of the skin. The tattooist holds the machine steady while guiding it along the skin. The electric current is controlled by a foot switch.

The needles protrude only a couple of millimeters from the tubes, so they don't penetrate deep into the skin. Each needle has its own tube, which enables the needle bar shaft to operate smoothly without damaging the needles. A single needle is used to make fine, delicate lines. A row of needles is used for shading and denser lines.

The end of the needle tube is dipped in a small amount of ink. As the tattooist guides the machine over the skin, the needle moves up and down, puncturing the skin and depositing ink along the way. Excess ink and the small amount of blood that oozes from the skin puncture are continuously removed with absorbent tissues.

Before beginning a tattoo, the tattooist, wearing medical latex gloves, inspects the customer's skin to make sure there are no open cuts or scrapes. The skin is sprayed with an antiseptic and the hairs in the area are shaved (the tattooist should immediately dispose of razors in a special container).

The tattooist then makes a stencil transfer of the tattoo outline onto the skin, or draws the outline on the skin with a pen. A thin layer of ointment such as petroleum jelly is spread over the area to be tattooed.

Getting a tattoo can be painful. The severity of the pain depends on the site of the tattoo and the person's level of pain tolerance. Small tattoos (up to 3 inches) can generally be completed within an hour. Larger ones may take several hours or more, and may be done in more than one sitting.

Once the tattoo is completed, the area is washed with mild soap and water and covered with an antiseptic ointment. Customers are instructed to keep the area clean with soap and water, leave it exposed to the air when possible, and apply a mild, hand cream to keep the tattooed area moist until healing is complete (usually 7 to 10 days).

The tattoo should not be exposed to direct sunlight for at least two weeks to prevent sunburn or pigment changes. Sunscreen should be applied during subsequent sun exposure to prevent fading of pigments. Swimming in fresh, salt, or chlorinated pool water is also discouraged during the first few weeks after the application of a tattoo to prevent the pigments from leaching out.

Tattoo Inks

The inks, or dyes, used for tattoos are considered "color additives" under the Federal Food, Drug, and Cosmetic Act.

The known incidence of adverse reactions or injury from tattoo ink is "minimal," says Allen Halper of FDA's division of cosmetics and colors. However, consumers should be aware that their safety has not been established. FDA is evaluating its role in the regulation of tattoo ink. At present, many states and local health departments regulate tattooing.

The colors used in temporary tattoos, which fade several days after application, also fall under FDA jurisdiction. Although no adverse reactions have been reported to FDA, the agency has issued an "import alert" for several foreign-made temporary tattoos, says Halper. These tattoos are not allowed into the United States because they don't carry the FDA-mandated ingredient labels or they contain colors not permitted by FDA for use in cosmetics.

Removing Tattoos

Although tattoos applied to the skin with needles are called "permanent," methods exist to remove them, according to Steven Snyder, M.D., a dermatologist in private practice in Owings Mills, Md.

These techniques include surgical removal; using tissue expanders (balloons inserted under the skin for six to eight weeks to stretch the skin, so when the tattoo is cut away there is less scarring); dermabrasion, which involves sanding the skin with a wire brush to remove the epidermis and dermis; salabrasion, the use of a salt solution to soak the tattooed skin (sometimes the solution can seep too deeply into the skin and leave an unsightly scar, according to Snyder); and scarification, which involves removing the tattoo with an acid solution and creating a scar in its place.

Three lasers, regulated by FDA, are also being used for tattoo removal:

- the Q-switched ruby laser,
- the neodymium YAG laser, and
- the Alexandrite laser.

These lasers can remove most color with very little scarring. However, the ruby laser does not work very well in removing red, yellow and orange colors, whereas the YAG laser does not work well on green pigment, according to Snyder.

Another problem with laser removal is called "paradoxical darkening," according to Ray Geronemus, M.D., associate professor of dermatology at NYU Medical Center in New York City. Light colors such as beige, pink and white may turn black when treated by the laser. To circumvent this problem, a small spot of color should be tested first to see whether darkening occurs, he says. If the tattoo ink is available, the laser-ink reaction can be tested in a laboratory dish.

Geronemus suggests that tattoo parlors or clients themselves keep records of the dyes used in their tattoos, including the lot number of each pigment, in case the client later wants the tattoo removed. "This would be like a medical record. Rather than dealing with a hodgepodge of inks, the dermatologist would know exactly what dyes were applied, which can assist in removal," he says.

People considering having a tattoo removed should make sure that the physician they select has training in the use of lasers and other removal techniques, Geronemus cautions. He suggests contacting a local hospital, the American Society for Laser Medicine, or the American Society for Dermatological Surgery for referrals.

Another way to "remove" an undesirable tattoo is to cover it up with another tattoo, notes Sperry. The new tattoo is usually larger than the tattoo it is replacing, incorporating and hiding the previous tattoo in new contours and colors.

Tattoos can also be covered with a special waterproof makeup foundation, according to cosmetologist Maurice Stein, founder of Cinema Secrets, a Burbank, California-based supplier to cosmetologists and medical facilities. Originally developed for use by burn victims and people with skin discolorations, the foundation is also used by people who feel their tattoos are inappropriate in certain situations. "The typical scenario is a woman with a tattoo on her bust line who wears a low-cut dress at a church wedding or other conservative setting. The tattoo can be covered for that particular occasion," Stein says.

Men also use the foundation. "My father had a tattoo he was embarrassed about, so he hardly ever wore short sleeves or went to the beach," Stein says. "Many men who got tattoos during the service are in a similar situation. The foundation allows them to feel more comfortable in public."

Health Risks

Contracting blood-borne illnesses such as hepatitis B or human immunodeficiency virus, which leads to AIDS, is a frequent worry of those considering getting tattooed.

According to Kris Sperry, M.D., a forensic pathologist in Atlanta, Ga., and co-founder of the Alliance of Professional Tattooists, based in Glen Burnie, Md., "If a tattooist follows appropriate cleanliness procedures, and the person who receives a tattoo takes proper care of it, the risk of infection at the site of the tattoo is minimal, and the risk of picking up any type of blood-borne pathogen is virtually nil."

Temporary inflammation around the tattoo is common for the first day or so. As part of the healing process, the skin that is tattooed crusts slightly and peels within the first week after application.

Some people occasionally have an adverse reaction to a particular pigment used in the tattoo, which may result in swelling or itching. This can usually be relieved by using a topical corticosteroid cream and keeping the tattoo out of direct sunlight (which may make the reaction worse).

Hepatitis B, a viral infection, can be transmitted from one customer to another if tattoo needles are inadequately sterilized, says Sperry.

Because HIV may be transmitted through the introduction of contaminated blood or blood products into the body through the skin, "it is theoretically possible that tattooing could transmit this viral disease," Sperry wrote in the January 1992 issue of *American Journal of Forensic Medicine and Pathology*. "To date, there has not been an unequivocally proven case where tattooing passed the human immunodeficiency virus from one individual to another. However, the prolonged incubation period of AIDS would make certain documentation of HIV transmission by tattoo difficult. The sterilization techniques commonly used by professional tattooists all adequately kill HIV, but the amateur tattooist who does not sterilize equipment could conceivably transfer HIV with dirty needles."

—by Marilynn Larkin

Marilynn Larkin is a medical writer in New York City.

Index

Index

Page numbers in italics refer to graphics and tables; the letter n following a page number refers to a note.

A

Aas, K. 186n97
abdominoplasty 118
Abel, E. A. 42n3, 47n1, 47n6, 55n17
ABMS Compendium of Certified Medical Specialists 112
abrasion treatment 77, 118
abrasive preparations 105
abscesses 434
Accreditation Association for Ambulatory Health Care, Inc. 119
accutane (isotretinoin)
  acne treatment 26, 496
  psoriasis treatment 127, 132
  side effects 26
acetic acid 401
Achromycin 418
acne 21-27, *22*, *24*, 59
  causes 21-23
  infants 3
  treatments 25-27
  triggers 23-24, 25

Acne, Morphogenesis and Treatment (Kligman) 75
acne medications 23-27, *250*
acne scars 478-79
acne vulgaris 21
acquired ichthyosis 236
acquired immune deficiency syndrome *see* AIDS
acrochordons (skin tags) 100
acromegaly 255
actinic assault 102
actinic cheilitis 328
actinic keratosis 100, 103, 327-31, 481
actinomyces 438
acupuncture 54, 606
acyclovir (Zovirax) 346, 370
  herpes 392-93, 395
  shingles 366
Adalat 269
Addison's disease 295
adenine 302
adhesions 410
Adinoff, A. D. 185n86
adolescents
  acne 21-24
  androgen 23
  atopic dermatitis 158
  dandruff 517
  obsessive-compulsive disorders 62

Skin Disorders Sourcebook

aeroallergens 168, 169, 175-78
African-Americans
  actinic keratoses 329
  photosensitivity 249
  psoriasis 125
  scarring 423
  see also race factors
age factor
  actinic keratoses 329
  dandruff 517
  lichen planus 239
  makeup 592
  psoriasis 125
  psychiatric disorders 64
  scarring 411
  scleroderma 266
  shingles 363-64, 371
  skin cancers 300
  skin treatments 99-109
  surgery 478
  varicose veins 96
  warts 385
  wrinkles 72, 497
  xeroderma pigmentosum 333
  see also adolescents; children; elderly population; young adults
Agency for Health Care Policy and Research (AHCPR) 450, 456, 475
age spots 77
agoraphobia 63
AHCPR *see* Agency for Health Care Policy and Research (AHCPR)
AIDS (Acquired Immune Deficiency Syndrome)
  genital herpes 395
  pruritus 42
  shingles 365
  tattoos 611
Albergo, R. 183n35
Albrecht, Renata, M.D. 31
alcohol
  cosmetics 600
  psoriasis 135
  rosacea 38
Aldomet 269
allergenic compounds 190
allergic contact dermatitis 190, 191, 193

allergies
  atopic dermatitis 167-81
  collagen treatments 118
  contact dermatitis 6, 564
  cosmetics 585-86, 587-88
  eczema 5
  hair loss 514
  lichen planus 240
Allergies Sourcebook (Omnigraphics) 197n, 564
Alliance of Professional Tattooists 606, 611
aloe vera 574
alopecia areata 67, 244, 245, 295, 514, 527-31, 533-38
  stress 59
alopecia totalis 527, 535
alopecia universalis 535
alpha-hydroxy acids 77, 232-33, 482
alpha interferon *see* interferon
Alpha Keri 52
alpha methyldopa (Aldomet) 269
Alprazolam (Xanax) 59, 60
Alternaria 176
aluminum acetate (Burrows solution) 199
American Academy of Cosmetic Surgery 552
American Academy of Dermatology 240, 242, 296, 313, 340, 531
American Academy of Facial and Reconstructive Surgery 552
American Academy of Pediatrics 16
American Association for Accreditation of Ambulatory Plastic Surgery Facilities 119
American Cancer Society 311, 340
American College of Obstetricians and Gynecologists 242
American Family Physician 351n
American Hair Loss Council 509, 510, 531, 533n, 542, 549n, 552
American Health Association (ASHA) 393
American Heart Association 17
American Pharmaceutical Association 417
American Podiatric Medical Association 85, 86, 87

Index

American Rheumatism Association 267-68
American Society for Dermatologic Surgery (ASDS) 477n, 502, 552, 610
American Society for Laser Medicine 610
amitriptyline HCl (Elavil, Endep) 59, 64
ammonium hydroxide 603
amniocentesis 212, 235
amniotic liquid 575
Amonette, Rex A., M.D. 331
amoxicillin 376, 443
anabolic hormones 43
Anacardiacaea family 202
Anafranil 59
anagen effluvium 510, 535, 536
anchoring fibrils 221-23
Anderson, J. A. 183n38
Andersson, K. 174, 184n66
Andrews, Alan D., M.D. 340
androgen hormone 23
androgenic alopecia 510, 533-38
anemia 82, 218
anesthetic gels 52
angel's kiss 7
animal bites 429-46
animal ringworm 362
animal skin, grafts 503
animal testing 589-90
antacids 270
anthralin 127, 130, 529
anthranilates 251
antianxiety medications 59, 60, 163
antibacterial medications 39, 366
antibiotic medications
  acne treatment 23, 25, 26
  atopic dermatitis treatment 163
  bite wounds 442-44
  calcinosis 270
  canker sores 348
  cephalosporins 15
  erythromycin 15
  herpes simplex 345
  penicillin 15
  prophylactic doses 17, 442-43
  pruritus 46, 50, 51, 53
  rheumatic fever treatment 14, 17, 377

antibiotic medications, continued
  rosacea treatment 39
  scar abrasions 412-13
  strep throat treatment 15-16, 376
  tetracyclines 39
  toxic streptococcal syndrome 20
  urticaria 282
  vaginal yeast infections 31
antidepressant medications
  pruritus treatment 54, 60
  skin disorders 61
  tricyclic 289
anti-fibrotic agents 269
antihistamine medications 260
  atopic dermatitis treatment 163
  lichen planus 240
  poison ivy infections 200
  pruritus 51, 53
  skin rashes 320
  urticaria 284-87, *288*
anti-hypertensive agents 269
anti-inflammatory medications 269
  aspirin 17
  atopic dermatitis 157
  psoriasis 152
  steroids 17
antimalarial medications
  lupus treatment 243
  pruritus 43
  psoriasis 134
antimicrobials 416, 602
antineoplastic medications 44
antiperspirants 50, 52
antiprotozoal medications 39
anti-Ro (SSA) antibodies 245, 246
antiseptics 415-21, 466
anti-viral therapies
  acyclovir 346
  genital herpes 400
  shingles 365, 369-73
anxiety
  skin disorders 58, 60
aphthous stomatitis (canker sores) 347-49
Arlen, David I. 87
Arshad, S. H. 184n69
arthritis 270
  foot problems 82
  psoriatic 127

arthritis, continued
  scleroderma 267
artificial light 249
aspirin 17, 270
  pruritus 43, 46, 54
  shingles 366
  urticaria 282
astemizole 287
asthma 157, 169, 190, 353
Atherton, D. J. 173, 178, 184n55, 186n98
athlete's foot 83, 360
atopic dermatitis 59, 157-65, 353, 354
  allergies 167-81
  see also eczema
Auerbach, Robert, M.D. 511
Aureomycin 418
Auspitz's sign 124
Austin, H. A. 150n
autoimmune disorders 354, 529
  pityriasis rosea 259
  psoriasis 139-40
  urticaria 279-80
autosomal dominant diseases 206-8
autosomal dominant inheritance 209-10, *210*
autosomal dominant Lamellar ichthyosis 236
autosomal recessive inheritance *211*, 211-12
Aveeno 199
Avobenzone (Parsol 1789) 251
azathioprine (Imuran) 269

B

Baciguent 418
bacitracin 417, 418
Backinger, Cathy, Ph.D. 606
Backman, G. 174, 184n63
bacteremia 375, 378-79
bacteria growth
  acne 24
  diaper area 4-5, 10
  nails 563
bacterial conjunctivitis 10

bacteroides fragilis 434, 438
Baden, H. P. 307
Baer, Harold 199
Baerlocher, K. 186n106
Bailes, J. A. 173, 184n56
Bailey, John, Ph.D. 524, 526, 564, 571, 575, 576, 585-86, 595-96
Baker, P. B. 69n11
Baker, S. G. 109n12
baldness 478
  see also hair loss
Ban Reijsen, F. 185n77
barefoot walking 86
Bark, Joseph P., M.D. 517
Barlock, A. L. 47n10
Barton, S. P. 109n8
basal cell carcinomas 102, 103, 108, 303, 477, 486
basal cells 299, 300
Basis 52
Bauer, Eugene, M.D. 223
Beasley, Mick Michieli- 606, 608
Beck H. I. 178, 186n95
Bedard, P. 291
bed sores *see* pressure ulcers
Bennich, H. 181n4, 182n21
benzocaine 418
  canker sores 348
  poison ivy infections 200
benzodiazepine 60
benzophenones 251
Bergbrant, I. M. 186n110
Berger, P. A. 182n23
Berman, Stuart, M.D. 403
Bernhard, J. D. 47n3, 49n1, 54n1
Bernhisel-Broadbent, J. 183n42
Bertolino, Arthur P., M.D. 511
beta blocker medications 134
Beutner, Karl 369, 370
bichoroacetic acid 402
Bickers, D. R. 108n1
Bieber, T. 185n78, 185n81, 185n83
Bihova, Diana, M.D. 510, 511, 512
Bina, P. 186n104
biologic response modifiers 46
biothionol 572, 591
Birchall, N. 153n
Birnbaum, J. 185n84

618

Index

birth control pills
  acne 24
  hair loss 512, 536
  skin rashes 320
  see also oral contraceptives
birth defects 137-38
birthmarks 3, 7-9, 498
bites 429-46
Blachley, J. D. 42n2
blackheads (comedo) 23
  extractors 25
  infants 3
Blank, L. 55n6
Blankenship, D. M. 42n2
bleaching creams 77, 482, 540
bleomycin 265, 489
blepharoplasty 116, 480-81
blisters 3
  epidermolysis bullosa 205-6, *222*
  friction 205, 207, 214, 216
  ichthyosis 227
  shingles 364
  see also fever blisters
blood eosinophila 158
blood infections
  Group A streptococcus 14, 15, 19
  impetigo 18
Bock, S. A. 183n40
Boden, G. 186n99
body lice 557
body ringworm 359, 360-61
Boland, G. 185n77
bone disease 253, 256
bone marrow transplantation 46
Bord, M. A. 49n3, 54n5
Borel, J. F. 150n
Bos, J. D. 182n17, 185n80
Boss, E. 291
Bostwick, Dave 519
Boulton, P. 173, 184n58
Bowling, Marcia, M.D. 401
Brash, Douglas E. 307
Braun-Falco, O. 185n81
breast augmentation (enlargement) 117
breast feeding 174-75
  epidermolysis bullosa 217
  thrush 10

breast lift surgery (mastopexy) 118
breast reduction 118
brittle bone disease 580
Broadbent, K. R. 183n42
Broberg, A. W. 186n111
Brodell, Robert, M.D. 400, 403, 405
Brostoff, J. 183n51
Brown, Anne 224
brown birthmarks 8-9
Bruijnzeel, P. L. B. 185n76
Bruynzeel, P. L. B. 184n73
Bruynzeel-Koomen, C. A. F. M. 184n73
Buchanan, R. A. 69n7
bullous congenital ichthyosiform erythroderma 227, 236
bullous epidermatosis 207
bullous pemphigoid 354
bunions 81, 84-85, *85*
Buras, E. M., Jr. 109n9
Bureau of Consumer Protection 111n
Burke, John, M.D. 504
Burke-Yannas skin 504-5
Burkhart, C. G. 356n4
Burkitt, Denis 89, 97
Burks, A. W. 182n34
Burney, P. G. J. 182n15
burns 415-21
burn treatment 503-6
Burrows solution
  epidermolysis bullosa treatment 214
  poison ivy infections 199
Buspirone HCI (BuSpar) 59, 60
butoconazole nitrate (Femstat 3) 32
butterfly rash 244
butylene glycol 603

C

café-au-lait spots 8-9, 257
Calamine lotion 355
Calcagno, David, M.D. 94
calcinosis 263, 270
calcipotriene (vitamin D) 130, 145
calcipotriol 529
calluses 82
Camp, R. D. R. 186n102

cancer therapy 44-46
  see also skin cancers
candelilla 602
candida 10, 29-33, 563
candida albicans 30
canine scabies 353-54
canker sores 347-49, 349
capnocytophaga canimorsus 430, 436
Capoten 269
capsaicin (Zostrix) 366-67
carbomer 602
carbon dioxide laser 330
carcinomas 42-43, 44
  see also skin cancers
carditis (rheumatic heart disease) 377
Cardizem 269
care givers
  epidermolysis bullosa 213-14
  pressure ulcers 455, 460-62
carnauba 602
Carrier, William L. 304
Carter, C. M. 173, 184n58
Casciato, D. A. 55n16
case studies
  compulsive hair pulling 67
  contact dermatitis 194-95
  psoriasis 68
  trichotillomania 68
Casimir, G. J. A. 173, 184n57
Cassileth, B. R. 55n14
Cassileth, P. A. 55n14
Castelain, M. 185n84
Castelain, P. 185n84
cat bites 432, 434-36
catopril (Capoten) 269
CDC *see* Centers for Disease Control and Prevention (CDC)
ceftriaxone 443
cefuroxime 443
cell growth factors 150
cellulite 119
cellulitis 375, 378
Centers for Disease Control and Prevention (CDC)
  genital warts 399, 403
  melanoma deaths 309-13
  streptococcal infections 14

cephalosporins 15, 376, 443
cerebral palsy 84
cerebrosides 575-76
ceruse 585
cetyl alcohol 602
Chanarin-Dorfman Syndrome (neutral lipid storage disease) 236
Chapman, M. D. 185n89
chemical names, cosmetics 595-604
chemical peels 77, 118, 330, 482, 483-84, 500-502
chemotherapy 428, 487
  hair loss 539, 542
  pruritus 44-45, 46
  warts 387
Chen, J. A. 356n7
cherry angiomas (De Morgan's spots) 100
chickenpox 360, 363-68, 372
children
  atopic dermatitis 5-6, 59, 157-65, 169
  bone disease 256
  chickenpox 363
  dandruff 517
  epidermolysis bullosa 206, 216-18
  food allergies 171-74
  footwear 87
  hair loss 533-42, 541
  head lice 553-58
  herpes simplex 344
  household glue remover 565
  ichthyosis 231-32
  medical epidemics 14
  obsessive-compulsive disorders 62
  precocious puberty 254-55
  protection from sunlight 324-25
  ringworm 361
  scabies 353
  skin infections 17
  strep throat 15
  xeroderma pigmentosum 336-37
CHILD syndrome (unilateral hemidysplasia) 236
Chiron Corporation 396, 397
chlorambucil (Leukeran) 269
chloroform 591
chlorpheniramine 53

Index

chlorpromazine (Thorazine) 250
chlorpropamide (Diabinese) 250
chlortetracycline hydrochloride 417, 418
cholestasis 43
cholestyramine 54
cholinergic urticaria 64
chondrodysplasia punctata syndrome (Conradi-Hunermann syndrome) 236
chorea 377
Chrisman, D. A., Jr. 109n9
chronic idiopathic pruritus 64
chronic idiopathic urticaria (CIU) 275-91
chronic urticaria 59
chrysanthemum flowers *see* pyrethrum
cigarette smoking
  squamous cell carcinoma 103
  wrinkles 73
cimetidine 54
cimetidine (Tagamet) 270
citric acid 603
CIU *see* chronic idiopathic urticaria (CIU)
Clark, R. A. F. 185n86
clavulanic acid 443
clean rooms 178
Clemmensen, O. J. 187n113
clindamycin 163, 376, 379
clomipramine HCI (Anafranil) 59, 62-63
clostridium 438
clostridium tetani 438
cloth diapers 5
clothing
  after liposuction 119
  contact dermatitis treatment 194
  epidermolysis bullosa 216
  lupus 247
  poison ivy infections 199
  pruritus 49, 50, 53
  ringworm 361
  scabies 352
  sun exposure avoidance 104, 107
  varicose veins 95
  xeroderma pigmentosum 336-37
clotrimazole (Gyne-Lotrimin) 32

coal tar preparations 157, 599, 603
  atopic dermatitis treatment 163
  cancer 299
  dandruff 516, 518-19
  psoriasis treatment 127, 129, 145
Coca, A. F. 167, 180, 181n1
Cohn, J. B. 69n9
coin-shaped lesions 243-45
colchicine 268, 269
cold sores 6, 343, 502
Coleman, R. 182n33
collagen 409-13, 424, 504, 579-83
  scleroderma 266
collagen, bovine 479, 484, 575, 580-81
collagenase 223
collagen injections 74, 77, 118, 484
Collins, Jane 153
collodion babies 234
Colloff, M. J. 178, 185n92
colloidal oatmeal treatment 50
colposcopy 401
comedo 22, 23
compression stockings 93
compulsion, defined 62
condylomata acuminata (genital warts) 386, 399
Condylox (podofilox) 402, 405, 489
congenital ichthyosiform erythroderma (CIE) 227, 229, 231, 233, 234, 236
conjunctivitis 10
Conradi-Hunermann syndrome 236
constipation 89-90, 97, 218
contact dermatitis 6, 159, 189-95, 564, 586
contagious infections
  anogenital warts 386
  genital herpes 389
  genital warts 399
  herpes simplex 344
  human papilloma virus 399
  scabies 351
  skin infections 17
  see also noncontagious infections
Contie, Victoria L. 141
contractures 219, 410
  graft *versus* host disease (GVHD) 46

Cook, B. L. 69n11
Cooke, R. A. 167, 180, 181n1
Cookson, W. O. C. M. 182n31
Cooper, K. D. 182n16
Cornell skin 505-6
corns 81, 82
cornstarch
   pruritus treatment 52
corticosteroids 242, 269-70, 289
   atopic dermatitis treatment 162-63
   epidermolysis bullosa treatment 223
   pruritus 46, 51
   psoriasis treatment 145
   scars 413
   steroid-induced rosacea 37
cortisone medications
   cradle cap 6
   eczema 6
   shingles 365
corynebacterium 434-38, 438
Cosmetic, Toiletry, and Fragrance Association, Inc. 521, 573, 576, 587
cosmetics 571-77
   acne 24
   collagen 74, 582
   hair dyes 521-26
   labels 595-604
   port wine stain 8
   rosacea 38
   safety 585-93
   wrinkles 71-74, 76-79
   see also makeup products
cosmetic surgery 111-20
   see also plastic surgery
Cotran, R. S. 183n46
cow's milk allergies 173-74
crabs 557
cradle cap 6, 518
CREST syndrome (limited scleroderma) 262, 263-64
crotamiton cream 355
crusty bumps 327
cryosurgery 329, 482, 487, 488
cryotherapy 386-87, 403
   scars 427
cryptorchidism (undescended testes) 234

Cuprimine 269
curettage 329, 487
Cushing's syndrome 255-56
cutaneous disfigurment 63-64
cutaneous infections 158, 176
cutaneous innervation 100
cuts 415-21
cyclomethicone 603
cyclophosphamide (Cytoxan) 269
cyclosporine 138, 145, 529
   psoriasis study 147-50, 152-53
cyproheptadine hydrochloride 53
cystic acne 26
cysts 477
cytokines 150, 151, 152
cytosine 302
cytotoxic agents 44-45
Cytoxan 269

D

Daly, B. M. 55n18
dandruff 6, 598
dandruff control 515-19
Danese, P. 177, 185n85
Dangel, R. B. 47n2, 54n2
Daniel, Ralph, M.D. 566-67
Dannaker, C. J. 195n2
Dannenberg, B. 185n83
David, T. J. 184n59
DEBRA *see* Dystrophic Epidermolysis Bullosa Research Association (DEBRA)
De Conno, F. 55n8
Deeg, H. J. 48n21
De Groot, Anton C., M.D. 545
de Jong, E. 143
delusional conditions 61-62
Demodex folliculorum (mites) 37
De Morgan's spots 100
Dennie-Morgan infraorbital fold 158
dental problems 219-20
deoxyribonucleic acid *see* DNA
Depen 269
D'Epiro, Peter 69
depression
   disfiguring skin diseases 63-64
   skin disorders 58, 60, 61

Index

dermabrasion 77, 118, 330, 479, 484, 490, 493-94, 609
  acne scars 26
  rhinophyma 40
dermal circulation 100
dermatitis herpetiformis 353, 354
dermatologists
  acne 25, 26
  lichen planus 240
  lichen sclerosus 242
  moisturizers 75
  psychological factors in skin treatment 57
  rosacea 37
  rosacea treatment 39
  seborrheic dermatitis 517
  tretinoin 497
  xeroderma pigmentosum 337, 339
dermatophagoides *see* house dust mites
dermatophyte infections 359-62
dermatosis 53
dermis 504
  attachment to epidermis 99, 221
  described 72
desaquamation process 45
desipramine HCI (Norpamin, Pertofrane) 59, 61
Deslorelin 255
desquamation 376
Devlin, J. 173, 184n59
DHHS *see* U.S. Department of Health and Human Services
diabetes
  foot care 86
  foot problems 82
  pruritus 42
dialysis 18
  see also kidney disease
Diamond, M. I. 426
diaper rash 4-5
diazepam 54
Dibenzyline 269
dicloxacillin 163, 376, 443
Diepgen, T. L. 181n8
diet
  elimination 173, 282
  ichthyosis treatment 233

diet, continued
  pregnancy 175
  psoriasis 133
  urticaria 278-79
  varicose veins 97
  see also nutrition and diet
diffuse systemic sclerosis 262
Diflucan (fluconazole) 29
dihydrotestosterone (DHT) 533
diltiazem (Cardizem) 269
dimethicone 602
diphenhydramine hydrochloride
  poison ivy infections 200
  pruritus treatment 53
diphenylcyclopropenone (DPCP) 529
Directory of Medical Specialists 112, 232, 241, 296
discoid lesions 243-45
discoid lupus erythematosus 243, 244
disposable diapers 4
dithranol 145
diuretics 18
DNA (deoxyribonucleic acid) 73, 248, 257, 404
  skin cancers 302-6
  sunlight damage 299
  xeroderma pigmentosum 334-35, 336
doctors *see* dermatologists; physicians
Doekes, G. 186n109
dog bites 431, 434-36
dominant dystrophic epidermolysis bullosa 208, 221
dopamines 62
Doppler probe 95
double-bind placebo-controlled food challenges (DBPCFC) 171-75
Dove 52
Downey, D. 186n101
doxepin HCI Cream 5 percent topical (Zonalon Cream) 59
doxepin HCI (Sinequan) 59, 61, 64, 66
doxycycline 443
D-penicillamine (Cuprimine, Depen) 268, 269
Draelos, Zoe, M.D. 542
Draize Eye Irritancy Test 590
drooping of lower eyelid 116

dry eye syndrome 116, 481
dry skin
  elderly population 105-6, 108
  ichthyosis vulgaris 227
  pruritus 41
  radiation therapy 45
  wrinkles 73
Dubowitz, M. 182n32
Duchateau, J. 173, 184n57
Duke, A. M. 172, 183n53
Dunagin, W. G. 47n7
Duncan, W. C. 42n1, 47n5
dysesthesia 370-71
dysphagia 217
dystonia 62
Dystrophic Epidermolysis Bullosa Research Association (DEBRA) 205, 221, 223-24

E

EB *see* epidermolysis bullosa
EB letalis 207
Ebling, F. J. G. 69n1
eccrine glands 106
ECG 62
ectropion 231
eczema (atopic dermatitis) 5-6, 59, 157-65
education
  atopic dermatitis treatment 164
  care givers
    epidermolysis bullosa 213
    pruritus 49-50
  patients
    pruritus 49-50
Edwards, B. K. 313n6
Edwards, J. H. 69n6
Eiermann, Heinz 74
eikenella corrodens 430, 438
Eisen, A. Z. 47n3, 47n4, 49n1, 54n1
Elais, J. 291
elastic stockings 93
elastin 424
Elavil 59
elderly population
  bruises 100
  foot care 85-86

elderly population, continued
  pruritus 41
  see also age factor
electrocautery (burning) 387, 403
electrodesiccation 329, 492
electrotherapy 473, 488, 606
Elias, P. M. 108n2
elimination diets 173
Elimite 355
Ellis, Charles N., M.D. 109n13, 147-49, 149n, 150n
emollients 105-6
  pruritus 51
  psoriasis treatment 127, 128, 136
emotions 50, 58
  acne 24
  atopic dermatitis 160
  disfiguring skin diseases 63-64
  ichthyosis 231-32
  pruritus 43, 48, 51
  psoriasis 125, 126
  rosacea 38
  scarring 410
  scleroderma 272-73
emulsifiers 603
enalapril (Vasotec) 269
En Coup de Sabre 262, 264
Endep 59
endocrine abnormalities 253, 254-56
endoscopic forehead lift 78
endoscopic surgery 78
Engman, M. F. 183n43
Engman, W. F. 183n43
enkephalins 43
environmental irritants 189-90
epidemics
  acute glomerulonephritis 18
  scabies 351-52
  strep throat 15
epidermal barrier dysfunction 169
epidermis 228, 504
epidermolysis bullosa 205-25, 207
epidermolysis bullosa simplex—generalized 206
epidermolysis bullosa simplex—localized 207
epidermolytic hyperkeratosis 227, 230, 233, 235, 236

Index

epidermothyton 359
Epidermothyton floccosum 83
erysipelas 375, 378
erythema (redness) 158, 251
erythrocyte sedimentation rate (ESR) 282
erythrodermic psoriasis 124, 126
erythrokeratodermia heimalis 236
erythrokeratodermia progressiva symmetrica 236
erythrokeratodermia variabilis 236
erythromycin 15, 376, 380-83
   atopic dermatitis treatment 163
   pruritus 43
esophageal dysfunction 263
Estelle, F. 291
estrogen 254
ethanol 603
etretinate 498
Eucerin 52
Eurax 355
EURO-PSO 143
Evans, Carnot, M.D. 22, 24, 25
excoriations
   antidepressant medications 61
   case history 66-67
exercise
   liposuction 119
   varicose veins 93, 96
exotoxin production 178-79
external beam therapy (radiation) 45
eye cancers 333-34
eyelid surgery (blepharoplasty) 116, 480-81
eye problems
   cosmetics 585, 587
   epidermolysis bullosa 219
   ichthyosis 231
   ophthalmic shingles 364, 365
   xeroderma pigmentosum 338
eye protection 322

F

face lifts (rhytidectomy) 78, 116, 484
facial pallor 158
facial redness 39
facial tightness 231, 235, 481

fadrozole 255
Faergemann, J. 186n110-11
Fair Packaging and Labeling Act (1973) 596
famciclovir 369, 371-72
familial pemphigus 236
Farber, E. M. 42n3, 47n1, 47n6, 55n17, 69n4
Farley, Dixie 421, 506
Fartasch, M. 181n8
fatty tumors 478
Faux, J. A. 182n31
Fawcett, J. 69n6
FDA *see* Food and Drug Administration
FDA Consumer 13, 21n, 29n, 35n, 71n, 81n, 123n, 197n, 399n, 503n, 509n, 515n, 521n, 543n, 553n, 559n, 571n, 579n, 585n, 595n, 605n
Federal Trade Commission (FTC) 120
   tanning devices 319, 323
Federman, D. D. 42n3, 47n1, 47n6, 55n17
Femstat 3 *see* butoconazole nitrate
Fenske, Neil A., M.D. 42n1, 47n5, 108n3, 109, 109n10
fetoscopy 212, 235
fever blisters 343-47
fibrel 479, 484
fibroblast cells 256
fibroblasts 266, 411, 424, 504, 527
fibrosis 266, 267, 580
Fields, W. C. 36
filiform warts 386
Finbloom, David, M.D. 400, 403
fingernail problems 32, 144, 559-67, 600
Finn method patch tests *192*
F.I.R.S.T. *see* Foundation for Ichthyosis and Related Skin Types
The First Five Years (Schultz) 11
Fischer, Alexander, M.D. 589
Fitzpatrick, T. B. 47n3, 47n4, 49n1, 54n1
5-fluorouracil cream 330, 387, 402
flap surgery 117, 550
flat feet 84
flat warts 386
Flieger, Ken 368

625

fluids in skin 73, 75, 229
fluoxetine HCI (Prozac) 59, 61, 63, 67
fluvoxamine maleate (Luvox) 59, 63
Folkenberg, Judy 548
follicles 527-28, 533
  mites 38
  transplanting 117, 478, 511-12, 549-52
folliculitis 354
fomites 359
food allergies 5, 6
  acne 24
  atopic dermatitis 158, 159, 168, 169, 171-75
  canker sores 348
  contact dermatitis 6
  herpes simplex 346
  rosacea 38
  skin rashes 320
  see also nutrition and diet
Food and Drug Administration (FDA)
  acyclovir 370
  antibiotics 15, 415-16
  baldness 510-12
  collagen 581
  cosmetics 71-72, 591, 598
  dandruff medications 516
  genital herpes 346
  hair dyes 522-23
  interferon 400
  nail products 560-62
  over the counter medications 415-21
  psoriasis treatment 124
  retinoids 496
  tanning devices 321, 323
  tattoo needles 608
  tetracycline 348-49
foot problems 81-88, 230
foot ringworm 359, 360
Forton, F., M.D. 38
fosinopril (Monopril) 269
fos-jun proteins 425
Foulke, Judith E. 577, 604
Foundation for Ichthyosis and Related Skin Types, Inc. 227n, 230, 236, 238
Fox, Michael D., M.D. 356, 357
Fradin, Mark S., M.D. 149n, 150

freckles 8, 312
friction and blisters 205, 207, 214, 216
Frogge, M. H. 49n2, 54n4
FTC see Federal Trade Commission
Fu, K. K. 47n16
fumaric acid 145
fungal infections
  athlete's foot 83
  nails 563
  seborrheic dermatitis 517
fusion of fingers and toes 219
fusobacterium 434, 438

G

Gage, Andrew A., M.D. 94
Gage, Andrew M., M.D. 94
Galli, S. J. 182n18
Gallico, G. Gregory, M.D. 506
gamma benzene hexachloride 355
gangrene 375, 379
Gant, C. 184n69
Gate theory 44
Gawkrodger, D. J. 174, 184n67
Geller, B. 165n4
Geltman, R. L. 55n13
gender factor, skin cancers 309, *310*
generalized morphea 262, 264
genetic blistering diseases 205
genetic counselors 212, 224
genetic defects
  ichthyosis 230, 235
  skin cancers 302
genetic inheritance 209
  hair loss 510, 528
  see also heredity
genetic markers 139
genetic research
  interferon 404-5
  scarring 424-25
  skin cancers 301-4
genital herpes 344, 346, 366, 389-98
genital warts 386, 399-405, 487-89
geographic factors
  photosensitivity 250
  poison ivy 202
  skin cancers 103, 301-2
  varicose veins 97

Index

Geronemus, Ray, M.D, 610
Gilleaudeau, P. 141
Giroux-Barbeay syndrome 236
Gleich, G. J. 183n44-45
glomerulonephritis 18, 378
　see also kidney disease
Glover, M. T. 178, 186n98
gloves 193, 194, 608
glucose 52
glyceral monostearate 603
glycerine 603
　ichthyosis treatment 233
　psoriasis treatment 136
glycol 136
glycolic acid 233
Goeckerman regimen 131
goiter 255
Goldstein, A. M. 313n7
Gomez, M. 356n8
Gondo, A. 184n75
Good, R. A. 182n26
Goodman, M. 49n2, 54n4
Gossart, B. 173, 184n57
Gottlieb, Alice B., M.D. 140, 150-53, 153n
Gottlieb, S. L. 141
Grabbe, J. 185n82
grafts 46
　hair 117, 485, 549-52
　skin 337, 428, 479, 503-6
graft versus host disease (GVHD)
　pruritus 46
Graham-Brown, R. A. C. 183n54
gramicidin 417
Grammer, L. C. 182n19
Granelli-Piperno, A. 153n
granulation tissue 409
Grayson, Leonard, D., M.D. 109
Greaves, M. U. 47n4
Green, Sidney, Ph.D. 590
Greigo, Robert D., M.D. 429n, 446
Groenwald, S. L. 49n2, 54n4
Grossman, Rachel M., M.D. 151-52, 153n
Grove, G. L. 109n4
Grulee, C. G. 174, 184n60
guanine 302
Guillet, G. 171, 177, 182n14

Guillet, M. 171, 177, 182n14
Gullo, S. M. 47n9
Gustafsson, D. 174, 184n66
guttate morphea 264
guttate psoriasis 124
GVHD see graft versus host disease
Gyne-Lotrimin see clotrimazole

H

Haas, N. 185n82
Haddad, Z. 165n4
Hadley, K. 186n101
Hailey-Hailey disease (familial pemphigus) 236
hair dyes 521-26, 540, 599, 603, 605
hair loss 59, 67, 231, 244, 245-46, 485-86, 509-14, 527-31, 533-42, 543-48
hair pulling, compulsive 60, 62, 67
　see also trichotillomania
hair transplants 117, 478, 511-12, 549-52
Halbert, Anne R., FACD 187
Halken, S. 174, 184n65
Hall, Peter A. 305
hallux valgus (bunions) 84
halogenated salicylanilides 572, 591
Halper, A. J. 307
Halper, Allen 609
Halpern, S. R. 174, 184n62
Halpert, Anne R. 167n
halporogin 84
Hamann, K. 185n82
Hammar, H. 183n52
Handbook of Nonprescription Drugs 417, 420
hand dermatitis 189
hand eczema 189
Hanifin, J. 164n2
Hanifin, J. M. 171, 183n39
Hankey, B. F. 313n6
Hansen, L. G. 174, 184n65
Hansen, R. C. 356n8
Harbeck, R. 186n104
Harlequin ichthyosis 235, 236
Harper, J. I. 182n33
Harras, A. 313n6
Harris, Natalie 559

Harris, Susan 138
Hartman, A. M. 313n7
Hassey, K. M. 47n12, 47n15, 55n9
Hassy, K. M. 55n11
Hay, R. J. 182n15
hay fever 190, 353
H2 blockers 289
Headington, J. T. 109n13
head lice 553-58
heart disease
　CREST syndrome 265
　rheumatic fever 14, 16-17, 377
heat rash 4
　See also prickly heat
Hecht, Annabel 88, 203
Heck, M. T. 184n71
Hefton, John, Ph.D. 505
Heller, S. 174, 175, 184n68
hemangiomas 498
hematologic disorders 42
　see also blood infections
hemodialysis 42
hemorrhoids 89
Heneson, Nancy 150
Henricksen, Ole, Ph.D. 141
Henson, Jim 14, 19-20
hepatic disease 54, 283
　see also liver diseases
hepatitis 438
　nail salons 562
　tattoos 606, 611
herald patch 259
heredity
　atopic dermatitis 167, 168
　bunions 84
　canker sores 348
　contact dermatitis 190
　epidermolysis bullosa 206-8, 209-12
　hair loss 528-29
　ichthyosis 230
　lichen planus 240
　male pattern baldness 485, 509, 510
　psoriasis 125
　scaly skin 235
　scarring 411
　skin cancers 312
　varicose veins 96
　xeroderma pigmentosum 333, 335

Herlitz disease 207
　see also epidermolysis bullosa
herpes hestationis 354
herpes simplex virus (HSV) 344-46,
　389-98, 438, 502
　eczema 6
　stress 59
herpes varicella (chickenpox) 363
herpes zoster 363
Herxheimer, Andrew, M.D. 545
hexachlorophene 572, 591
hickey 7
Hide, D. W. 175, 184n70
Hilderley, L. 55n7
Hill, D. 313n8
Hill, D. J. 172, 183n53
Hill, L. W. 168, 181n3
Hill, S. 109n8
Hill, Suzette 560
Hingley, Audrey T. 519
Hirose, R. 109n4
histamines
　atopic dermatitis treatment 172
　pruritus 43, 44
Histerelin 255
HIV (human immunodeficiency virus)
　bites 438-39
　nail salons 562
　scabies 351-52
　shingles 371
　tattoos 611
　vaginal yeast infections 30
Hjorth, N. 187n112-13
HLA see human leucocyte antigens
　(HLA)
Hodgkin's disease 42, 44, 54
Hoffman, D. R. 165n4, 181n11
Hogan, C. M. 55n12
Hogan, D. J. 195n2
Hogan, M. B. 182n19
Holbrook, M. M. 181n5
Holohan, Thomas, M.D. 505
homeostatic environment of body *101*
Hood, A. F. 47n8
hormonal agents 269-70
　estrogens 43, 46, 510
　gonadotropins 254

Index

hormonal agents, continued
  growth 255
  hair loss 536, 537
  progestins 43, 46
  testosterone 43, 46, 242, 254, 510, 533
hormone therapy
  canker sores 348
Hosking, C. S. 172, 183n53
Host, A. 174, 184n65
hot baths
  psoriasis treatment 136
  vasodilation 52
hot flashes 37
hotlines
  American Society for Dermatologic Surgery 502
  Federal Drug Administration 119
  Herpes Resource Center 393, 398
  LUNG LINE 165
  minoxidil 531
  National Center for Nutrition and Dietetics 476
  rabies 445
house dust mites 168, 169, 176-78
Howley, Peter M. 303
Howser, D. M. 47n10
Hubbard, S. M. 47n10
human bites 429-46, 432-34, 436-39
human leucocyte antigens (HLA) 139, 529
human papilloma virus (HPV) 399-405, 487
  see also papillomaviruses
human placenta 574-75, 582
humectants 73
  see also moisturizers
humid environments
  athlete's foot 83
  pruritus 51, 53
  during winter 106
humidifiers 76
humidity
  atopic dermatitis 159, 162
  occupational skin disease 190
  ringworm 361
Hurwitz, Sidney, M.D. 3
Hutchison, P. E. 183n54

hydration
  atopic dermatitis treatment 160-62
  ichthyosis treatment 233
  psoriasis treatment 135-36
hydrochlorothiazide (Hydrodiuril) 250
hydrocortisone 105, 106, 425
  poison ivy infections 200
Hydrodiuril 250
hydrophilic creams 260
hydroxychloroquine (Plaquenil) 243, 247, 269
hydroxyzine 53
hydroxyzine hydrochloride 53
hyperkeratotic cutaneous lupus lesions 244
hypersensitivity 167, 176-78, 417
  IgE-mediated 168, 172
  see also allergies
hyperthyroidism 295, 514
hypertrophic cutaneous lupus lesions 244
hypertrophic scars 411, 423-28
hypoallergenic cosmetics 588-89
hypothyroidism 295, 514

I

IBIDS syndrome 237
ichthyosis 158, 227-38
ichthyosis hystrix (Curth-Maklin type) 237
ichthyosis linearis circumflexa 237
ichthyosis vulgaris (common ichthyosis) 227, 229, 233, 235, 237
IgE antibodies 179
IgE receptors 168, 169-71, 176-78
immune dysregulation 169
immune system 19, 139-40, 151-53
  kidney disease 18
  lichen planus 240
  scleroderma 265
  shingles 365
  vitiligo 294
immunizations 220
  see also vaccines
immunosuppression 269
  actinic keratoses 329

immunosuppression, continued
  canker sores 349
  cyclosporine 147-48, 152-53
impaired vision 36
impedance plethysmography (IPG) 95
impetigo 14, 17, 355, 375, 377-78
incontinence 449-50, 454, 474-75
inderal 134, 269
indomethacin (Indocin) 270
infants
  acne 3
  collodion babies 234
  epidermolysis bullosa 207, 208
  formulas 217
  genital herpes 392-93, 394
  ichthyosis 234-35
  infection treatment 9-11
  lupus 245
  psoriasis 125
  scabies 353
  seborrheic dermatitis 518
  skin protection 3-6
  sunlight 315-16
  viral conjunctivitis 10
"Infants: The New Knowledge" (McCall) 9
infection avoidance
  atopic dermatitis 157, 178-80
  epidermolysis bullosa 214-15
  psoriasis treatment 137
  yeast infections 33
infections
  bites 429-46
  infant rashes 4
  lichen planus 240
  pressure ulcers 472
  pruritus 47
  tattoos 606
ingrown toenails 84
inhalant allergens *see* aeroallergens
injection therapy 129, 479, 494-96, 499, 581
  facial wrinkles 118
  scars 427
  varicose veins 93, 94-95
inosiplex 529
Inouye, J. C. 182n22
insect infestations 354

insomnia 66-67
insurance
  cosmetic surgery 111, 115
  hair prosthesis 542
interferon 400, 403-5, 489
interferon-gamma treatment 428
interleukin-4 170
interleukin-2 (IL-2) 140
interleukin-6 (IL-6) 150-52
intermittent claudication 93
International Association of Enterostomal Therapy 455
International Cosmetic Ingredient Dictionary 573, 597
intralesional steroid injections 129
inverse psoriasis 124
iodine preparations 419
iodochlorhydroxyquin 83
IPG *see* impedance plethysmography (IPG)
iron oxides 603
Irons, J. 181n10
irritant contact dermatitis 190, 191, 193
Irwin, M. M. 48n20
Irwin, R. 313n5
Ishizaka, K. 181n5
Ishizaka, T. 181n5
ISIS Pharmaceuticals 405
isopropyl lanolate 602
isotretinoin (Accutane) 496
itching
  candida 29
  elderly population 105
  epidermolysis bullosa 214
  pruritus 41
  psoriasis 133
  see also pruritus

J

Jacks, Tyler 305, 307
Jacobs, Alvin H. 7, 8
Jacques, P. 291
Janniger, Camila Krysicka, M.D. 356, 356n5
Johansson, S. 186n111
Johansson, S. G. O. 181n4, 182n21, 182n24-25, 186n103

Index

Johnson, E. 181n10
Johnson, R. 141
Johnson, R. B. 174, 184n62
Johnson, Richard 370-71
Joint Commission for the Accreditation of Healthcare Organizations 119
joint pain 267
jojoba oil 106
Jolie, P. L. 183n41
Jonason, Alan S. 305, 307
Jones, H. E. 182n22
Joost van Neerven, R. J. 185n79
Jordan, R. E. 183n45
Journal of American Academy of Dermatology 167n
Juhlin, L. 182n21

K

Kahonen, K. 185n87
Kajosaari, M. 174, 184n63-64
Kaplan, A. P. 291
Kaposi's sarcoma
  pruritus 42
  see also AIDS
Kapp, A. 183n47, 185n76
Karlsrud, Katherine, M.D. 11
Kastans, Michael B. 305
Katz, Bruce E., M.D. 412
Katz, S. I. 109n4
Kay, A. M. 183n48
Kay, J. 174, 184n67
Keller, F. D. 69n7
keloids 410, 423-28
Kemp, A. S. 177, 185n91
Kennedy, R. Z. 426
keratin 228
keratinocytes 140, 150-52, 527, 528
keratits-ichthyosis-deafness syndrome 236, 237
keratolytics 232-33
keratosis 328
keratosis follicularis spinulosa decalvans 237
keratosis palmaris 158
kerion 359
ketoconazole 180

kidney diseases 14, 514
  CREST syndrome 265
  Group A streptococcal infections 18
  impetigo 18
  scleroderma 268
  see also glomerulonephritis; renal disease
KID syndrome 236, 237
Kieffer, M. 186n110
Kihiczak, George, M.D. 356, 356n5, 357
Kimmelman, J. 307
Kimura, C. 182n30
Klein, L. 54n3
Kligman, A. M. 109n4, 181, 186n100, 187n114
Kligman, Albert, M.D. 72, 74-75
Kligman, L. H. 109n6
Koblenzer, C. S. 69n3
Kobren, Gerri 409n, 410
Koebner phenomenon 126, 249
Koh, H. K. 313n2
Koj, A. 153n
Konig, W. 186n105, 186n108
Koo, John Y. M., M.D. 69, 69n5
Korsgaard, J. 178, 186n95
Kosary, C. L. 313n6
Kost, Ronda 370
Kozar, Rose 530
Kraemer, Kenneth H., M.D. 340
Kramer, M. S. 184n61
Kravits, H. M. 69n6
Kricker, Anne 301
Kripke, M. L. 109n7
Krown, S. E. 48n18
Krueger, James G., M.D. 139-41
Krueser, J. 153n
Kuijper, P. H. M 185n76
Kunala, Subrahmanyam 304
Kupper, T. S. 153n
Kurtzweil, Paula 383, 567
Kwell 355

L

Lachapelle, J. M. 186n99
LactAid 218
lactase deficiency 218-19

631

lactic acid 73, 106, 136, 233
lactose intolerance 218-19
Lamellar ichthyosis 227, 229, 230, 231, 233, 234, 237
Lane, David P. 305
Langerhans cells 100, 102, 176, 179, 190
Lanigan, S. W. 69n4
lanolin 51, 73, 106, 233, 602
Larkin, Marilynn 612
laser surgery 330, 477, 480, 482, 487, 488, 490, 492
 described 498-99
 genital warts 403
 rosacea treatment 39
 scars 427
 tattoo removal 610
late phase reactions (LPR) 172, 175
laundry detergent
 atopic dermatitis 159
 pruritus 50, 53
 see also soaps
lauramide DEA 603
Lavoie, A. 291
Leffell, David J., M.D. 307, 331
leg cramps 92
lentigines 481
lentigos 481
Leroy, B. P. 186n99
lesions see skin lesions
leukemia 42, 44
Leukeran 269
Leung, D. Y. M. 183n46, 186n104, 186n107
Leung, Donald Y. M., M.D. 165
Lever, R. 186n101
Lever, R. S. 178, 185n92
Levine, Robert, M.D. 424
Levy, M. 55n14
Lewis, Ricki, Ph.D. 405
Leyden, J. E. 186n100
Li, A. 182n32
lichen planus 239-41, 354
lichen sclerosus 241-42
lidocaine 52, 200, 419
Lier, J. G. 185n88
Lin, A. 307
lindane 355, 555

Lindgren, L. 186n103
linear IgA bullous dermatosis 354
linear scleroderma 262, 264
Lipicky, Raymond, M.D. 545
lipids 75, 228
lipoinjection 479, 482-83, 484, 494-96
liposomes 573
liposuction (suction-assisted lipectomy) 118-19, 494-96
lisinopril (Prinivil, Zestril) 269
liver diseases 514, 580
 CREST syndrome 265
 pruritus 42
liver spots 481-83
living epidermis 228
Lober, C. W. 108n3
localized sclerodermas 262
logistical regression tests 169
loratidine 287
Love, Audrey 415, 417
Lovell, Christopher, M.D. 579, 582
Lowe, Nicholas, M.D. 39
Lowhagen, R. 174, 184n66
Lowitz, B. B. 55n16
Lubriderm 52
Lumpkins, Debbie 419-20
Lupron 255
lupus 243-52, 514
lupus erythematosus 243, 247, 262
Lupus Foundation of America 243n, 248
lupus profundus 244
Luvox 59
Lydon, J. 49n2, 54n4
Lyell, A. 356n3
lymphomas 42, 44
lysine 346

M

macules 293
Madden, Michael, M.D. 505
Magnan, M. A. *469*
magnesium aluminim silicate 603
Mahoney, Mike 542
Maienza, J. 55n10

Index

makeup products
  acne 24
  rosacea 38
  skin cancers 103
  see also cosmetics
Maklebust, J. *452, 469*
malaria *see* prickly heat
Malbach, H. I. 195n2
Malbin, Irene 587
male pattern baldness 485, 509, 510, 533-42
Mallory, S. B. 182n34
malnutrition 100
Manzini, B. M. 177, 185n85
Marfan's syndrome 580
Marks, R. 109n8, 313n8
Marks, Robin 301
Marples, R. R. 186n100
Marsden, R. A. 173, 184n56
masoprocal cream 330
mastopexy 118
Mathews, K. P. 290
Mathias, C. G. T. 190, 195n1
matrix proteins 424
Matthews, L. 175, 184n70
Matthews, S. 175, 184n69-70
May, L. 153n
May, L. T. 153n
Mayer, D. K. 48n17
Mayo Clinic Health Letter 76
McCall, Robert B. 9
McCaskill, C. C. 182n12
McCray, N. 49n3, 54n5
McCune-Albright syndrome 253-57
McEwen, Gerald, M.D. 586-87, 589, 592
McFadden, J. P. 186n102
McGerity, J. L. 182n22
McIntyre, R. 182n23
McKenna, G. J. 307
McNally, J. C. 49n3, 54n5
McSharry, C. 178, 185n92
MCTD *see* mixed connective tissue disease (MCTD)
Meharry Medical College 424-25
Meinking, T. L. 356n6-7
melanin 23, 249, 294, 299
melanocytes 100, 102, 294, 299, 300

melanoma, malignant 100, 103, 108, 300, 477, 486
  deaths 309-13
  see also skin cancers
Mellon, M. H. 174, 175, 184n68
Menter, A. 42n2
The Merck Manual of Diagnosis and Therapy 359n
mercury compounds 572, 591
Merthiolate antiseptic 415
Messana, Joseph M., M.D. 149, 149n
Methimazole 255
methotrexate 269
methotrexate (MTX)
  birth defects 137-38
  psoriasis treatment 127, 132, 145
methyline chloride 572, 591
methyl methacrylate 564
metoclopramide 270
Metrogel (metronidazole) 39
Meyer, Marcia 35-36, 40
Miaskowski, C. 47n13
mica 603
Michieli-Beasley, Mick 606, 608
miconazole (Monistat 7) 32
miconazole nitrate 84
micro lipoinjection *see* lipoinjection
microsporum 359
migraine headaches 37
military service 135
Miller, B. A. 313n6
Milstein, Stanley R., Ph.D. 573-74
Min, K. 153n
Miner, J. N. 426
mineral oil 51, 73, 106, 233
Minipress 269
minoxidil (Rogaine) 269, 486, 510-11, 529, 534, 537, 543-48
Minus, Harold R., M.D. 588
Mitchell, E. B. 182n13, 185n89
mites 37, 38
  scabies 351-52
  see also house dust mites
mixed connective tissue disease (MCTD) 262
Mizutani, H. 153n
Mohs micrographic surgery 477, 487

633

moisturizers
  collagens 582
  contact dermatitis treatment 194
  dry skin 105-6, 230
  infants 6
  oil in water creams 74
  pruritus 51-52
  psoriasis treatment 127, 136
  side effects 251, 602
  wrinkles 73, 79
  see also humectants
moles 8, 499
  elderly patients 103
  skin cancers 312
  surgery 477
Monafo, William W., M.D. 411
mongolian spots 9
monilia 10
monilia diaper rash 5
Monistat 7 *see* miconazole
monoclonal antibodies 43, 223
Monopril 269
monosymptomatic hypochondriacal psychosis 61-62
Monroe, E. W. 291
Morbidity and Mortality Weekly Report 309n
Morelli, Joseph G., M.D. 167n, 187
Moriarity, Dan 588-89
morphea 262, 264
morphine 46, 50
Mortimer, M. J. 174, 184n67
mosaic warts 386
mottled pigmentation 100
mRNA 150, 152
Mudde, G. 185n77
multiple sulfatase deficiency 237
Munro, A. 69n10
Murphy, D. P. 153n
muscle atrophy 219
Mustoe, Thomas A., M.D. 412-13
Myciguent Cream 418
mycobacterium tuberculosis 438
Myers, J. C. 426
myositis 270, 375, 379
myths
  acne 24
  hair loss 538

myths, continued
  poison ivy 198, 199
  tanning devices 320-22
  warts 385

N

nail psoriasis 143-45
nail ringworm 359, 360
NAIMS *see* National Institute of Arthritis and Musculoskeletal and Skin Diseases
naproxen (Naprosyn) 250, 270
Naproxyn 270
Nater, Johan P., M.D. 545
National Alopecia Areata Foundation 527n, 530
National Cancer Institute 41n, 340
The National Center for Education in Maternal and Child Health 224
The National Ichthyosis Foundation, Inc. *see* Foundation for Ichthyosis and Related Skin Types, Inc.
National Information Center for Handicapped Children and Youth 224
National Institute of Allergy and Infectious Diseases (NIAID) 345, 375n, 386, 389n, 392
National Institute of Arthritis, Diabetes and Digestive and Kidney Diseases 205n, 221
National Institute of Arthritis and Musculoskeletal and Skin Diseases (NIAMS) 239n, 240, 242, 293n, 296, 527n
National Institute of Dental Research 343, 345, 346, 348, 373
National Institutes of Health (NIH) 205n, 221, 253n, 343n, 385n, 521n
  Pain Research Clinic 373
National Interstate Council of State Cosmetology Boards 562
National Jewish Center for Immunology and Respiratory Medicine 157n, 165, 189n, 275n
National Pressure Ulcer Advisory Panel 455, 475

Index

National Professional Society of Pharmacists 417
National Psoriasis Foundation 123n, 138, 143n
National Rosacea Society 36
National Weather Service, Ultraviolet Index 312
nayad 573
NCRR Reporter 139n, 423n
necrotizing fasciitis (gangrene) 375, 379
Neild, V. S. 173, 184n56
neomycin 417, 418
neonatal acne 3
neonatal lupus syndrome 245
neoplastic diseases 44, 49
nerve damage 116
Netherton's syndrome (ichthyosis linearis circumflexa) 237
Neuber, K. 186n105, 186n108
neurological examinations 338
neurotic excoriations 60
neurotransmitters 58
neutral lipid storage disease 236
Neutrogena 52
Newcomer, Victor D., M.D. 109
NIAID *see* National Institute of Allergy and Infectious Diseases (NIAID)
Nicol, Noreen H., R.N. 165
nicotinic acid 269
nifedipine (Procardia, Adalat) 269
Nigra, Thomas, M.D. 547
NIH *see* National Institutes of Health (NIH)
Nims, J. W. 48n22
nitrogen mustard 529
nitroglycerin 37
Nivea 52
Nix cream 355
NMDA blockers 372
Noble, W. C. 186n102
nodular prurigo 354
non-bullous congenital ichthyosiform erythroderma (CIE) 227
noncontagious infections
  ichthyosis 230
  pityriasis rosea 260

noncontagious infections, continued
  poison ivy 198
  vitiligo 293
  see also contagious infections
Nonprescription Drug Manufacturers Association (NDMA) 516
nonprescription medications
  acne 25
  poison ivy infections 200
  see also over the counter medications
Nordwall, S. L. 186n103
Norpamin 59
North American Contact Dermatitis Group 587
Norwegian scabies 351-53
Norwood classifications *534*
nose surgery (rhinoplasty) 116
NPF *see* National Psoriasis Foundation
nucleotide bases 302-4
nutrition and diet
  acne 24
  canker sores 347
  epidermolysis bullosa 216-18
  hair loss 513, 536
  pruritus 50
nystatin 84

O

oatmeal baths 260
  poison ivy infections 199
  psoriasis treatment 130
oatmeal preparation (Aveeno)
  poison ivy infections 199
obsession, defined 62
obsessive-compulsive disorder 58, 60, 62-63
occlusives
  atopic dermatitis treatment 162
  ichthyosis treatment 233
occupational dangers
  lupus 249
  scleroderma 265
occupational skin disease (OSD) 189
occupational therapy 271-72
octyl dodecanol 602

Ogawa, M. 182n23
Ohman, S. 182n24
oil in water creams 74
oleic acid 602
oleoresins 201
Olsen, Elise, M.D. 545, 547
omeprazole (Prilosec) 270
oncogenes 302, 425
onycholysis 144
Oohashi, M. 178, 186n94
ophthalmic shingles 364, 365
opium derivatives 43, 46, 50
opportunistic infections 42
oral contraceptives 42
  see also birth control pills
oral disorders 10, 32, 343
Orap 59
Oren, Moshe 305
Orengo, Ida F., M.D. 429n, 446
O'Rourke, M. E. 47n14
orthopedic shoes 87
OSD see occupational skin disease
osteogenesis imperfecta 580
osteomylitis 432-33
OTC see over the counter medications
ovarian cysts 254
over the counter medications
  acne 25
  antibiotics 415, 418-20
  athlete's foot treatment 83
  capsaicin 366-67
  corns and calluses 82
  dandruff control 515-19
  head lice 555
  labelling rules 419-21
  plantar warts 83
  poison ivy infections 200
  vaginal yeast infections 29, 30
  warts 387
  wrinkle treatment 79
Oxman, Michael 370, 371
oxybenzone 104, 250
oxytetracycline hydrochloride 417, 419
ozone layer, skin cancers 108

P

PABA see para-aminobenzoic acid (PABA)
Pace, K. B. 49n3, 54n5
Padimate 251
Page, A. R. P. 182n26
Paige, R. L. 55n13
pain control
  pruritus 43, 46
  varicose veins 95
Palestine, A. G. 150n
palmar hyper-linearity 158
Palmer, Kenneth, Ph.D. 503
palmoplantar keratoderma ichthyosis 237
panthenol 602
papillomaviruses 303, 386
papular urticaria 353
papules 239, 240, 241
papulosquamous lesions 259
para-amino benzoic acid (PABA) 104, 247, 251
paranychia 433
parasitosis 58, 60, 61-62
parchment-like skin 99
Parents 3n
Parlette, H. L. 356n1
Parsol 1789 104, 251
Pasternack, B. 181n6
pasteurella multocida 430, 434
patch tests 176-77, 191, 192-93
  hair dyes 525
  poison ivy 201
Patient Care 57n
Patlak, Margie 20, 40, 526
Patterson, R. 181n10, 182n19
peaches and cream complexion 36
pediculosis 355
pediculosis corporis 354
pediculosis pubis 354
pediculus capitis humanus 553
pediculus humanus corporis 557
peeling skin syndrome 237
penicillins 15, 268, 282, 376, 379, 443
peptostreptococcus 434, 438
perforator veins 92
permethrin 355, 555

Index

permethrin cream 351
pernicious anemia 295
Perry, M. C. 47n11
Pertofrane 59
Pessar, Arlene, R.N. 224
Peterson, R. D. A. 182n26
petrolatum (petroleum jelly) 51, 105-6
  ichthyosis treatment 233
  red veterinary 250
  wrinkles 73
Pfeifer, Gerd P. 304
p53 gene 299, 302-6
Pham, C. T. 69n5
phantom feelings 370-71
pharmacologic therapy 53
phenothiazines 43, 46
phenoxybenzamine (Dibenzyline) 269
phenytoin (Dilantin) 213, 223
Phillips, T. L. 47n16
phlebitis 89, 95, 491
PHN *see* post-herpetic neuralgia (PHN)
phospholipids 573
photoaging 102, 104-5
photon therapy (radiation) 45, 529
  see also ultraviolet light
photoprotection 249-50
photosensitivity
  coal tar 519
  lupus 245, 246-47, 248-51
phthirius pubis 557
physical therapy 219, 271-72
physicians
  board certified 113
  choice of for cosmetic surgery 112-15
  genetic counseling 212, 224
  psoriasis treatment 137
pigmentation
  skin cancers 312
  vitiligo 293, 605
Pike, G. 173, 184n58
pilosebaceous units in skin *22*, 23
pimozide (Orap) 59, 62
pimples
  causes 38
  infants 3
  pink 4
  red 4

pimples, continued
  white 4
  see also acne; rosacea
pimples and pustules 23
Pine, Devera 514
pitrosporum ovale 178
pituitary gland 255
pityriasis rosea 259-60, 354
pityriasis rubra pilaris 237
Pityrosporum IgE antibodies 179
pityrosporum ovale 517
plantar warts 82-83, 385-86
Plaquenil 243, 269
plaque psoriasis 124, 147, 150
plaques, scleroderma 264
plaques of pregnancy 354
plastic surgery
  acne scars 26
  scars 410, 413
  wrinkle treatment 78
  see also cosmetic surgery
Platts-Mills, T. A. E. 182n13, 182n20
PM/DM disorders 118
pneumonia 375, 379
Pober, J. S. 183n46
Podocon-25 402
podofilox 402
Podofin (podophyllin) 402
podophyllin 488, 489
podophyllotoxin 387
podophyllum 387
poikiloderma of Civatte 100
poison ivy dermatitis 197-203
  see also urushiol
poison oak 200, 201, 202-3
poison sumac 200, 201, 202-3
poliomyelitis 84
pollen allergies 175-76
polyarthralgia 267
polycythemia vera 42, 54
polyethylene 602
polymyositis 262
polymyxin B sulfate 417, 418
polyostotic fibrous dysplasia 256
polysorbates 603
Polysporin 419
Pontén, Jan 303, 307
Pope, F. M. 185n89

porphyromonas 434, 438
port wine stain 8, 498, 605
post-herpetic neuralgia (PHN) 64, 363-68, 369, 371
Potaba 269
potassium hydroxide solutions 353
potassium para-aminobenzoate (Potaba) 269
Pott, Percivall 299, 300
Potts, R. O. 109n9
Powell, Frank, M.D. 38
prazosin (Minipress) 269
precancer 327
precocious puberty 254-55
Prednisone 243
pregnancy
  canker sores 348
  diet 175
  genital herpes 392, 394
  genital warts 488-89
  psoriasis 133, 137-38
  scabies 354
  varicose veins 96
prenatal detection
  epidermolysis bullosa 212
  ichthyosis 235
  xeroderma pigmentosum 339
prescription medications
  acne 23
  athlete's foot treatment 84
  wrinkle treatment 77
  see also *individual medications*
pressure points *448*
pressure therapy 427-28
pressure ulcers 447-56
  treatment 457-76
prevotella 434, 438
Price, J. F. 186n96
Price, P. 186n106
prickly heat (milaria) 4
Prilosec 270
Prinivil 269
Prinz, J. C. 185n83
Procardia 269
pro-drugs 370
Professional Guide to Diseases 259n
progressive systemic sclerosis (PSS) 261

propanolol (Inderal) 269
propylene glycol 233, 603
Propylthiouracil 255
prostaglandins
  pruritus 43
  urticaria 277-78
proud flesh 409
Provera 254-55
Prozac 59
pruritic urticarial papules and plaques of pregnancy (PUPPP) 354
pruritus (itching) 41-55
  atopic dermatitis 157-58
  pityriasis rosea 260
  scabies 355
pseudomonas bacterial infection 563
pseudo-parkinsonism 62
psoralen (PUVA) 127, 131, 145, 295
psoriasis 59, 498, 515, 518
  case study 68
  cyclosporine study 147-50
  immunity study 139-41, 150-53
  psychiatric disorders 63-64
  understanding 123-38
  see also nail psoriasis
Psoriasis Treatment Center 68, 69
psoriasis vulgaris (plaque psoriasis) 124, 147
psoriatic arthritis 127, 135, 144
PSS *see* progressive systemic sclerosis (PSS)
psychiatric disorders 60
psychodermatologic disorders classification *65*
psychodermatology 57-69
psychological factors
  ichthyosis 231-32
  lichen planus 240
  pruritus 51
  see also emotions
  psoriasis 126
  skin disorders 57-69
psychophysiologic disorders 59-60
psychosis, skin disorders 58, 60, 61-62
psychosomatic disorders 59-60
psychotropic medications 58
puberty abnormalities 253
pubic lice 557

Index

punch grafting 117, 485
PUPPP *see* pruritic urticarial papules and plaques of pregnancy (PUPPP)
Purl, S. 49n2, 54n4
pustular psoriasis 124, 126, 129
PUVA *see* psoralen
pyloric atresia 207
pyrethrum 354-55, 555
pyrimidine bases 302-4
pyritione zinc 516

Q

Quaternium 15 195
quinidine
   pruritus 43
   psoriasis 134

R

rabies 444-46
race factors
   actinic keratoses 328-29
   lichen sclerosus 241
   photosensitivity 249
   scarring 411, 423
   skin cancers 301, 309-11, *310*
   vitiligo 294
radiation treatment 428
   pruritus 45, 46, 53
   topical skin care 51
radioallergosorbent tests (RASTs) 169, 171
Rajka, G. 164n1, 181n9, 182n27
Rand, Seymour, M.D. 39
Rapoport, J. L. 69n12
rashes 3
   contact dermatitis 189
   infants 3-4
   linear 199
   lupus 243
   shingles 364
Ray, A. 153n
Raynaud's phenomenon 263, 267, 269
RCMI Program 424-25
RDEB *see* recessive dystrophic epidermolysis bullosa (RDEB)

recessive dystrophic epidermolysis bullosa (RDEB) 208-9, 223
recessive X-linked ichthyosis (steroid sulfatase deficiency) 237
recombinant technology 396, 404
red birthmarks 7-8
red mask *see* rosacea
Rees, Jonathan L. 305
Refsum's disease (phytanic acid storage ichthyosis) 237
Rein, G. 69n4
Reitamo, S. 185n87
Remick, R. A. 69n7
Remington, L. 307
renal disease
   pruritus 42, 54
   scleroderma 268, 270
   see also kidney diseases
Research Resource Reporter 147n, 150
respiratory atopy 170-71, 175, 177
Retin-A
   acne treatment 23, 25, 496
   lupus treatment 250
   photoaging 104-5
   wrinkle treatment 77
retinoic acid 77, 428
retinoid medications 127, 132, 137-38, 145, 496
rhabdovirus (rabies) 430
rheumatic fever 14, 16-17, 377
rheumatic heart disease (carditis) 14, 16-17, 375, 377
rhinitis, allergic 157, 169, 177
rhinophyma 36, 39
rhinoplasty 116
Rhodes, Athur R. 340
rhytidectomy 116
Richey, H. K. 109n10
rickets 256
Rid shampoo 355
Ries, L. A. G. 313n6
ringworm 359-62
Rius, F. 356n2
Roberts, D. L. L. 185n93
Roberts, Rosemary, M.D. 14, 16
Robins, Perry, M.D. 331
Rockefeller University 139-41, 151

Rogaine 269, 486, 510-11, 529, 534, 537, 543-48
Romeu, J. 356n2
Rook, A. 69n1, 164n3
Rops, R. 143
rosacea 35-40, 59, 498
Rose, C. M. 47n12
Rosen, Ted, M.D. 413, 429n, 446
Ross, C. M. 55n11
Rowntree, S. 182n13
Rubenstein, E. 42n3, 47n1, 47n6, 55n17
Rudolph, J. A. 307
Rud's syndrome 237
Russell, James, M.D. 424
Russell, Shirley, M.D. 424-26

S

Saarinen, U. M. 174, 184n63-64
Sabnis, S. G. 150n
Saeki, N. 184n75
Safety and Efficacy of Topical Drugs and Cosmetics Symposium (1982) 73
Saita, L. 55n8
salabrasion 609
salicylates 269
salicylic acid 232, 516
  corns and calluses treatment 82
  plantar warts treatment 83
  psoriasis treatment 130, 136
saline-filled breast implants 117
saline (salt) solutions
  epidermolysis bullosa treatment 214
  poison ivy infections 199
  pressure ulcers 466
salmon patch 7
Sampson, H. A. 165n5, 172, 173, 182n12, 183n35-37, 183n41-42, 183n49-50
Sanchez, R. 356n7
Sanda, T. 178, 186n94
Sanders, J. E. 48n21
Sanders, John 74-75
Sandimmune (cyclosporine) 138
sandpapering skin *see* dermabrasion
Sanford, H. N. 174, 184n60

saphenous veins 90, 94
sarcoptes scabiei mites 351-52
Sasaki, K. 185n90
Sawaya, Marty, M.D. 547-48
scabies 351-57
scales
  dandruff 515-19
  ichthyosis 229-30, 231
  lichen planus 239
  psoriasis 124, 135-36, 147, 498
scalp reduction 117, 485, 550
scalp ringworm 359, 361
scaly bumps 327
scarification 610
scarlet fever (scarlatina) 14, 16, 376
scarring 409-13
  abnormal 423-28
  cosmetic surgery 116
  epidermolysis bullosa 208
  surgery 478
  treatment 118
schizophrenia 61
Schnyder, U. W. 182n29
Schoen, Linda Allen 572
Schopfer, K. 186n106
Schultz, Dodi 11
Schultz, M. W. 356n8
Schwartz, Robert A., M.D. 356, 357
Scientific American, Inc. 299n
sclerodactyly 263, 267
scleroderma 46, 261-73
scleroderma renal crisis (SRC) 270
sclerotherapy 93-94, 491-92
scrapes 415-21
  scabies 353
scratching 43-44
scybala 352
sebaceous glands 22, *22*, 23, 26, 106
seborrheic dermatitis 354, 515, 517
seborrheic keratoses 100
sebum 22, *22*, 26
Sehgal, P. 153n
Sehgal, P. B. 153n
Seidenari, S. 177, 185n85
selective serotonin re-uptake inhibitors (SSRI) 63
selenium sulfide 516
Sellar, B. 181n11

Index

Sellars, W. A. 174, 184n62
senile ectasia 100
sepsis 375
septic arthritis 432-33
septicemia 19
  see also blood infections
Setlow, Richard B. 304
Sewell, M. 173, 184n55
sexually transmitted diseases 399-400, 557
Seys, B., M.D. 38
shampoo *see* soaps
Sharma, H. W. 307
Sharp, P. A. 182n31
shave removal 329
Sherman, Elisabeth J., Ph.D. 425
Shike, Moshe 307
shingles 363-68, 369-73
Shirakawa, T. 182n32
shoes, choice of 85, 87
Shupack, Jerome, M.D. 509, 513
Shuster, S. 55n18
Silastic 504
silastic gel sheeting 427
silica 603
silicone implants 117, 479, 484
Simon, Jeffrey A. 305, 307
Simon, Nissa 6
Simons, K. J. 291
Simons, R. 291
Sinequan 59
Sirera, G. 356n2
Siridavong, Kim 559
Sjögren-Larsen Syndrome 235, 236, 237, 270
skin
  body weight percentage 41
  described 228
  Group A streptococcal infections 17-18
skin biopsy
  lichen planus 240
  lichen sclerosus 242
The Skin Cancer Foundation 327n
skin cancers 100-103, 107-8, 326, 481-82, 486-87
  hair dyes 522-24
  sunlight 299-307

skin cancers, continued
  tretinoin 497
  xeroderma pigmentosum 333, 334, 337-38
  see also *individual carcinomas*
skin care 49-50, 591
  epidermolysis bullosa 214-15, 216
  face washing 74-75
skin deterioration *101*
skin eruptions, lichen sclerosus 242
skin grafts 337, 428, 479, 503-6
skin lesions
  acrochordons 100
  actinic keratosis 327-28
  atopic dermatitis 157, 176
  basal cell carcinoma 103
  elderly patients 103
  genital herpes 390
  lichen sclerosus 241
  lupus 243
  papulosquamous 259
  psoriasis 124, 152
  urticaria 276-78, 280
skin mites 38
skin prick tests 171, 179
skin tags (acrochordons) 100
skin types 249, 252
SLE *see* systemic lupus erythematosus (SLE)
Sloper, K. S. 183n51
Smalley, R. V. 48n17
Smitt, J. H. S. 182n17
smoker's face 73
Snider, Sharon 27
Snyder, Steven, M.D. 609, 610
soaps
  atopic dermatitis 159
  contact dermatitis 193
  cosmetics 591, 599
  drying effect 75
  hair loss 513
  poison ivy infections 199
  pressure ulcers 450, 474
  pruritus 50, 52
  psoriasis 136
social factors
  disfiguring skin diseases 63-64
  ichthyosis 231-32

Social Security Administration (SSA) 135
sodium bicarbonate (baking soda) 199
sodium lauryl sulfate 603
sodium tetradecyl sulphate 93
soft tissue augmentation 479, 482, 484
solar keratoses 333
solar lentigines 100
solar rays *see* sunlight
Solley, G. O. 183n45
somatopsychic disorders 59-60
somatostatin 255
Somerville, E. T. 49n3, 54n5
Soothill, J. F. 173, 184n55, 186n96
sore throat 13
Sperry, Kris, M.D. 606, 611
SPF *see* sun protective factor (SPF)
spiderbursts 90, 93
spider veins 478, 491, 499
Spiegel, R. J. 48n19
splints 428
splotchy pigmentation treatment 118
squames 228
squamous cell carcinomas 102, 103, 108, 303, 328, 477, 486
squamous cells 299, 300
Squires, Sally 373
SRC *see* scleroderma renal crisis (SRC)
SS *see* systemic sclerosis (SS)
Staberg, B. 109n11
Stair, J. C. 49n3, 54n5
Stanford University School of Medicine 7
Stanton, R. H. J. 173, 184n59
staphylococcus aureus 163, 178
staphylococcus infections
  bites 434-38
  eczema 6
  impetigo 18
  infants 9-10
stearic acid 602, 604
stearyl alcohol 602
Stehlin, Dori 76, 593
Stein, Maurice 610-11

Steinbeck, John 21
Sterling, Glenn B., M.D. 356, 356n5
Stern, R. S. 109n12
Stern, Robert, M.D. 546
steroid-induced rosacea 37
steroids
  hair loss 512
  lupus treatment 243
  pruritus 52
  psoriasis treatment 127, 128
  see also corticosteroids; systemic steroids; topical steroids
steroid sulfatase deficiency 237
Stewart, L. A. 195n1
Stewart, Leslie, M.D. 195
Stifler, W. C. 181n7
stockings
  elastic 93
  wet dressings *161*
Stone, Katherine, M.D. 399, 400, 401, 404
stork bite 7
Storrs, Frances, M.D. 513-14
stratum corneum 75, 106, 228, 233
Straus, Stephen E., M.D. 394-95
Straus, Walter 19
Strauss, J. S. 181, 187n114
strawberry marks 7-8
strep infections *see* streptococcal infections
strep throat (streptococcal pharyngitis) 14, 15-16, 375-77
streptococcal infections
  bites 434-38
  eczema 6
  Group A 13-15, 20, 375-83
    symptoms 13
  Group B 20
  Groups C, D, G, H, K 20
  psoriasis 125
  streptococcus mutans 20
  streptococcus pneumoniae 20
  treatments 417
streptococcal pharyngitis *see* strep throat
streptococcus mutans 20
streptococcus pneumoniae 20
streptococcus pyogenes 375

Index

stress
  acne 24
  atopic dermatitis 160
  cold sores 346
  hair loss 512, 528, 536, 537
  lichen planus 240
  management therapy 59
  psoriasis 125, 136
  skin disorders 59
  vitiligo 294
  see also emotions;
    psychodermatology
stricture 410
Strom, S. 48n22
subacute cutaneous lupus lesions 245
subcutaneous fat 90
substance P 367
suction-assisted lipectomy 118-19
Sugiura, H. 185n90
sulfa drugs 250
Sullivan, K. M. 48n21
sulphur preparations 355, 516
Sulzberger, M. B. 167, 168, 180, 181n2-3
sunlight
  acne 24
  actinic keratoses 328
  lupus 246, 248-51
  psoriasis treatment 127, 134, 136
  Retin-A 25
  rosacea 38
  skin cancers 102, 248, 315
  skin lesions 100
  skin protection 104, 107
  skin types 249
  tattoos 609
  tretinoin 497
  vitiligo 294
  wrinkles 72-73
  xeroderma pigmentosum 333
  see also photosensitivity; ultraviolet light
sun protection factor (SPF) 315, 316-17, 330
sun protective factor (SPF) 251
sunscreens 75, 79, 104, 315-18, 330, 482, 591, 598
  children 324-25

sunscreens, continued
  herpes simplex 346
  lupus 247-48, 250-51
  psoriasis 134
  vitiligo 295
  xeroderma pigmentosum 336-37
surgery
  bunions 85
  dermatologic 477-502
  endoscopic 78
  genital herpes 402, 403
  tattoo removal 609-10
  varicose veins 94-95
  warts 387
  see also cosmetic surgery; plastic surgery
swallowing problems 217-18
sweating inability 231
symptoms
  actinic keratoses 328
  anticholinergic 61
  athlete's foot 83
  basal cell carcinoma 103
  blood infections 19
  cellulitis 378
  CREST syndrome 263-64, 265
  Cushing's syndrome 255-56
  epidermolysis bullosa 206, 213
  erysipelas 378
  genital herpes 390, 401
  Group A Streptococcal infections 13
  head lice 554
  herpes simplex 344
  impetigo 17, 377
  kidney disease 18
  lichen planus 239
  lupus 243, 246
  McCune-Albright syndrome 253
  pruritus 48-49
  psoriasis 124, 126
  rheumatic fever 16, 377
  rosacea 36, 37
  scabies 352-53
  scarlet fever 16
  scleroderma 266-67
  shingles 372
  skin cancer 108
  strep throat 15, 376

symptoms, continued
  thrush 32
  toxic streptococcal syndrome 19-20
  vaginal yeast infections 30
  yeast infections in men 31
syndactyly 219
synthetic skin 503-6
syphilis 354
systemic corticosteroids 260, 529
systemic lupus erythematosus (SLE)
    243, 244-45, 248
systemic sclerodermas 262
systemic sclerosis (SS) 261, 262
systemic steroids 134
  atopic dermatitis 170
  contact dermatitis 194
systemic therapies
  atopic dermatitis treatment 163
  ichthyosis treatment 233-34

T

tachykinins 43
Tagamet 270
talc 604
Tandy, Jack *452*
tanning 248, 249, 252, 315-26
tanning parlors 319-23, 330
Taplin, D. 356n6-7
tardive dyskinesia 62
Task Force on Xeroderma
    Pigmentosum 340
Tatter, S. B. 153n
tattoos 478, 489-91, 499, 605-12
Tay's syndrome (trichothiodystrophy;
    IBIDS syndrome) 237
T-cell function 100, 102
T-cells 140, 172, 176, 179, 190
  lupus 245
Tegison (etretinate)
  birth defects 132, 137-38
  lupus treatment 247
  psoriasis treatment 127, 132
tegretol 372
telangiectasia 263, 264, 267, 498
telogen effluvium 59, 510, 535, 536
terfenadine 287
testolactone 255

testosterone 46, 254, 510, 533, 548
testosterone ointment 242
tetracaine 200
tetracycline hydrochloride 417, 418
tetracyclines 250
  canker sores 348
  rosacea treatment 39
tetrasodium edetate 602
thalamus 43
theophylline 37
therapies
  atopic dermatitis 160-63
  biopsychosocial treatment 58
  bite wounds 440-44
  pruritus treatment 50-51, 53-54
  psoriasis treatment 127-28
thimerisol 415
Thompson, Richard 583
Thorazine 250
throat infections 13, 15
  see also strep throat
thrombophlebitis 89, 95
thrombosis 491
thrush 10, 32
thymine 302
thymopentin 529
thyroid function
  povidone-iodine 419
  urticaria 283
  vitiligo 295
thyroid gland abnormalities 255
  dry skin 106
  hair loss 536
thyrotoxicosis 42
tinea capitis 359, 361
tinea corporis 359, 360-61
tinea fungus 359-62
tinea pedis 359, 360
tinea unguium 359, 360
titanium dioxide 250
titanium oxide 247
tobacco, xeroderma pigmentosum 335
  see also cigarette smoking
tocopherol *see* vitamin E
toenail problems 144
Tokuda, Y. 184n75
tolbutamide 43
tolnaftate 83

Index

Tolypocladium inflatum 148
topical medications
  actinic keratoses 330
  genital herpes 392
  ichthyosis 232-33
  ingrown toenails 84
  lichen sclerosus 242
  pruritus 51-52, 53
  psoriasis treatment 128-30, 145
topical steroids 260
  atopic dermatitis treatment 162-63
  contact dermatitis treatment 194
  epidermolysis bullosa treatment 214
  hair loss 514
  lichen planus 240
  lupus treatment 247
  poison ivy infections 200
  psoriasis 134
torsades de pointes 287
toxic shock-like syndrome 375, 379
toxic streptococcal syndrome 14, 19-20
traction alopecia 535
tranquilizing agents 54
Transcutaneous Electronic Nerve Stimulators (TENS) 54
trauma
  lupus 249
  psoriasis 134
Trembath, R. C. 182n33
trenchfoot 87
trephine 485
treponema pallidum 438
tretinoin 104-5, 250, 482, 496-98, 529
  see also Retin-A
trichloroacetic acid 387, 402, 488
trichophyton 359
Trichophyton mentagrophytes 83
Trichophyton rubrum 83
trichothiodystrophy 237
trichotillomania (compulsive hair pulling) 60, 62, 68
tricyclic antidepressant medications 61, 62, 64
triethanolamine 603
tripelennamine hydorchloride 200
trisodium edetate 602
true lamellar ichthyosis 227

Trupin, Joel S., M.D. 424, 425, 426
Trupin, K. M. 426
Tsushima, W. T. 69n2
Tuffanelli, Denny, M.D. 266
Tuft, L. 184n71-72
tummy tucks (abdominoplasty) 118
tumor suppressor genes 302-4
Twain, Mark 71
Tyring, Stephen K., M.D. 369, 371, 403

U

Uehara, M. 170, 182n28, 182n30, 185n90
Uenishi, T. 182n30
ultrasonography 254
ultraviolet light
  atopic dermatitis treatment 164
  DNA (deoxyribonucleic acid) 302
  lupus 245, 246-47, 248-51
  pruritus treatment 54
  psoriasis treatment 68, 127, 129
  skin damage 99, 102
  tanning 317
  type A (UVA) 104, 317, 320-21
    psoriasis treatment 131
  type B (UVB) 104, 317, 320
    psoriasis treatment 127, 129, 131
  vitiligo 295
  xeroderma pigmentosum 333, 336-37
  see also sunlight
undecylenic acid 83
unilateral hemidysplasia 236
United Scleroderma Foundation 261n
University of Michigan 147
Updike, John 123
Upjohn Company 531, 543-46
urea 73, 106, 136, 232
urecholine 270
urticaria 173, 275-91
urticarial vasculitis 281-83
urticaria pigmentosa 281
urushiol 197-98
U.S. Bureau of Labor Statistics 189
U.S. Department of Health and Human Services (DHHS) 447n, 457n, 571n, 585n

UVA *see* ultraviolet light: type A
UVB *see* ultraviolet light: type B
uveitis 295

V

vaccines
  herpes 394-98
  herpes simplex 345
  poison ivy infections 201
vaginal yeast infections 4-5
  candida 29
  causes 30-31
valacyclovir 369-70
valves in veins *91,* 92-93, 94
Van Asperen, P. P. 177, 185n91
Van Bever, H. P. 184n74
van de Kerkhoff, P. C. M. 143
Van der Heijden, F. L. 185n79-80
Van Ieperen-Van Dijk, A. G. 186n109
van Katwijk, M. 185n79
Van Voorst Vader, P. C. 185n88
varicella-zoster virus (VZV) 363-68, 369, 372
varicose veins 89-97, 478, 491
Varney, V. 183n48
vascular disorders
  rosacea 37-38
  scleroderma 265
  varicose veins 89-97
vascular nevi 7
vasculitis 246
Vaseline *see* petrolatum
vasoactive peptides 43
vasodilators 269, 277, 512
Vasotec 269
Vaughn, Chris 574
veillonella parvula 434, 438
vein construction 90-92, *91*
venereal warts 386
venous stasis ulcers 491
Ventafridda, V. 55n8
vinyl chloride 572, 591
viral agents 259
Visa, K. 185n87
vitamin A 573
  hair loss 513, 536
  ichthyosis treatment 233

vitamin B12 347
vitamin B complex
  pruritus 43
vitamin D 130, 145, 256, 573
  psoriasis treatment 127, 130
vitamin E 573, 574, 595-96, 602
  hair loss 513
vitamin K 573
vitiligo 293-96, 605
Voorhees, John J., M.D. 150n
VZV *see* varicella-zoster virus (VZV)
VZV Research Foundation, Inc. 370, 373

W

Wadsworth, J. 183n51
Waersted, A. 187n112
Warner, J. O. 186n96
warts 385-87
  surgery 477
  see also genital warts
waterless cleansers 193
waxes 602
The Wayward Bus (Steinbeck) 21
weather
  psoriasis 134
Webber, S. A. 183n54
Weber-Cochayne disease 207
  see also epidermolysis bullosa simplex - localized
Weinstein, M. C. 109n12
Weiss, J. S. 109n13
Weiss, R. 183n43
Weiss, R. B. 47n11
Wessels, M. W. 186n109
Weston, William L., M.D. 167n, 187
wheals 275, 280
wheal tests 168
whiteheads 3, 22, 35
Wickham's striae 239
Wierenga, E. A. 182n17, 185n80
Wilcox, C. S. 69n9
Wilcox, Neil, D.V.M. 589, 590
Wiley, H. E. 313n8
Wilkin, Jonathan, M.D. 35, 36, 37, 40
Wilkinson, D. S. 69n1

Index

Williams, H. C. 182n15
Williams, L. W. 182n34
Williams, Scott, M.D. 424, 425
Willis, Judith Levine 32, 558
Winawer, Sidney J. 307
Winkelman, R. D. 55n15
Wise, F. 167, 168, 180, 181n2
Wiskur, Lois 562
Wnokur, G. 69n11
Woest, T. E. 185n88
Wolf, John, M.D. 429n, 446
Wolff, K. 47n3, 47n4, 49n1, 54n1
women
   canker sores 348
   hair loss 533-42
   lichen sclerosus 241
   occupational skin disease 190
   scleroderma 266
   vaginal yeast infections 4-5, 10, 29
   varicose veins 96
Wound Ostomy and Continence Nurses Society (WOCN) 476
wrinkles 71-79, 495, 581
   tanning 315-16
Wulf, H. C. 109n11
Wuthrich, B. 182n29

X

Xanax 59
Xeroderma Pigmentosum Registry 339
xeroderma pigmentosum (XP) 333-40
xerosis 105-6, 158
X-linked ichthyosis 227, 229, 230, 233, 234, 235
XP *see* xeroderma pigmentosum (XP)

Y

Yale University School of Medicine 3
Yamamoto, F. Y. 165n4, 181n11
Yamamoto, K. R. 426
Yannas, Ioannis, Ph.D. 504
Yarbro, J. W. 47n11
Yasko, J. 55n12
Yasko, J. M. 55n12
Yasue, T. 178, 186n94
yeast infections 4-5, 10
   candida 29
   seborrheic dermatitis 517
   see also vaginal yeast infections
Ying, S. 183n48
Yoder, Ida I. 516
Yoshinaga, S. K. 426
Young, Teresa A. 558
young adults
   acromegaly 255
   melanoma 103
Yourish, D. 153n

Z

Zamula, Evelyn 97
Zeiger, R. S. 174, 175, 184n68
Zestril 269
Ziegler, A. 307
zinc oxide 250
zinc stearate 604
zirconium salts 572, 591
zits *see* acne
Zonalon Cream 59
Zostrix 366-67
Zovirax 366
zyderm collagen 484
zyplast collagen 484

LIBRARY
WEST GEORGIA TECHNICAL COLLEGE
303 FORT DRIVE
LAGRANGE, GA 30240